Liver and Environmental
_____ Xenobiotics

Liver and Environmental Xenobiotics

Editors
S.V.S. Rana
K. Taketa

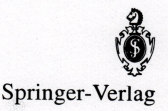

Springer-Verlag

Narosa Publishing House

EDITORS
S.V.S. Rana
Department of Zoology
Ch. Charan Singh University
Meerut 250 004, India

K. Taketa
Department of Public Health
Okayama University Medical School
Okayama 700, Japan

ISBN 3-540-62690-5 Berlin Heidelberg New York
ISBN 0-387-62690-5 New York Berlin Heidelberg
ISBN 81-7319-121-2 Narosa Publishing House, New Delhi

Printed in India

Foreword

Today the general populations are incidentally exposed to a wide variety of xenobiotics as a consequence of the pollution of the environment by industrial and agricultural chemicals. The action of these xenobiotics on the body shows certain specificity, depending upon the compound's chemical structure and reactivity. Further, the final exposition of cytotoxicity and genetic injury is determined by receptors, enzyme active or regulatory sites, structural elements and ion channels as well as covalent interactions with tissue macromolecules including nucleic acids. The consequences of metabolism for the pharmacological and toxic activity of a compound may involve a number of possibilities. It may form reactive species and cause oxidative stress. Free radicals are important in tissue damage, e.g., in inflammation, ageing and chemical injury so that their formation as a consequence of xenobiotic metabolism is noteworthy.

Hepatocellular degeneration and death are amongst the most important effects caused by these xenobiotics. There are well accepted mechanisms for a few of them. However, we have to update our knowledge on many others. Therapeutic advances are also to be considered. There have not been sufficient attempts to study liver protective mechanisms.

I am happy to go through this book that not only describes general aspects of toxic liver injury but also deals with the involvement of liver in handling the industrial and environmental xenobiotics.

Dr. S.V.S. Rana studied toxic liver injury in the Department of Public Health, Okayama University Medical School, Japan as a Senior JSPS scientist when I worked as Professor and Chairperson. In 1991, Dr. Kazuhisa Taketa took over as Professor and Chairman of the Department of Public Health. Dr. Rana worked in that Department again in 1995. They worked together on this book. In my opinion this colabortion has been successful and I wish them success in their future endeavours.

MASANA OGATA
MD
Kawasaki University of Medical Welfare
Japan

Preface

The general populations are incidentally exposed to a wide variety of xenobiotics as a consequence of the pollution of the environment by industrial and agricultural chemicals. Xenobiotics entering the animal will undergo one or more of the following fate: (a) elimination unchanged, (b) metabolism by enzymes, (c) spontaneous chemical transformation and (d) remain unchanged in the body. The actions of xenobiotics on the body exhibit certain specificity depending upon the compound's chemical structure and reactivity. Since the processes of metabolism change these chemical properties of a xenobiotic, bewildering number of reactions continue to pose new challenges to toxicologists and pharmacologists. It necessitates periodic and precise revision of the subject.

This book contains invited contributions from learned colleagues that offer an excellent survey of and profound insight into the disposition and metabolism of a few environmentally and industrially significant xenobiotics. The topics range from an assessment of drug metabolising enzymes in the liver, DNA damage by reactive oxygen species generated by pesticides, role of NO in liver injury, hepatotrophic growth factor in liver regeneration, extracellular matrix in the liver, oncogene expression in liver injury, the hepatocarcinogenesis to oxidative stress and undifferentiated gene expression. Detailed analysis of the validity of liver function tests has been included. Last Chapter addresses the problem of apoptosis, which plays a key role in the signal transduction system of xenobiotics-induced liver injury.

The reader should appreciate that overall exposure to this field is expanding at a rapid pace and selections had to be made.

During the development of this book, we received help and advice from many colleagues for which we are thankful. We gratefully acknowledge the understanding, care and precision of the publisher that made this book possible.

EDITORS

Contents

Liver and Environmental Xenobiotics
S.V.S. Rana and K. Taketa (Eds)
Copyright © 1997, Narosa Publishing House, New Delhi, India

1. Extracellular Matrix in Liver

P.R. Sudhakaran, N. Anil Kumar and Anitha Santhosh

Department of Biochemistry, University of Kerala, Trivandrum, India

Introduction

The extracellular matrix is a complex network of macromolecules that interact with one another as well as with cells in tissues. It comprises both interstitial stroma and the basement membrane that surround the epithelial tissues, nerves, fat cells and muscle. The major components of the extracellular matrix (ECM) in various tissues are collagen, elastins, proteoglycans and glyco-proteins such as fibronectin, laminin, nidogen, entactin, tenascin etc. Apart from providing physical support to hold cells and tissues together, the ECM provides a highly organised lattice within which the cells can migrate and interact with one another. The interactions of cells with the ECM are critically important in the embryonic development, growth regulation and differentiation. The composition of ECM interacting with cell surface has important regulatory and structural consequences for cells and an extensive literature now documents these biological roles. The proportion of the ECM and the connective tissue in relation to the parenchymal tissue is very small in liver. Nevertheless, the tasks which the ECM of the liver have to fulfil are complex. It has to combine maximum mechanical stability with minimum hindrance to the free transport of proteins and metabolites between parenchymal cells and the blood stream. In this chapter a brief review on the composition and distribution of extracellular matrix in liver, the interaction of liver cells with the components of the ECM and the biological consequences of these interactions, is presented.

Hepatic Parenchyma

Liver is a vital organ involved in a series of physiological functions in vertebrates. Some of the major functions include: synthesis and secretion of plasma proteins and bile; absorption, utilisation, storage and redistribution of nutrients derived from diet; detoxification of potentially harmful xenobiotic substances. By virtue of its unique and strategic positioning between blood plasma and bile, hepatocytes, the main epithelial type of cell in liver is carrying out these diverse group of activities [1]. The organisation of hepatic parenchyma is different from other epithelia and is described as a continuum of hepatocytes arranged in 1-cell thick plates separated by blood sinusoidal spaces. In the livers of birds, amphibians and certain fishes, the hepatocytes are arranged in 2-cell thick plate instead of one. In human liver, the plates are several cell thick at birth forming what is known as a muralium multiplex, which then gradually remodels to a 1-cell thick muralium simplex within the first several years of postnatal life [2].

Hepatocytes constitute more than 90% of the liver mass in most mammalian species. It is a polyhedral cell whose shape ranges from heptahedral to dodecahedral, depending upon its placement within the liver muralium [2]. Unlike simple epithelial cells, hepatocytes in adult liver is structurally and functionally polarised and has three distinct membrane domains, sinusoidal (basal), lateral and canalicular (apical). Functional polarisation of hepatocytes is evident in the secretion of bile into bile duct by traversing the apical surface whereas albumin is secreted into circulation by traversing the sinusoidal surface [3, 4]. Sinusoids are modified capillaries which carry blood from portal vein and hepatic artery to the central vein and are lined by discontinuous, fenestrated endothelium. Other than endothelial cells, the major type of nonparenchymal cells are Kupffer cells (resident macrophages in sinusoidal lumen) and fat storing Ito cells residing in peri-sinusoidal space of Disse. Canalicular surfaces form the bile canalicular network that transports bile. Lateral plasma membrane fuse along side bile canaliculi to form tight junctions that occlude the apical domain from the basolateral surface. Intermediate junctions, desmosomes and gap junctions on lateral domains provide cohesive strength and functional communication between hepatocytes.

Hepatic Matrix

Unlike the classical epithelium, hepatocytes have a belt of apical surface dividing the two basolateral surfaces that are in contact with the ECM. Although there is no morphologically identifiable basement membrane close to the putative basal surface of the hepatocytes, the sinusoids contain typical matrix components that appear to contact the sparse endothelial cells as well as the hepatocytes and these components are found elsewhere through the tissue indicating that the ECM is a structurally important component in liver [5–9]. Characterisation and distribution of ECM in liver have been studied by biochemical and immunocytochemical methods [5–8, 10–11]. The major types of collagens are Col. I, III and IV. The matrix glycoproteins, fibronectin and laminin and heparan sulphate proteoglycan are also present. Ultrastructural localization studies in mouse liver revealed the presence of typical collagen fibrils and small bundles in portal tracts and Disse's space. Col. I is present in liver capsule, portal stroma and in the perisinusoidal space indicating a structural role supporting the hepatocyte layer at the intralobular regions. Col. type III appears to be present only in stroma in liver and is not in direct contact with hepatocyte surface. Basal surface of hepatocytes are in contact with typical basement membrane components such as Col. IV, laminin, fibronectin (Fn) and heparan sulphate proteoglycans. Fibronectin is present on all cell surface domains of hepatocytes [12] in contrast to the exclusively basal distribution of this protein in other epithelia. It is most prominent in perisinusoidal space where it is in direct contact with hepatocyte microvilli and separated from the endothelial surface [5, 9, 12, 13]. It is also present in liver capsule and portal stroma and was detected in bile ducts and at lateral surfaces between contacting hepatocytes. Heparan sulphate proteoglycan has been located in close proximity to the sinusoidal surface of hepatocytes [14, 15]. In addition to heparan sulphate, biochemical analyses have shown the presence of relatively less amount of glycosaminoglycans such as chondroitin sulphate and dermatan sulphate and trace amounts of hyaluronic acid and keratan sulphate in extracellular sites in liver tissue [16, 17]. Col. IV and laminin are present in ductal, neural and vascular membrane and also as small discrete deposits between hepatocytes and endothelial sinusoids [7]. As the discontinuous distribution argues against a simple supporting role, it has been suggested that, the basement membrane that is probably formed transiently during parenchymal development may initially perform a supporting role, but is degraded once the tissue modelling is accomplished so as to facilitate rapid exchange of plasma metabolites [5].

The cellular source of these extracellular matrix components in liver appears to be of mixed origin. Primary cultures of hepatocytes have been shown to synthesise various components of the extracellular matrix which are either secreted into the medium or are deposited into the pericellular layer. *In vivo* and *in vitro* studies with liver tissue or isolated hepatocytes in culture have demonstrated the synthesis of acid glycosaminoglycans by liver. Whereas isolated rat hepatocytes synthesise almost exclusively heparan sulphate in a proteoglycan form [18] liver tissue synthesises chondroitin 4 and 6-sulphates, dermatan sulphate and hyaluronic acid [17, 19–21]. Heparan sulphate proteoglycans are secreted into the culture medium as well as distributed on the hepatocyte surface. Part of this is associated with the cell surface through electrostatic interactions with heparan sulphate side chains, while another form of HSPG is intercalated into the membrane through the protein core [22].

Primary cultures of hepatocytes synthesise and secrete fibronectin [23–25]. There is a progressive increase in the expression of cellular form of fibronectin at the expense of the soluble plasma form of Fn with increase in the duration of culture [25, 26]. This may reflect the progressive dedifferentiation process which is typical of hepatocytes *in vitro*. Evidence in support of this comes from the observation that in liver, transcripts bearing the additional ED-A and ED-B segments characteristic of cellular fibronectin are not detectable but ED-A expression does occur in fetal liver and tumours [27]. Type IV collagen is also synthesised by hepatocytes in culture [25]. Immunofluorographic analysis using specific antibodies against laminin showed that rat hepatocytes in culture produced Ln peptides which migrated as a single band corresponding to β chain apparently indicating that either they produce only β chains *in vitro* or it may represent an isoform of laminin (Ln) (P.R. Sudhakaran, unpublished data).

Although, hepatocytes in culture do synthesise Col. IV, Fn and HSPG, the precise cellular source of the various components of basement membrane and details of its biogenesis in liver are not known. Nearly 5% of the total [35] (S) -HSPG synthesised by hepatocytes was found to be present in a soluble form beneath the cell layer [28]. This basal HSPG bound to basement membrane Col. IV while its binding to Col. 1 was less, indicating a possible role for hepatocytes in producing the components for the organisation of basement membrane in liver. When heparan sulphate chains were initiated on artificial acceptors such as p-nitrophenly-β-D-Xyloside, these chains were not detected in the basal side of the hepatocyte monolayers indicating that the protein core is probably required for targeting the HSPG to the basal side (Sudhakaran, unpublished data). Details of the basolateral sorting processes in hepatocytes have not been known fully.

Influence of Matrix on Cell Function

The nature and influence of adhesive interactions of liver cells with the various components of the ECM have been studied using isolated rat liver cells. Hepatocytes *in vitro* attach, spread and adapt significantly different morphologies, on noncollagenous components such as fibronectin and laminin [29–33], on collagens including type IV [29–34] and on isolated liver biomatrix which is a mixture of glycoproteins, proteoglycans like HSPG and collagens [35, 36]. They bind directly to collagen, Fn and Ln coated substrata by apparently different mechanisms. Distinct and saturable kinetics of attachment of hepatocytes to different matrix protein substrata also indicated the presence of specific cell surface receptors for each matrix protein or shared receptors of having different affinities for each ligand (to be discussed later).

Hepatocytes can be maintained in culture on the matrix substrata and the possibility of their maintenance in a serum free medium make it a useful system to study the influence of the ECM on cellular activity. Hepatocytes in culture have a tendency to lose the transcription of liver specific mRNA, but the transcription of mRNAs for most of the housekeeping activities remain unaffected. Addition of hormones [37] or hepatic plasma membrane [38], or coculture with biliary epithelial cells [39] could maintain the expression of certain liver specific functions. Growth of cells inside hydrated collagenous matrices [40] on Engel breth-Holm Swarm (ESH) tumour derived gel matrix [41], specific tissue biomatrix [36] or even specific matrix protein substrate [25] could counteract the retrodifferentiation to varying degrees. Cells cultured on Col. IV retained differentiated phenotype more efficiently than those maintained on laminin substrata as measured by the synthesis of albumin and the production of a dedifferentiation marker, α-fetoprotein [25]. The viability and metabolic activity of hepatocytes from various sources have likewise been shown to be enhanced when the cells are cultured on collagen or biomatrix rich in laminin, Col. IV and HSPG [25, 35, 42, 43]. We have investigated further in detail the influence of the matrix substratum on the metabolic activity of hepatocytes in culture by analysing the various differentiated, dedifferentiated, constitutive and inducible functions in cells cultured on different tissue biomatrix or on different matrix protein substrata (A. Santhosh, Ph.D. Thesis). Synthesis of lipids, a major house keeping activity appeared to be similar in cells maintained on different matrix substrata; like albumin, synthesis of apo B, the major apoprotein of VLDL also lost progressively when cells were maintained in culture. The rate of loss of this differentiated function was also significantly low in cells cultured on homologous hepatic biomatrix than those maintained on connective tissue rich aortic biomatrix. Another hepatocyte specific function examined was the induction of cyt P450 a major constituent in hepatic microsomal system involved in the oxidative metabolism of a wide variety of xenobiotics and endogenous substrates. Cyt. P450 declines rapidly to low levels in primary cultures of hepatocytes. A few iso forms of the Cyt. P450 such as P450 IAI and P450 IIIAI are induced in the primary cultures with suitable inducers. When rat hepatocytes were maintained on Matrigel substrata, and treated with phenobarbital, induced expression of a new form of the protein viz. P450 IIBI occured [44]. However, constitutive form of Cyt. P450 including P450 II C II, could not be maintained in these cells. We found that the cells maintained on matrix proteins such as Fn, Col. IV and Ln retain the production of Cyt. P450 with an average molecular size of 47 kDa, while those maintained on tissue biomatrix produced, in addition to this, another form of Cyt. P450 with an average molecular size of 58 KDa. But in response to phenobarbital, Cyt. P450 induction occured only in cells maintained on tissue biomatrix; an inducible 53 KDa Cyt P450 protein appeared in significant amounts in cells maintained on homologous hepatic biomatrix (A. Santhosh, Unpublished data).

There is also indication that the effect of extracellular matrix on the phenotypic expression of cells may, among other factors be due to its influence on cell shape and on specific cytoskeletal pattern [45]. Hepatocytes attach to the matrix substrata and develop cytoskeletal structures which also contribute to the morphology of the cells. Cell adhesion sites have been identified ultrastructurally as areas of cell surface thickening adjacent to the ECM components [46]. A large number of molecules have been identified as components of these organised structures. They include actin, α-actinin, fibronectin, talin, vinculin, vimentin and cytoskeleton-associated molecules which are believed to link actin filaments to the cell surface [47–50]. SEM analysis showed that the morphology of the hepatocytes maintained on different substrata during the early stages of culture are different [29]. But it is not known whether this difference in early stages can contribute to the various effects described above. We investigated this further by maintaining hepatocytes on collagen coated plastic where the cells are normally attached along their basal surface to the substrata and on the three dimensional gel forms of collagen where the cells can penetrate the gel fibre and remain spherical. Albumin synthesis was significantly high in cells maintained on collagen gels while the synthesis of cytoskeletal protein was lower than that in cells maintained on the two dimensional substrata indicating that the morphology of the cells as influenced by the matrix can be one of the factors contributing to the matrix effect on hepatocyte behaviour [51]. The organisation of the cytoskeleton which is dictated by the extent of cell-cell and cell-matrix interaction is intimately associated with mechanisms that regulate tissue specific gene expression. A differential regulation of the expression of the cytoskeletal genes for actin, tubulin and cytokeratin and several liver specific genes has been suggested from studies carried out with hepatocytes maintained on EHS-derived matrix gel [41]. We investigated this further by studying the synthesis of various components of the cytoskeleton such as cytokeratin C_8, C_{18} and actin in cells maintained on different tissue biomatrices and individual matrix protein substrata and found a reciprocal relationship between the synthesis of albumin and that of cytoskeletal protein by analysing the same set of cultures (A. Santhosh, Unpublished data). Pulse labelling studies in cells maintained on different substrata for different length of time showed that in cultures where the albumin synthesis was high, that of C_8, C_{18} and actin was relatively less and vice versa. In general, these studies indicate that the rate of loss of differentiated functions was less when the cells were maintained on homologous hepatic biomatrix than on connective tissue rich heterologous tissue biomatrices.

Although availability of a suitable substratum improves the survival and metabolic activity of hepatocytes, the elaboration of an endogenous extracellular matrix also seems to be an important factor. D-Penicillamine which inhibits matrix collagen fiber formation, strongly inhibits the induction of DNA synthesis in primary cultures of rat hepatocytes [52]. Similarly, ascorbic acid which stimulates production of mature collagen, enhanced DNA synthesis [52]. Likewise, in mammary epithelial tissue, on inhibition of collagen synthesis, hormonal induction of milk protein synthesis was blocked suggesting that matrix synthesis in general, and collagen synthesis in particular, may be required for optimal expression of differentiated functions [53]. These observations indicate the importance of extracellular matrix in the control of the metabolic activity of hepatocytes.

Control of Matrix Synthesis

A number of observations indicate the existence of precise regulatory mechanisms controlling the composition of the extracellular matrix in liver. These include: (a) the fact that hepatocytes which constitute more than 90% of the liver cell mass can synthesise various components of the ECM, (b) the relatively low amount of the ECM in liver under physiological conditions and their accumulation in liver in response to acute and chronic liver injury and under pathological conditions such as liver fibrosis [54–56] and (c) the ability of the ECM to influence the metabolic activity of hepatocytes. There are several reports demonstrating regulatory effect of extracellular agents of hormonal and nonhormonal nature in the biosynthesis of matrix components [57–61]. Apart from the general mechanisms known to operate in the regulation of the synthesis of matrix components such as collagen and proteoglycan, two specific regulatory mechanisms in the synthesis of extracellular matrix macromolecules appear to exist in liver. These are: (a) hormonal control of HSPG synthesis and (b) feed back control by matrix itself. Liver is a major target organ for different hormones and drugs. Dibutyryl cyclic AMP and hormones and drugs which increase the intracellular concentration of cyclic AMP were found to inhibit the synthesis of HSPG in primary cultures of rat hepatocytes apparently by affecting the initiation of HS chains on the protein core [57].

Another possible regulatory mechanism in matrix synthesis is through a feed back control by the matrix component itself. This is evidenced by the reduced synthesis of Fn by hepatocytes maintained on fibronectin substrata and a decrease in synthesis of Col. IV by cells maintained on Col. IV substrata when compared to the synthesis of these components by cells maintained on heterologous matrix protein substrata [25]. This appeared to be dose dependent as the rate of synthesis of endogenous Fn and Col. IV is inversely related to the amount of the respective exogenous protein used to coat culture substrata. Although these observations suggest a negative feed back mechanism, we cannot, of course, exclude the possibility of a positive regulatory mechanism operating concurrently on heterologous matrix proteins as indicated by the observation that collagen synthesis by ARL-6-cells, a cell line derived from rat liver was enhanced by whole serum, but not by fibronectin depleted serum [62]. Our studies on cell surface HSPG further suggest feed back regulatory mechanism. The pericellular form of HSPG can be released by treatment with heparin. Depletion of pericellular HSPG by heparin or more specifically by heparitinase caused an increase in the synthesis of HSPG by hepatocytes in culture suggesting a possible regulatory role for cell surface HS in its production (Sudhakaran, Unpublished data). This further indicated the possibility of the occupation of saturable cell surface binding sites by HS leading to a control of the production of HSPG. Interaction of HSPG with the cell surface and the extracellular matrix may therefore serve as a regulatory mechanism in the control of the composition of the matrix as well as in maintaining a proper balance between the cells and the matrix. In conditions of liver injury which are associated with a change in the balance between parenchyma and stroma, there is an alteration in cellsurface HSPG [63]; similarly, in liver regeneration after CCl$_4$ or [63] thioacetamide injury [64] or after partial hepatectomy [65], there is a biphasic change in plasma membrane HS. HSPG also has the ability to self associate as well as to interact with Fn, Ln and Col. IV of the basement membrane [66]. It therefore appears that cell surface heparan sulphate proteoglycan has an important role in the regulation of hepatocyte matrix interaction and matrix assembly. Of particular interest is the observation that cell surface heparan sulphate synthesised by virally transformed cells and by transformed cell lines are under sulphated [67]. HSPG produced by cultured rat hepatoma cells that also do not deposit a pericellular matrix were under sulphated and had a lower affinity for fibronectin than HS isolated from normal liver [68]. Studies with transformed cells in culture also suggested that HSPG is essential for matrix assembly.

There also appears to exist an interrelation between the synthesis and assembly of certain components of the ECM. Treatment of hepatocytes with D-penicillamine, an inhibitor of collagen synthesis, caused a reduction in the synthesis of HSPG. Similarly, ascorbic acid which increases collagen synthesis caused an increase in the synthesis of HSPG. Although, studies with transformed cells in culture suggested that HSPG is essential for matrix assembly, it is not known whether there exists any mechanisms for intracellular coordination of the synthesis of these components or is a consequence of the extracellular assembly of the matrix on events at the cell surface/ intracellular sites. Experiments carried out in other systems, particularly mammary epithelial cells also indicate a relationship between nature of the matrix substrata and ability of the cells to synthesise matrix proteins; for instance, mammary epithelial cells cultured on type I collagen expressed lower levels of mRNAs and proteins of basement membarane than cells cultured on plastic [69]. Similarly, smooth muscle cells grown on Fn produced less amount of Fn than those cultured on albumin [70] or laminin [71]. Although the presence of matrix dependent elements in the promoter region of the β-casein gene in mammary epithelial system has been demonstrated [71a], the existence of such mechanism in the transcription of genes in hepatic system is not known. The above described observations primarily made in liver derived cells indicate the existence of apparently complex regulatory mechanisms controlling the composition and assembly of extracellular matrix in liver. An alteration in these regulatory mechanisms may lead to changes in the composition of ECM which can cause alteration in hepatocyte specific activity and behaviour in pathological conditions.

ECM in Liver Regeneration and Disease

In response to chronic hepatic injury the components of the ECM accumulate considerably. The synthesis of collagen enhanced promptly after acute liver damage. An increase in the activities of several of the collagen biosynthetic enzymes occurred early after injury [72] and preceded an increase in the collagen content of the liver [73]. After partial hepatectomy or drug induced injury, the liver is capable of complete regeneration, restoring normal hepatic size, architecture and function. Localisation of Col I, III, IV., Ln and Fn subsequent to hepatectomy was done by immuno histochemical techniques [74]. There was a brisk mitosis of hepatocytes with dramatic changes in ECM components. In 24 hrs, Ln appeared in the hepatic sinusoids, reaching a maximum staining intensity at 48 hrs; on completion of regeneration, there was no incidence of any substantial changes in the ECM/cell mass ratio. Thus the prominent expression of Ln and its proposed functions in morphogenesis suggest a critical role for this ECM component in the formation and reorganisation of the regenerating liver. The attachment of hepatocytes from regenerating liver to Ln was significantly more than adult rat liver cells [75, 76]. A 67 KDa Ln binding protein was isolated from regenerating rat liver [75]. This protein which binds to Laminin with very high affinity recognises YIGSR sequence in Ln and is apparently similar to the LB 67 isolated from tumour tissues [77].

Since hepatocytes are in close contact with the ECM, any alterations in ECM under pathological conditions can lead to altered hepatocyte-matrix interaction. Fibrosis is a rare event during liver disease, whether of toxic, viral or parasitic origin. From the available clinical and experimental data, the deterioration of hepatocellular function associated with fibrosis may be ascribed in part to the loss of biologic support provided by a normal ECM. In fibrosis, there is accumulation of collagen and PGS particularly CS/DS PGS, in liver. This appears to be due to enhanced rate of their production. Although the nature and origin of the cells which are activated to produce ECM components during liver fibrosis are not fully understood, Ito cells appear to play a major role. The recruitment of matrix producing cells, their proliferation, the secretion of matrix constituents, the remodelling and degradation of the matrix are some of the major events involved in fibrotic process. In areas of necroinflammation, the fat storing cells (perisinusoidal lipocytes, Ito cells) proliferate and transform into desmin and smooth muscle α actin positive myofibroblast—like cells which can synthesise significant amounts of collagens, PG, and matrix glycoproteins [78]. These cells appear to have a central role in the pathogenesis of fibrosis. β-D-xyloside induced abrogation of synthesis of PG, resulted in a reduction in the rate of proliferation and transformation of cultured liver fat storing cells and, deposition of matrix glycoproteins such as Fn, Ln and tenascin was reduced, further suggesting an interrelation between the synthesis of various matrix components and also cytoskeleton [79]. Apart from their role in the production of ECM components, the hepatic lipocytes may also play a role in the pathogenesis of liver fibrosis through the secretion of netural matrix metalloproteases. Activation through plasminogen activator mediated proteolytic cleavage and inhibition by tissue inhibitor of metalloproteinase, constitute two possible mechanisms for the control of the matrix/cell mass ratio. Hepatic lipocytes, by controlling the expression and release of TIMP-1 also may play a role in the pathogenesis of liver fibrosis [80].

Hepatosplenic Schistosomiasis is of interest, being an immune cell mediated granulomatous disease [81]. Fn and other macromolecules such as HSPG deposition occurs concomitantly with the development of granulomatous inflammation in the mouse liver infected with *Schistosoma mansoni*. An alteration in the metabolism of ECM components has also been reported in cirrhosis [82]. In experimental hepatocarcinogenesis apparently some humoral factors have been suggested to influence the hepatocyte to "turn on" the genes encoding the basement membrane components and further stimulate their assembly and deposition [83].

Matrix Receptors in Liver

As indicated above, macromolecules of the ECM play important positioning effects in the anchorrage, polarity and migration of cells. They also regulate their synthesis in a feed back manner and influence metabolic activity of the cells. These diverse biological effects are apparently mediated through interaction of the matrix macromolecules with specific cell surface components generally referred to as matrix receptors. More recently the focus of research in matrix biology has shifted to matrix receptors and the generation and transduction of signals intracellularly. Cell-cell and cell-matrix interactions in liver are also mediated by cell surface receptors. Affinity chromatography with extracellular matrix adhesive glycoproteins such as Fn and laminin, use of antibodies to inhibit cell adhesion to matrix glycoproteins and demonstration of the adhesion perturbing antibodies in blocking binding of matrix molecules to membrane proteins led to the identification and localisation of receptors for matrix molecules on the cell surface [84–85]. A group of integral membrane proteins that bind with varying specificity to various matrix proteins, belonging to a super family of gene called "integrins" have been characterised. Various types of integrins that bind with firbonectin, collagen, laminin and other adhesion proteins have been identified. The functional receptor is a non-covalently linked heterodimer of α and β subunits that can mediate cell-matrix as well as cell-cell interaction. Hepatocyte adhesion to Fn is mediated by $\alpha_5\beta_1$ integrin in a Ca^{++} dependent manner apparently through the RGD sequence in the cell binding domain of Fn [85, 86]. Heterodimeric $\alpha 1\beta 1$ integrin isolated from rat liver cells has been shown to bind to laminin [87], collagen I [88] and collagen IV [89]. Proteolytic fragments of Ln have been shown to promote attachment of adult rat hepatocytes and the $\alpha_1\beta_1$ integrin appears to bind to two structurally distinct domains of laminin, viz pepsin fragment P1 from the central region and elastase fragment E8 from the distal arm of the cross shaped Ln molecule [87]. Although it was suggested that the cell recognition sequence YIGSR is not involved in the attachment of hepatocytes to Ln, Clement et al [90] showed the presence of a group of laminin binding proteins on the hepatocyte surface which include a 68 kDa protein that may recognise the YIGSR sequence. However, the absence of any competitive inhibition of attachment of hepatocytes to PI fragment of Ln by peptides having the pentapeptide sequence suggests that either the 68 kDa nonintegrin receptor is not directly involved in attachment to Ln or that some other recognition sequence is involved.

Comparison of the attachment of adult and fetal hepatocytes and the cells from regenerating liver showed that fetal hepatocytes [75] and those from regenerating liver [76] adhere more to Ln and suggested the occurance of more number of laminin binding cell surface molecules in fetal liver. $\alpha_1\beta_1$ integrin isolated from human fetal liver appears to be a common receptor for laminin and Col. IV. Another protein with an average mol. wt. of 230 kDa consisting of two polypeptide chains each of average mol. size 110 and 130 kDa and linked through disulphide bonds has also been isolated from fetal liver. It binds to Ln in a Ca^{++} dependent manner [91]. The role, if any, of this protein in mediating hepatocyte adhesion and liver growth is yet to be established.

At least three other integrin α subunits have been detected in adult rat liver in association with β_1 sub units. Histochemical studies have shown the presence of α_2, α_3 and α_6 subunits, β_4 subunit and the receptor for vitronectin viz. $^{\alpha}_{vn}\beta_1$ in normal bile duct epithelium and their ectopic expression in neoplastic human parenchymal biopsies [92]. Apart from these integrin receptors, non-integrin receptors for matrix proteins have also been identified . By successive affinity chromatography of the membrane extracts of rat hepatocytes on WGA sepharose and fibronectin-sepharose, a 110 KDa protein (AGp 110) that binds to Fn with high affinity in a Ca^{++} dependent and RGD independent manner has been isolated [93]. AGp 110 is an extensively glycosylated integral membrane glycoprotein. Double label immunofluoresence and interference reflection microscopy studies using hepatocytes attached to fibronectin showed colocalisation of termini of actin filaments and vinculin and fibronectin receptors $\alpha_5\beta_1$ and AGp 110 at focal contact sites [94]. Similarly in Hep G_2 cells $\alpha_1\beta_1$ integrin appears to be concentrated in the basal area (Fig. 1).

Apart from adhesion receptors involved in cell matrix interaction, molecules involved in cell-cell interaction have also been identified in liver. E-Cadherin, a major molecular component of intermediate junction has been detected in hepatocytes [95]. Similarly DGl, a desmosomal component is also shown in hepatocytes (95); C-CAM, a developmentally regulated cell adhesion molecule has also been identified in normal rat liver [96]. Low level expression of intercellular adhesion molecule (I-CAM-I) and leukocyte function associated antigen (LFA-3) have also been found on sinusoidal cells [97].

Hepatocyte adhesion to the matrix proteins mediated by the transmembrane integrin type receptors may have important consequences for the cell. Two

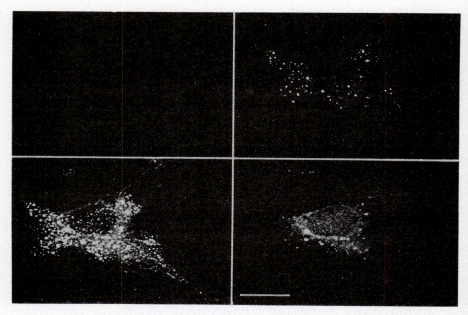

Fig. 1. **Laser Scanning Micrograph. HepG$_2$ cells were treated with antibodies against α_1 integrin and FITC labelled secondary antibodies and signals were monitored by laser scanning microscopy. Signal intensity was more towards basal area (bottom panel) than the top surface (top-left panel) Bar-25 μM. Similar pattern was seen for β_1 integrin staining.**

general views on the mechanism of integrin mediated signalling are currently being held. It is suggested that integrins transmit signals by organising the cytoskeleton, thus regulating cell shape and internal cellular architecture [98, 99]. Cytoplasmic domain of intergins in fact interact with cytoskeletal components [100, 101] and sites of ECM-integrin mediated adhesion serve as nucleation foci for cytokeletal assembly [101]. As indicated before, ECM, in fact influences the cell shape and the synthesis and assembly of cytoskeletal components in hepatocytes. Appropriate cell shape and cytoskeletal organisation might regulate the biosynthetic capabilities of the cell and thus may contribute to cell growth or differentiation [41, 102, 103].

Another view is to consider integrins as true receptors capable of generating biochemical signals within the cells. Binding of ligands to integrins has been shown to alter cellular pattern of tyrosine phosphorylation in a number of systems. In human carcinoma cells, clustering of integrins caused enchanced tyrosine phosphorylation of a complex of proteins of 120–150 kDa [104]. One of the components of the 120–130 KDa tyrosine phosphorylated complex in human carcinoma cells reacts with antibodies to a 125 kDa protein [104, 105] which had previously been identified as a substrate for src family of tyrosine kinases [106]. Integrin stimulated tyrosine phosphorylation of the 125 kDa protein has also been demonstrated in a number of other systems [107, 108] and based on its focal contact localisation [105, 109], the 125 kDa protein, which has got the capacity to autophosphorylate, has been termed pp125 Focal Adhesion kinase (pp125 FAK) [109]. It has been suggested that activation of pp125 FAK is related to anchorage dependence of cell growth [110]; another possibility is that this kinase regulates the cytoskeleton [111]. It is likely that integrin mediated activation of pp125 FAK is an early step in a signal transduction cascade that permits the flow of information. Using phosphotyrosine antibodies, the appearance of a protein of molecular size 120 kDa on the attachment of hepatocytes to matrix protein substrata has been found in our laboratory. The relation to 125 FAK and the role if any in integrin mediated signalling in hepatocytes are to be established.

In addition to changes in tyrosine phosphorylation, a number of other integrin-related signalling events have been described. These include changes in calcium activated proteases [112], $Na^+ \mid H^+$ antiporter [113] and subcellular distribution of phosphoinositide-3-kinase [114]. Integrin mediated events induce calcium transients in monocytes [115], and osteoclasts [116] while both cAMP [117] and calcium [118] are affected by $\beta2$ integrin mediated events in neutrophils. The occurrance of diverse group of adhesion proteins and their receptors in liver cells, their selective distribution and expression in embryonic and adult and regenerating conditions and their alteration in inflammatory conditions suggest the importance of cell-matrix interaction and molecular mechanisms thereof in the development and maintenance of hepatic parenchymal architecture and in liver functions relating to xenobiotic metabolism and stress related conditions. Apart from inflammatory conditions [97], other forms of stress such as oxidant stress, hyperthermia and heavy metals appear to cause alteration in hepatocyte adhesion [119]. These stress conditions apparently cause alteration in the cytoskeletal arrangement and cell surface distribution of matrix receptors. Liver being the major site of detoxification of drugs, the xenobiotic metabolism may also cause stress conditions *in vivo* and can affect cell-matrix interaction.

Summary

Biochemical and immunochemical studies have demonstrated the presence of various components of ECM such as proteoglycans, different types of collagens and glycoproteins such as fibronectin and laminin in liver. Distribution pattern of the various components of the basement membrane-like structure in liver suggests that they serve more than a simple structural function. Unlike the classical epithelium, hepatocytes have a belt of apical surface dividing the two basolateral surfaces that are in contact with the components of the basement membrane. These components apparently have an important role in maintaining the structural and functional polarity of hepatocytes. During tissue development, hepatic regeneration and under pathological conditions such as liver fibrosis, the composition of the ECM in liver changes. *In vitro* studies reveal that the metabolic activity and the morphology of the hepatocyte are influenced by the ECM. Similar studies also reveal that the synthesis and assembly of the matrix components are regulated by hormonal and nonhormonal factors as well as by a feed back control by the matrix itself. Matrix receptors belonging to the transmembrane integrins as well as the non-integrin group of receptors for matrix proteins such as collagen, fibronectin and laminin are present in liver. Although the matrix receptors mediate interaction of hepatocytes with the matrix components, precise mechanisms by which these interactions can lead to generation of specific intracellular effect to influence the metabolic activity of the cells, are not known.

Acknowledgement

Financial support from Department of Science and Technology, Government of India and University Grants Commission, New Delhi is gratefully acknowledged. Financial assistance from German Academic Exchange Service, is also gratefully acknowledged. Laser scanning microscopy was done while the author (P.R.S.) was a guest professor in Prof. K. von Figura's laboratory in Gottingen, Germany.

References

1. Arias I.M., Jakoby W.B., Popper H., Schachter D. and Schafritz D.A. (eds). (1988). The Liver-Biology and Pathobiology 2nd edn. Raven Press, New York.
2. Elias H. and Sherrick J.C. (1969). Morphology of the Liver. Academic Press, New York.
3. Evans W.H. (1980). Biochem., Biophys., Acta. **604**, 27–64.
4. Dunn J.C.Y., Yarmush M.L., Koebe H.G. and Tompkins R.G. (1989). FASEB. J. **3**, 174–177.
5. Hahn E., Wick G., Pencer D. and Timpl R. (1980). Gut. **21**, 63–72.
6. Rojkind M. and Ponce-Noyola P. (1982). Col. Relat. Res. **2**, 151–175.
7. Martinez-Hermandez, A. (1984). Lab. Invest. **51**, 57–74.
8. Clement, B.M., Rissel S., Peyrol Y., Mazurier Y., Grimaud J. and Guillouzo A. (1985). J. Histochem. Cytochem. **33**, 407–414.
9. Hughes R.C. and Stamatoglou S.C. (1987). J. Cell Sci. **8**, 273–291.
10. Wishes M.H. and Evans W.H. (1975). Biochem. J. **146**, 375–388.
11. Bartles J.R., Braiterman L.T. and Hubbard A.L. (1985). J. Biol., Chem., **260**, 12792–12802.
12. Enrich C., Evans W.H. and Gahmberg C.G. (1988). FEBS Lett. **228**, 135–138.
13. Enrich C. and Gahmberg C.G. (1985). Biochem. J. **227**, 565–572.
14. Höök M., Woods A., Johansson S., Kjellen L. and Couchman J.R. (1986). In: Functions of the Proteoglycans. CIBA. Symp. **124**, 143–151.
15. Stow J.L., Kjellen L., Unger E., Höök M. and Farquahr M.G. (1985). J. Cell Biol. **100**, 975–980.
16. Nakamura N., Hurst R.E. and West S.S. (1978). Biochem., Biophys., Acta. **538**, 445–457.
17. Gressner A.M., Pazen H. and Greiling H. (1977). Hoppe Seyler, Z. Physiol. Chem. **358**, 825–833.

18. Prinz R., Klein U., Sudhakaran, P.R., Sinn. W., Ullrich K. and Von Figura K. (1980). Biochem., Biophys. Acta. **630**, 402–413.
19. Delbrück A. (1968). Z. Klin. Chem. Klin. Biochem. 6, 460–466.
20. Suzuki S., Suzuki S., Nakamura N. and Koizumi T. (1976). Biochem. Biophys. Acta. **428**, 166–181.
21. Dietrich C.P., Sampaio L.O. and Toledo O.M.S. (1976). Biochem. Biophys. Res. Commun. **71**, 1–10.
22. Höök M., Kjellen L., Johansson S. and Robinson J. (1984). Ann. Rev. Biochem. **53**, 847.
23. Voss B., Allam S., Rauterberg S., Ullrich K., Gieselman V. and Von Figura K. (1979). Biochem., Biophys. Res. Commun. **90**, 1348.
24. Tamkun J.W. and Hynes R.O. (1983). J. Biol., Chem., **258**, 4641.
25. Sudhakaran P.R., Stamataglou S.C. and Hughes R.C. (1986). Exp. Cell. Res. **167**, 505–516.
26. Odenthal M., Neubauer K., Baralle F.E., Peters H., Meyer-Bushenfelde K.H. and Ramadori G. (1992). Exp. Cell. Res. **203**, 289–296.
27. Oyama F., Horihashi S., Shimosato Y., Titani K. and Sekijuchi K. (1989). J. Biol. Chem. **264**, 10331–10341.
28. Babu P.B.S. and Sudhakaran P.R. (1991). J. Cell, Biochem., **46**, 48–53.
29. Bissell D.M., Stamatoglou S.C., Nermut M.V. and Hughes R.C. (1985). Eur. J. Cell. Biol. **40**, 72–78.
30. Gjessing R. and Seglen P.O. (1980). Exp. Cell. Res. **129**, 239.
31. Johansson S. and Höök M. (1984). J. Cell Biol. **98**, 810–817.
32. Johansson S., Kjellen L., Höök M. and Timpl R. (1981). J. Cell Biol. **90**, 260–264.
33. Timpl R., Johansson S., Van Delden V., Oberbaumer I. and Höök, M. (1983) J. Biol. Chem. **258**, 8922–8927.
34. Rubin K., Höök M., Obrink B. and Timpl R. (1981). Cell. **24**, 463–470.
35. Reid L.M. and Jefferson D.M. (1983). Hepatology, **4**, 548.
36. Rojkind M., Gatmaitan Z., Mackensen S., Giambrone M.A., Proce P. and Reid L.M. (1980). J. Cell. Biol. **87**, 255–263.
37. Jefferson D.M., Clayton D.F., Darnell J.F., Jr. and Reid L.M. (1984). Mol. Biol **4**, 1929–34.
38. Nakamura T., Yoshimoto K., Nakayama Y., Tomita Y. and Chihara A. (1983). Proc. Natl. Acad. Sci. USA. **80**, 7229–7233.
39. Fraslin J.M., Kneip N., Vaulont S., Glaise D., Munnich A. and Guguen-Guilozo C. (1985). EMBO J. **4**, 2487–2491.
40. Dunn J.C.Y., Tompkins R.G. and Yarmush M.L. (1992). J. Cell. Biol. **116**, 1043–1053.
41. Ben-Zeev A., Robinson G.S., Bucher N.L.R. and Farmer S.R. (1988), Proc. Natl. Acad. Sci., U.S.A. **85**, 2161–2165.
42. Enat R., Jefferson D.M., Ruiz-Opazo N., Gatmaitan Z., Leinwand L.A. and Reid L.M. (1984). Proc. Natl. Acad. Sci. USA. **81**, 411.
43. Isom H.C., Scott T., Georgoff I., Woodworthic and Mummaw. (1985). Proc. Natl. Acad. Sci. USA. **82**, 3252–56.
44. Emi Y., Chijiiwa C. and Omura T. (1990). Proc. Natl. Acad. Sci. USA **87**, 9746–9750.
45. Spiegelman B.M. and Ginty. G.A. (1983). Cell. **35**, 657–666.
46. Abercrombie M., Heysman E.M. and Pegrum S.M. (1971). Exp. Cell. Res. **67**, 359–367.
47. Wehland J., Osborn M. and Webe K. (1979). J. Cell Sci., **37**, 257–273.

48. Burridge K. and Feràmisco J. (1980). Cell. **19**, 587–595.
49. Geiger B., Tokuyasu K.T., Dutton A.H. and Singer S.J. (1980). Proc. Natl. Acad. Sci. USA, **77**, 4127–4131.
50. Burridge K. and Connell L. (1983). J. Cell. Biol. **94**, 359–367.
51. Santhosh A. and Sudhakaran P.R. (1994). Mol. Cell. Biochem. **137**, 127–133.
52. Nakamura T., Teramoto H., Tomita Y. and Ichihara A. (1984). Biochem., Biophys., Res. Commun. 122, 884.
53. Wakimoto H. and Oka T. (1983). J. Biol., Chem., **258**, 3775–3779.
54. Gressner A.M. (1980). Med. Melt. **31**, 11–16.
55. Rauterberg J., Voss B., Pott. G. and Gerlach V. (1981). Klin. Wochenschr. **59**, 167–79.
56. Unnikrishnan V.S. and Sudhakaran P.R. (1985). Ind. J. Biochem., Biophys., **22**, 304–308.
57. Sudhakaran P.R., Sinn. W. and Von Figura K. (1980). Biochem. J. **192**, 395–402.
58. Gressner A.M. and Schultz W. (1981). Horm. Metab. Res. **13**, 649–650.
59. Kilgore B.S., McNatt M.L., Meador S., Lee J.A., Hughes E.R. and Elders M.J. (1979). Pediat. Res. **13**, 96–99.
60. Kato Y. and Gospodarowicz D. (1985). J. Biol., Chem., **260**, 2364–2373.
61. Roden, L. (1980). In "Biochemistry of Glycoproteins and Proteoglycans" (W.A. Lennarz, ed) p. 267–371. Plenum Press, N.Y.
62. Foidart J.M. Berman J.J., Paglia. L., Rennard S., Abe. S., Perantoni A. and Martin G.R. (1980). Lab Invest. **42**, 425.
63. Unnikrishnan V.S. and P.R. Sudhakaran (1989), J. Biosci., **14**, 163–172.
64. Gressner A.M., Cadenbach J.E. and Greiling H. (1981). J. Clin. Chem., Clin. Biochem., **19**, 465–469.
65. Edward M., Long. F.W., Watson H.K.H. and Williamson B.F. (1980). Biochem. J. **188**. 769–773.
66. Gallagher J.T., Lyon M. and Steward (1986). Biochem. J. **236**, 313–325.
67. Underhill C.B., Chi Rosso G. and Toole B.P. (1983). J. Biol., Chem., **258**, 8086.
68. Robinson J., Viti M. and Höök M. (1984). J. Cell. Biol., **98**, 946.
69. Streuli C.H. and Bissell M.J. (1990). J. Cell. Biol. **110**, 1405–1415.
70. Holderbaum D. and Ehrhart L.A. (1986). J. Cell. Physiol., **126**, 216–224.
71. Hedin U., Bottger B.A., Forsberg E., Johansson. S. and Thyberg J. (1988). J. Cell. Biol., **107**, 307–319.
71a. Schmidhauser C., Bissel M.J., Myers C.A. and Casperson G.F. (1990). Proc. Natl. Acad. Sci. USA. **87**, 9118–9122.
72. McGee J.O.D., O'Hare, R.P. and Patrick R.S. (1973). Nature (Lond) New Biol. **243**, 121.
73. Risteh J. and Kivirikko K.L. (1976). Biochem. J, **158**, 361.
74. Martinez, Hernandez A., Delgado M. and Amenta P.S. (1991). Lab. Invest. **64**, 157–166.
75. Anil Kumar N. and Sudhakaran P.R. (1993). Biochem., Mol. Biol., Int. **31**, 201–209.
76. Carlson R., Engvall E., Freeman A. and Rouslahti E. (1981). Proc. Natl. Acad. Sci. USA. **78**, 2403.
77. Steller-Stevenson W.G., Aznavoorian S. and Liotta L.A. (1993). Ann. Rev. Cell. Biol., **9**, 541–573.
78. Rumadori G. (1992). Z. Gastroenterol. **30**, 17–20.
79. Gressner A.M. (1991). Exp. Mol. Pathol. **55**, 143–69.
80. Iredale J.P., Murphy G., Hembry R.M., Friedman S.L. and Arther M.J. (1992). J. Clin. Invest. **90**, 282–287.

81. Grimaud J.A. (1987). Mem. Invest. Oswaldo, Craz. **82**, 55–65.
82. Jezequel A.M., Ballardini G., Mancini R., Paolucci F., Bianchi F.B. and Orlandi F. (1990). J. Hepatol. **11**, 206–214.
83. Albrechtsen R., Wewer U.M. and Thorgeirsson S.S. (1988). Hepatology **8**, 538–546.
84. Buck C.A. and Horwitz A.F. (1987). Ann. Rev. Cell. Biol. 3, 179–205.
85. Rouslahti E. (1988). Ann. Rev. Biochem **57**, 375–413.
86. Johansson S., Forseberg E. and Lundgreen B. (1987). J. Biol. Chem. **262**, 7819–7824.
87. Forsberg E., Paulsson M., Timpl R. and Johansson S. (1990). J. Biol. Chem. **265**, 6376–6381.
88. Gullberg D., Turner D.C, Borg T.K., Terracio L. and Rubin K. (1990). Exp. Cell Res. **190**, 254–264.
89. Stamatoglou S.C., Bawumia S., Johansson S., Forsberg E. and Hughes R.C. (1991). FEBS. Lett, **288**, 241–243.
90. Clement B., Segui Beat B., Savangner P., Kleinman H.K. and Yamada Y. (1990). J. Cell Biol. **110**, 185–192.
91. Anil Kumar N. and Sudhakaran P.R. Occurrence of a 230 kDa protein with affinity for laminin in fetal liver (Abstract) 16th Int. Cong. of Bioch. and Mol. Biol. (1994), New Delhi.
92. Volpes R., Van Den Oord J.J. and Desmet V.J. (1993). Am. J. Pathol. **142**, 1483–1492.
93. Stamatoglou S.C., Ge R.C., Mills, G., Butters T.D., Zaidi F. and Hughes R.C. (1990). J. Cell Biol. **111**, 2117–2127.
94. Stamatoglou S.C. and Hughes R.C. (1994). FASEB J. **8**, 420–427.
95. Stamatoglou S.C., Enrich C., Manson M.M. and Hughes R.C. (1992). J. Cell Biol. **116**, 1507–1515.
96. Obrink B. (1991). Bio Essays. **13**, 227–233.
97. Volpes R., Van den Oord J.J. and Demet. V.J. (1990). Hepatology. **12**, 59–65.
98. Fox J.E. (1993). Adv. Exp. Med. Biol. **344**, 175–183.
99. Fox J.E. (1994). Ann. N.Y. Acad. Sci. **714**, 75–87.
100. Otey C.A., Pavalko F.M. and Burridge K. (1990). J. Cell Biol. **111**, 721–729.
101. Burridge K., Fath K., Kelley T., Nuckolls G. and Turner C. (1988). Ann. Rev. Cell Biol. **4**, 487–525.
102. Ingber D.E. and Folkman F. (1989). Cell **58**, 803–805.
103. Ingber D.E. (1991). Chest. **99**, 34–40.
104. Kornberg L., Earp. H.S., Turner C., Prokop C. and Juliano R.L. (1991). Proc. Natl. Acad Sci. USA. **88**, 10222–10226.
105. Kornberg L., Earp H.S., Parsons J.T., Schaller M., and Juliano R.L. (1992). J. Biol. Chem. **267**, 23439–23442.
106. Kanner S.B., Reynolds A.B., Vines R.R. and Parsons J.T. (1990). Proc. Natl. Acad. Sci. USA. **87**, 3328–3332.
107. Guan J.L., Trevethick J.E. and Hynes R.O. (1991). Cell Regul. **2**, 951–964.
108. Shattil S.J. and Brugge J.S. (1991). Curr. Opin. Cell Biol. **3**, 869–879.
109. Schaller M.D., Borgman C.A., Cobb B.S., Vines R.R. Reynolds A.B. and Parson J.T. (1992). Proc. Natl. Acad. Sci. USA. **89**, 5192–5196.
110. Guan J.L. and Shallway D. (1992). Nature, 358, 690–692.
111. Burridge K., Turner C.E. and Romer L.H. (1992). J. Cell Biol. **119**, 893–903.
112. Fox J.E.B., Goll D.E., Reynolds L.C. and Phillips D.R. (1985). J. Biol. Chem. **260**, 1060–1066.
113. Banga H.S., Simons E.R., Brass L.F. and Rittenhouse S.E. (1986). Proc. Natl. Acad. Sci. USA. **83**, 9197–9201.

114. Zhang J., Fry M.J., Waterield M.D., Jaken S., Laao L., Fox J.E.B. and Rittenhouse S.E. (1992). J. Biol. Chem. **267**, 4686–4692.

115. Menon R.P., Pillai S. and Sudhakaran P.R. (1993). Biochem. Mol. Biol. Int. **31**, 833–840.

116. Mianchi A., Alvarez J., Grenfeld E.M. et al. (1991). J. Biol. Chem. **266**, 20369–20374.

117. Nathan C. and Sanchez E. (1990). J. Cell Biol. **111**, 2171–2181.

118. Ng-Sikorski J., Anderson R., Patarroyo M. and Anderson T. (1991). Exp. Cell Res. **195**, 504–508.

119. Mathew S. and Sudhakaran P.R. (1993). Biochem. Biophys. Acta. **1178**, 146–152.

Liver and Environmental Xenobiotics
S.V.S. Rana and K. Taketa (Eds)
Copyright © 1997, Narosa Publishing House, New D

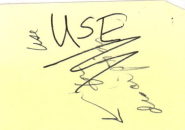

2. Drug Metabolizing Enzymes in the Liver

Mohammad Athar, S. Zakir Husain and Nafisul Hasan

Department of Medical Elementology and Toxicology, Jamia Hamdard
Hamdard Nagar, New Delhi 110062, India

Liver is the principal body organ which plays an important role in the metabolism of foreign (xenobiotic) compounds that enter into the body. Humans are exposed to these compounds through the environmental exposure or through the consumption of contaminated food materials or during the exposure in occupational environment. In addition, human beings consume a lot of drugs (medicinal preparations) during the disease states which are mainly synthetic product and are foreign for the body organs. All of these compounds produce a variety of toxic manifestations including carcinogenesis. Irrespective of the mode of exposure and toxic manifestations of these compounds, the objective of the body tissue is to eliminate such foreign compounds as early as possible. This is done through the normally existing biochemical mechanisms in the tissue. For this purpose, body tissues utilize certain enzymes and other endogenous biomolecules which are actually meant for the metabolism of endogenous substrates. However, a few of the similar enzymes/biomolecules are also induced in response to the exposure of the foreign compounds.

Biotransformation of a xenobiotic compound following its exposure can alter its distribution and action, usually leading to its detoxification and excretion. On the contrary, an enhancement in the toxicity may also be observed due to the bioactivation of xenobiotic compound. Compounds structurally similar to endogenous compounds may enter the body via active transport mechanism sharing sites meant for biochemical action and metabolism of endogenous compounds. Several organs, particularly liver, contain enzymes with very broad substrate specificity and capability to metabolize a wide range of lipid-soluble organic compounds. As a result, the generation of a more water-soluble product is resulted which is excreted fast thus decreasing its body burden, time of exposure and consequent toxic manifestations. However, similar enzymes can often bioactivate some of them to reactive intermediates that ultimately bind with the cellular macromolecules producing cytotoxicity and/or carcinogenicity. Figure 1 describes general picture of the fate of compounds usually that enter into the body till they are excreted.

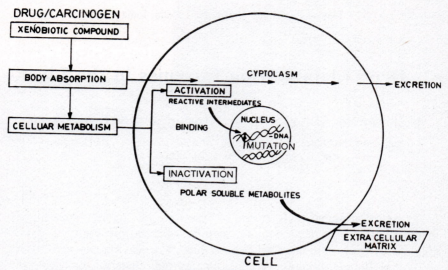

Fig. 1 Metabolic fate of drug/carcinogen entering into the body

When a reactive intermediate is formed during metabolism, often it exerts toxicity in the immediate vicinity. Many xenobiotics bioactivated by hepatic cytochrome P-450 system cause centrilobular necrosis. Incidently, the highest concentration of cytochrome P-450 is found in the centrilobular region. However, the centrilobular region is also rich in conjugating enzymes. The oxygen-rich periportal region contains mostly enzymes of intermediary metabolism for plasma protein synthesis and lipid and carbohydrate metabolism. Necrosis of the periportal region is associated with direct-acting hepatotoxins that enter the liver there, from the portal vein, and do not require bioactivation. Examples are hepatotoxic metals such as iron, manganese, arsenic, and phosphorus. Because the biliary tree drains from accumulation of biliary excretory products, cholestasis is first seen in the periportal region [1, 2].

Detoxification and Bioactivation

The biotransformation reactions can be classified into two phases. Phase I metabolism involves oxidative, reductive, and/or hydrolytic reactions that cleave substrate molecules to produce a more polar moiety. Sometimes, the reaction products generated at this stage being highly reactive produce toxic‘ manifestations before they enter into the Phase II reactions.

Phase II reactions also sometimes called as synthetic reactions involve conjugation or addition of certain endogenous molecules to the Phase I transformed xenobiotic compounds to make them still more polar and highly water soluble. While phase II metabolites have been considered as almost invariably nontoxic, the examples of exception to this rule are numerous and growing with increasing knowledge of basic metabolism of a variety of structurally different chemical compounds. Figure 2 represents the basic concepts of Phase I and Phase II xenobiotic metabolism. During Phase I metabolism, the formation of epoxy/hydroxy derivatives have been shown.

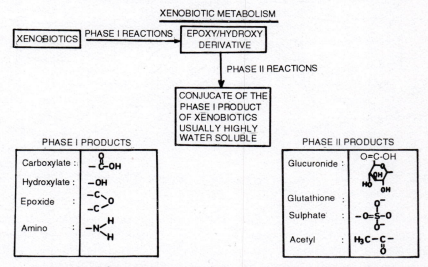

Fig. 2. Depiction of phase I and phase II products of a xenobiotics.

Other Phase I products include the formation of carboxylate and amino and hydroxylamine derivatives. The enzymes carrying out Phase I reactions are microsomal flavincontaining mono-oxygenase, alcohol dehydrogenases, amidases, monoamine oxidases, peroxidases such as of prostaglandin synthase and myeloperoxidase. Based on reconstitution studies, it has been demonstrated that microsomal flavin-containing monooxygenase require cytochrome P-450, NADPH-dependant P-450 reductase and phospholipid to perform catalytic action. Some of the mono-oxygenases reactions are summarized in Figure 3. Phase II products are usually the conjugates of Phase I products. The conjugating moieties in this reaction include glutathione, cysteine, glucuronide, sulfate or formation of acetyl derivatives. Phase II reactions are catalyzed by the enzymes, epoxide hydrolases, glutathione S-transferases, uridine diphosphate (UDP)-glucuronoyl transferases, cysteine conjugate β-lyase, γ-glutamyl transpeptidase, methylases etc. The other important enzyme in this category is quinone reductase which converts toxic quinones into relatively non-toxic phenols. Some of these enzymes are described in a greater detail below:

1. Phase I Metabolism

(I) Cytochrome P-450

The cytochrome P-450s are heme proteins and represent a multigene family of isozymes involved in oxidative biotransformation of lipid-soluble

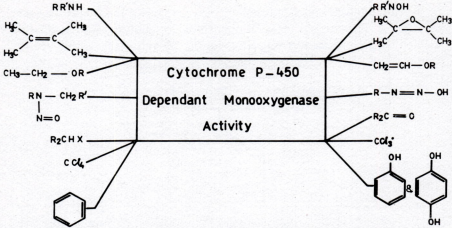

Fig. 3.   Some important phase I products generated by cyt. P450-dependent monooxygenase systems.

compounds to polar metabolites. The key enzymatic components of this membrane bound enzyme system are the flavo protein NADPH-cytochrome-P450-oxydoreductase and cytochrome P-450. The term cytochrome P-450 has been given to this protein because the visible spectra of reduced protein bound to carbon monoxide shows an absorption maximum at 450 nm as identified by Kilingenberg and Garfinkle in 1958. This pigment was further characterized as a cytochrome P-450 heme protein by Omura and Sato in 1962. Since this protein catalyzes the insertion of one oxygen atom from the oxygen molecule, the enzymes are broadly known as cytochrome P-450 dependant mono oxygenases. They are present in the highest concentration in liver, but in most other tissues, including kidney, lung, gut, skin and nasal epithelium their presence can also be demonstrated both biochemically and immunohistochemically. Several isozymes are dedicated for the metabolism of specific endogenous molecules such as kidney mitochondrial 1-alpha-hydroxylase is highly substrate specific and appears to metabolize 25-hydroxy cholecalciferol. However, isozymes in the hepatic endoplasmic reticulum show a rather broad substrate specificity, catalyzing oxidation of many structurally related chemicals. Furthermore, a single substrate may be metabolize by many isozymes. Substrate specificities, inducibilities, and amino acid sequences are highly conserved across species. Oxidative attack occurs at N, S, and C bonds, resulting in the insertion of one atom of molecular oxygen into the substrate, often producing an unstable intermediate that breaks down to yield the final product. For example, the N-alkylated compound N-methylaniline is metabolized to intermediate oxidation product that breaks down to formaldehyde and aniline. Occasionally, the oxidized products are highly toxic unstable electrophiles. A large number of isozymes of cytochrome P-450 have been isolated and many of them have been purified to homogenity. Their encoding genes have been identified and their regulation has been studied. At present, at least 70 different cytochrome P-450s have been purified from mammalian tissues whose protein sequences are known out of which at least 20 distinct P-450s have been identified in liver [3, 4]. The following isozymes in liver are described in a greater detail:

P-450a: This is a constitutive form which accounts for nearly all of the testosterone 2α-hydroxylase activity in rat liver microsomes. This isozyme has also been shown to be involved in 17β estradiol 2-and 4-hydroxylation and oxidation of acetaminophen, nifedipine etc. This is an isozyme which is not induced by the common xenobiotics and is sensitive to hormonal regulation.

P-450b: This is a phenobarbital inducible isozyme. It has high demethylase activity towards the d-benzphetamine and aminopyrine. It hydroxylases testosterone at the 16α, 16β and 17β position; however, only the 16β-hydroxylation is highly specific to this isozyme. The most specific substrate of P-450b is 7-pentoxyresourfin.

P-450c: Polycyclic hydrocarbons such as the 3-methylcholantherene, β-naphthoflavone, benzo(a) pyrene, etc. induce another P-450 isozyme which is known as P-450c. This isozyme can oxygenate at the sterically hindered positions and is supposed to be responsible for the activation of procarcinogens into carcinogens. 6β-hydroxylation is the major activity observed with testosterone 7-ethoxyresorufin is, probably the single most definitive substrate of this enzyme.

P-450d: The 3-methylcholanthrene and other hydrocarbons besides inducing P-450 also induce this isozyme.

P-450e: Phenobarbital besides inducing P-450b also induces this isozyme.

P-450p: Pregnenolone 16α-carbonitrile (PCN) preferentially induce this isozyme. Ethylmorphine N-demethylase activity is preferentially catalyzed by this enzyme.

P-450j: Many solvent like ethanol, acetone, pyridine etc. induce this isoform which is also known to catalyze the conversion of procarcinogens into carcinogenic reactive metabolites.

Besides, a large number of other isozymes are induced in response to both endogenous substrates and exogenous chemicals. Some of the substrates also called as suicidal substrates are the compounds which are metabolized to highly reactive chemical entity that binds irreversibly with the active site. This results in the deactivation of the enzyme protein. This is known as suicidal inactivation. The most important example of suicidal substrates of the cytochrome P-450 are carbon tetrachloride and chloramphenicol.

(ii) Other Phase I Reactions

1. Hydrolysis: The hydrolyzing enzymes are wide spread throughout the body, including the blood plasma, and have been shown to catalyze the hydrolysis of esters and amides. Classification of these enzymes is ill-defined due to the wide substrate distribution and overlapping specificities.

2. Reduction: A large number of nitro and azo compounds undergo anaerobic NADPH-dependent reduction reactions that can be inhibited by carbon monoxide, implicating a role of cytochrome P-450 in this process. However, a separate flavin nitroreductase has also been shown to exist. Carbon tetrachloride and halothane are the examples of the chemical that are metabolized both oxidatively and reductively by cytochrome P-450. Reduction of these compounds results in the their bioactivation leading to the formation of toxic intermediates, while oxidation reaction is a detoxification step. It has been shown that the oxygen tension in liver determines the route of metabolism. In addition the reduction reactions can be carried out by a number of aldehyde reductases, and alcohol dehydrogenases which are distributed throughout the body. Alcohol dehydrogenase catalyzed conversion of chloral hydrate to trichloroethanol is one such example.

3. Non-P450 Oxidation: A number of oxidases other than cytochrome P-450 dependent microsomal enzyme exist in the body which catalyze various oxidation reactions. Such non-P450-dependant microsomal oxidation system which is present in many tissues including liver but is more versatile for kidney, is prostaglandin synthase which is a glycoprotein with a heme containing centre. This enzyme produces prostaglandins from arachidonic acid oxidatively. In this reaction, a peroxide byproduct is also generated. A number of xenobiotics have been shown to be co-oxidized to toxic metabolites during prostaglandin synthase dependent reactions. The other oxidases present are monoamine oxidases (MAO) and diamine oxidases (DAO). Both of these enzymes are widely distributed. Monoamine oxidases are mitochondrial flavoproteins which are responsible for the catabolism of monoamine neurotransmitters such as dopamine, norepinephrine, epinephrine etc. These enzymes can also oxidize a number of xenobiotic amines. Similarly, diamine oxidases are Vitamin B_6-dependent cytosolic enzymes that preferrentially metabolize short chain aliphatic diamines. It may also convert amines to aldehyde in the presence of oxygen. In addition, alcohol dehydrogenases, another, another group of cytosolic enzymes can oxidize a variety of alcoholic compounds [5, 6].

2. Phase II Metabolism

Phase II metabolism has been known for the last 200 years when the conjugation of benzoic acid with the glycine has been demonstrated. Phase II metabolism involves a number of reactions usually on the products which are formed as a result of Phase I transformation of both endogenous and xenobiotic compounds. A large group of enzymes capable of performing diverse nature of reactions participate in this process. However, the ultimate objective of such reactions as already discussed is to make more polar and water soluble metabolites which may easily be excreted usually through urine. Though, as has been observed during Phase I reactions, certain Phase II products become highly toxic instead of becoming non-toxic and produce a variety of adverse responses. The detailed description of various groups of these enzymes is given below.

(a) Epoxide Hydrolase

Epoxide hydrolase catalyses the hydrolysis of epoxide of xenobiotics including carcinogens and drugs to form the corresponding dihydrodiols. These epoxy products are formed through the mono-oxygenase activity of cytochrome P-450. Epoxide hydration is associated with the detoxification of reactive epoxides to less reactive, water soluble dihydrodiols, which may be excreted fast.

First rigorous demonstration of the formation of epoxides of arenes in liver done by Jerina and his group in 1968 using benzene oxide showed that it serve as a precursor for the formation of phenol, catechol etc. and later demonstrated the formation of epoxide intermediates of naphthalene using hepatic microsomes. The enzymes that regulate tissue concentrations of these reactive epoxides are known as epoxide hydrolase (E. C. 3. 3. 2. 3). The other synonyms of this enzyme are epoxide hydrase and epoxide hydrolase. Although, this is ubiquitous enzyme present in most of the tissues, liver is one of the organs in which its highest activity has been demonstrated. Immunohistochemical studies suggest that centrilobular region of liver contains higher levels of this enzyme as compared to mid zonal and periportal regions. Similarly, highest staining has been observed in hepatocytes than in Kupffer and endothelial cells. In subcellular fractions, the epoxide hydrolase activity was found in the microsomal fraction. All other membranes such as the nuclear envelope, plasma membrane etc. also contain demonstratable enzyme activities. Though there are remarkable differences in nuclear and microsomal inducibility of epoxide hydrolase by 3-methyl cholanthrene, metyrapone and phenobarbital but the two enzymes have identical molecular weight of 49 KDa and are also immunologically identical.

Hammock and co-workers demonstrated the epoxide hydrolase activity in soluble fraction of liver and kidney homogenates. They also showed that trans β-ethyl styrene is an excellent substrate of this enzyme. In another study, Watabe et al showed cis-hydrogen stilbene oxide is hydrated

700-times faster as compared to its trans-isomer by the microsomal epoxide hydrolase where as trans-stilbene oxide is an excellent substrate for cytosolic enzyme. It has also been shown that liver microsomal and cytosolic isozymes are immunologically distinguishable from each other. Similarly, mitochondria also shows the presence of epoxide hydrolase. Its activity is mainly located in the matrix and intermembrane space of mitochondria and shows similarity with cytosolic epoxide hydrolase in substrate specificities, molecular weight and inhibitors.

Similar to other drug/carcinogen metabolizing enzymes, epoxide hydrolase has been shown to be induced by a large number of xenobiotics. Some important examples include trans-stilbene oxide, benzyl, butylated hydroxy toluene, butylated hydroxyanisole and 2-aminoacetyl fluorene which are effective inducers of microsomal isoform. Effect of various compounds on the relative induction of microsomal epoxide activity towards styrene 7, 8, epoxide hydrolase has been shown in Figure 4. Microsomal epoxide hydrolase has been shown to metabolize some steroids. C_{16}-unsaturated steroids, estratetraenol and androstadienone are metabolized to corresponding 16α, 6α-epoxide which is formed both in humans and in mice is hydrated by a microsomal enzyme distinct from epoxide hydrolase [7, 8].

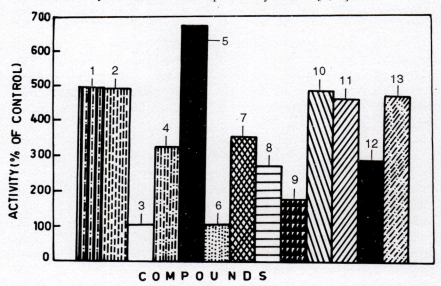

Fig. 4. **Effect of the various compounds on the relative induction of microsomal epoxide hydrolase activity towards styrene 7, 8, epoxide. 1—Anisil, 2—Benzil, 3—Bis (2-Naftyl)-etendion, 4—Chalcone epoxide, 5—Clotrimazole, 6—Dinitrobenzil, 7—Elipticine, 8—Flavone, 9—9-Fluorene, 10—Harmane, 11—Isoquinoline, 12—Metyrapone, 13—1-(2-Naftyl)-2-phenyletandion.**

The mechanism of naphthalene-mediated cataractogenesis involves its cytochrome P-450-dependent conversion to dihydrodiol. In the eye, this product is reduced to catechol by the lenticular catechol reductase. Catechol auto-oxidizes to 1,2 naphthoquinone with the release of hydrogen peroxide. The naphthoquinone is then again reduced to catechol at the expense of GSH. This cycle depletes orbital GSH, causing oxidative damage to lenticular proteins which are denatured and precipitated. This decreases the opacity of the lens that results in cataract formation.

(b) Glucuronidation

The glucuronide and sulfate conjugation reactions are known since 1870. Glucose is readily available in the tissues and is utilized for the glucuronidation reactions. The tissue pool of sulfate or glycine available for conjugation is relatively smaller in comparison to glucose and therefore, conjugation with sulfate or glycine constitute only minor part of the Phase II metabolism. The family of enzymes that are responsible for catalyzing glucuronide conjugation are known as glucuronyl transferases, which are present in the microsomal fraction of liver and other tissues. These enzymes catalyze the transfer of UDP-glucuronic acid to a variety of endogenous and xenobiotic compounds having hydroxyl, amino and sulfhydryl groups. Thus, N-, O-, and S-glucuronides are formed which are excreted into bile and urine.

At least 20 different isozymes are known to exist. Many of them have been purified to homogeneity from liver of different animals including humans. A list of commonly occurring UDP-glucuronidase in rat and human liver is given in Table 1. Broadly, these isozymes have been differentiated on the basis of their differential inducibility, substrate specificity and their ontogenic and perinatal development. Based on their ability to form conjugates with different substrates, three broad categories of isoforms have been identified. Isoforms that catalyze glucuronidation of bulky substrates such as morphine, 4-hydroxy biphenyl, terpentenes etc. have been shown to be stimulated by phenobarbital. Similarly, another group include isozymes that can catalyze UDP-glucuronide conjugation of planar molecules such as 1-naphthol or 4 methyl lumbelliferone is induced by 3-methyl cholanthrene whereas clofibrate and some other aryl carboxylic acids administration increases selectively the glucuronidation of bilirubin. It has also been shown that triphenylacetic acid is an effective and selective inhibitor of bilirubin glucuronidation in rat liver microsomes.

Besides, providing higher water solubility, a few glucuronide metabolites may be more active than parent drug or may show higher toxic potential than the parent xenobiotic compound. For example, morphine 6-0-glucuronide is more potent analgesic than morphine. Although, this metabolite is not formed in high concentration in rat liver but human liver produces its high concentrations. The examples of exacerbation of toxic responses include the covalent binding of N-hydroxy phenacetin glucuronide with proteins, inhibition of canicular bile flow and bile acid secretion by estrogen D-ring glucuronides and anaphylactic reaction of protein bound glucuronides of non-steroidal anti-inflammatory drugs [9, 10].

Table 1

UDP Glucuronyl transferase	Substrate specificity (exogenous)
Rat Liver	
1. 17β-OH steroid	p-Nitrophenol, 1-naphthol, α- and β-naphthylamine
2. 3-OH steroid	4-Aminobiphenyl, α- and β-naphthylamine
3. p-Nitrophenol	p-Nitrophenol, 1-naphthol, 4-methylumbelliferone
4. Bilirubin	4-OH-dimethylaminoazobenzene
5. Morphine	Naloxone
6. DT-1	Digitoxigenin monodigitoxoside, digitoxigenin bisdigitoxoside
7. 4-OH-biphenyl-1	4-OH biphenyl, 4-methylumbelliferone, p-Nitrophenol
8. 4-OH-biphenyl-2	4-OH-biphenyl, chloramphenicol
9. Serotonin Human Liver	p-Nitrophenol, 1-naphthol, eugenol
10. Estriol (pl 7.4)	p-Nitrophenol, 4-methylumbelliferone, α-naphthylamine
11. Phenol (4-amino-biphenyl)	Phenols, 4-aminobiphenyl
12. HLUGP1	Phenols

(c) Sulfation

The xenobiotics or their metabolites containing phenolic, alcoholic, hydroxylamine, hydroxamic acid, amino and sulfhydryl groups may undergo sulfate conjugation reactions. These conjugates are excreted in urine and by (faeces) of animals. This path of Phase II reactions represents only a minor pathway. Before sulfate an be transferred to an acceptor substrate, it is required to be activated to form adenosine 3′-phosphate, 5′-sulfophosphate. This is also known as active sulfate. The formation of active sulfate is a two step process. Step 1 is ATP dependent and requires an enzyme known as sulfurylase and step 2 is catalyze by another enzyme known as APS kinase. Under normal conditions, rat liver contains about 30 nmole/gm liver of activated sulfate though rate of its formation in isolated perfused rat liver has been estimated to be 100 nmol/min/gm liver. The sulfur transferases unlike glucuronide transferases are soluble cytosolic enzymes [11, 12]. Their selective and potent inhibitors include 2,4 diachloro-4-nitrophenol (DCNP) and penta-chlorphenol which are effective both *in vitro* (μ1M concentration) and *in vivo* (DCNP-26m mol/kg, i.p.).

(d) Glutathione conjugation

Glutathione has a capability to spontaneously form conjugates with electrophiles. However, the rate of spontaneous reactions is quite slow.

Same reaction can be catalyzed by a group of enzymes konwn as glutathione S-transferases. Usually, the resultant conjugate gets metabolized further to cysteinyl conjugate by the removal of glutamine and glycine part of the tripeptide. The cysteinyl conjugate after acetylation is converted into mercapturic acid derivative which is readily excreted in urine. A number of workers consider that conversion of glutathione conjugate into mercapturic acid is the III Phase of metabolism.

The versatility of glutathione S-transferases is evident from the fact that they are present in microorganisms, plants and animals. In animals, their presence is almost in all the body organs. In liver, they constitute about 10% of the soluble proteins. There are several isoforms in which this enzyme exists. Well characterized mammalian cytosolic glutathione S-transferases have been classified into alpha (basic) Mu (neutral) and Pi (acidic) forms which can be differentiated by their distinct physical, chemical, enzymatic, and structural properties. These classes of glutathione S-transferase are products of distinct genes. However, all of these isozymes are dimeric proteins with subunit molecular weights of about 25 KDa. These isozymes are differentially inducible by a variety of drugs/xenobiotics. Their over expression has also been found in a variety of cancers. Therefore, the over expression of some isoforms is the characteristic future of preneoplastic lesion[13, 14].

(e) Metal Metabolism

Liver is capable of removing chemicals from blood in one pass through it. This is known as first pass effect or presystemic hepatic elimination. Among the list of chemicals which are removed by the liver, heavy metals constitute one important category . Usually, these chemicals removed during first pass effect, are metabolized before they are again released into blood. Unlike the organic chemicals which are metabolized and are converted to a number of different compounds with different properties and reactivities, metals cannot be converted metabolically into other forms. However, like reactive intermediates of organic compounds, metal ions can bind with a wide variety of cellular components. Such a binding with biomacromolecules may alter their configurations and many of these molecules loose their activity becoming glucosidically non-functional. While relatively little is known about the metabolism of metals, the interaction of metal ions with biomolecules has been studied in a greater detail. The uptake of metal ions usually occur in a bi-phasic manner. Many metal ions such as zinc and cadmium are transported within the tissues through a simple diffusion as well as through the carrier mediated mechanisms. In case of iron, ferrous iron is taken up by the hepatocytes through simple diffusion mechanism whereas the uptake of ferric iron is receptor mediated. Similarly, the transferrin bound iron at low concentration is taken up by the receptor-mediated mechanism whereas at high concentration diffusion becomes the dominant mechanism. The interaction of metal ions with biomolecules has been shown to play a regulatory role in the storage and transport of these metal ions. Several metal ions form excretable complex with GSH. For example, methyl mercury, copper, silver and zinc glutathione complexes play role in the excretion of these metal ions into bile. Infusion of glutathione has been shown to enhance biliary excretion of methyl mercury. Similarly, glutathione depletors have been show to inhibit biliary excretion of these metal ions. Metallothionein are induced in response to various heavy metal ions and function primarily as metal storage proteins. The primary inducers of metallothionein are zinc, cadmium, mercury etc. Whereas these and a number of other metal ions can bind with it. The examples of metal ions which can bind with metallothionein include Cd, Hg, Cu, Au, Ag, Zn, Pt etc. Therefore, metallothionein serves as sequester protein and solely functions to divert the metals from binding with other crucial molecules [15]. A few metals, most notably among them are the oxyanions of chromium and arsenic which undergo reduction to form ions that are no longer able to penetrate the cell membrane [16]. Organic compounds of metal ions are highly lipid soluble, allowing their access to the brain where they produce a number of toxic responses. The best example is methyl mercury which crosses blood brain barrier to reach in the brain and manifesting neuro-toxicity [17].

References

1. Klaassen, C.D. and Watkins III, J.B., Pharmacolo Rev., **36**, 1–67 (1984).
2. Popper, H., Hepatology, **1**, 187–191 (1981).
3. Guenogerich, F.P. and Turry, J. Pharmacol. Exp. Therap., **256**, 1189–1194 (1991).
4. Wolf, C.R., Trends In Genetics, **209**, 309–314 (1986).
5. Conney, A.H., Cancer Res., **42**, 4875–4917 (1982).
6. Bresnick, E., In: Enzymatic basis of detoxication. Ed. W.B. Jakoby, Academic Press, New York, pp. 69–81 (1980).
7. Alworth, W.L., Dang, C.C., Ching L.M. and Viswanathan, T., Xenobiotica, **10**, 395–400 (1980).
8. Seidegard, J. and DePierre, J.W., Biochim. Biophys. Acta, **695**, 251–270 (1983).
9. Puig, J.F. and Tephly, T.R., Mol. Pharmacol., **30**, 558 (1986).
10. Tephly, T.R., Townsend, M. and Green, M.D., Drug Metabol. Rev., **20**, 689–695 (1989).
11. Adams, J.B., Biochem. Biophys. Acta, **83**, 127 (1964).
12. Bircher, J. and Preising, R., In: Concepts in drug Metabolism, Marcel Dekker, New York, pp. 377–422 (1983).
13. Warholm, M., Guthenberg, C., and Mannervik, B., Biochem., **22**, 3610–3617 (1983).
14. de Waziers, I., Cugnenc, P.H., Yang, C.S., Lerouse, J.P. and Beaune, P.H., J. Pharmacol. Exp. **253**, 387–394 (1990).
15. Webb, M., Biochem. Pharmacol., **21**, 2767–2771 (1972).
16. Athar, M. and Vohora, S.B., Heavy metals and environment, Wiley Eastern, New Delhi, 1995.
17. Siegel, H., Metal ions in biological systems, Vol. 20, Mercel Dekker, New York, 1986.

Liver and Environmental Xenobiotics
S.V.S. Rana and K. Taketa (Eds)
Copyright © 1997, Narosa Publishing House, New Delhi, India

3. Liver Injury: Genetic factors in alcohol and acetaldehyde metabolism

Mikihiro Tsutsumi and Akira Takada

Division of Gastroenterology, Department of Internal Medicine,
Kanazawa Medical University, Uchinada, Ishikawa 920-02, Japan

The number of patients with alcoholic liver disease (ALD) has increased recently in parallel with the increase in alcohol consumption in Japan as it is throughout the world [1]. However, heavy drinkers do not always develop ALD, indicating that genetic factors may be involved.

Although many factors related to the pathogenesis of ALD have been considered, one of the most important factors is the toxic effect of acetaldehyde a product of ethanol metabolism in the liver [2]. Only 2 to 10% of the ethanol absorbed is eliminated through the kidneys and lungs. The rest must be oxidized in the body, principally in the liver, which contains the bulk of the body's enzymes capable of ethanol oxidization. The relative organ specificity probably explains why, despite the existence of intracellular mechanisms to maintain homeostasis, ethanol disposal produces striking metabolic imbalances in liver. These effects are aggravated by the lack of a feedback mechanism to adjust the rate of ethanol oxidation to the metabolic state of the hepatocytes.

The hepatocyte contains three main pathways for ethanol metabolism, each located in a different subcellular compartment: the alcohol dehydrogenase (ADH) pathway in cytosol, the microsomal ethanol-oxidizing system (MEOS) located in endoplasmic reticulum, and catalase located in peroxisomes. In the normal state, approximately 75% of absorbed ethanol is metabolized by ADH and the rest is metabolized by the non-ADH pathway [2]. However, following chronic ethanol consumption, the amount of ethanol metabolized by the non-ADH pathway is increased, because MEOS is significantly induced by ethanol [2]. Recently, it has become clear that cytochrome P4502E1 (CYP2E1) is the main enzyme which oxidizes ethanol in the non-ADH pathway (3). Consequently, acetaldehyde produced from ethanol through the ADH and CYP2E1 system is metabolized by aldehyde dehydrogease (ALDH). The ALDH family of isozymes with broad substrate specificity has been grouped into three classes according to their catalytic and structural characteristics and subcellular localization. Only class 1 ans 2 isozymes, which are encoded by the ALDH1 and ALDH2 loci, respectively, are thought to be involved in acetaldehyde oxidation. ALDH1 is the isoenzyme with a high K_m (30 μM) for acetaldehyde that is constitutively expressed in the cytosolic subcellular fraction, and ALDH2 has a low K_m (3 μM) for acetaldehyde that is present in mitochondria [4].

Recently, genetic polymorphism of enzymes, ADH, CYP2E1 and ALDH, have been discovered [5–7]. This review focuses on recent gains in our knowledge of the biochemical genetics of ADH, CYP2E1 and ALDH, the principal enzymes of ethanol oxidation in liver, and discusses the relationship between the genetic polymorphism of these enzymes and ALD.

ADH

It has long been known that there exist multiple molecular forms of human liver ADH, which can be identified by starch gel electrophoresis of liver extracts and staining for ethanol oxidizing activity. All ADH forms are dimeric molecules with subunits of 40,000 D, which contain 2 g-atom of zime par mole of enzuyme subunit. At present, seven diferent ADH genes and five classes of enzymes have been identified (Table 1). In seven ADH genes, polymorphism occurs at ADH2 and ADH3, giving rise to the β_1,

Table 1. Genetic medel of human ADH liver isoenzymes

Class	Locus	Peptide
I	ADH1	α
I	ADH2	β_1
		β_2
		β_3
I	ADH3	γ_1
		γ_2
II	ADH4	π
III	ADH5	χ
IV	ADH7	σ
V	ADH6	?

β_2, and β_3 and γ_1, γ_2 subunits, respectively. The three β subunits differ by one amino acid each; β_2 has a His for Arg_{47} substitution and β_3 has a Cys for Arg_{369} substitution. Both of these substitutions are in the coenzme binding site and affect directly the coenzyme kinetic constants and V_{max} for ethanol oxidation (Table 2). Ethanol- metabolizing activity of the homozygous ADH2^2 gene product ($\beta_2\beta_2$ isoenzyme) is 20 times higher than that of the homozygous ADH2^1 gene ($\beta_1\beta_1$ isoenzyme) (6). Recently, Xu, et al [8] reported that the incidence of ADH2^2 gene in patients with ALD was significantly higher than that in normal subjects, suggesting that the polymorphism of ADH2 may be related to the development of ALD. On the other hand, Bosron and Li [9] and Yamamoto et al [10] reported that both ethanol and acetaldehyde

Table 2. Steady-state kinetic constants of homodimeric isoenzymes

	Isoenzymes							
	Class I				Class II			
	$\alpha\,\alpha$	$\beta_1\beta_1$	$\beta_2\beta_2$	$\beta_3\beta_3$	$\gamma_1\gamma_1$	$\gamma_2\gamma_2$	$\pi\,\pi$	
K_m ethanol (mM)	4.2	0.05	0.94	36	1	0.63	34	
K_m acetaldehyde (mM)	4.3	0.1	0.2	3.4	0.3	0.2	30	
K_m NAD (μM)	13	7.4	180	710	7.9	8.7	14	
Km NADH (μM)	11	6.4	105	260	7	—	2.5	
Vmax (unit/mg)	0.6	0.23	8.6	7.9	2.2	0.87	0.5	

levels in blood after ethanol administration in subjects with ADH2[2] gene did not differ from those in subjects with the ADH2[1] gene, and that those levels were related to the genotypes of ALDH2. Harada et al [11] also reported that there was no difference in the incidence of different ADH2 genotypes in patients with ALD. These results suggest that polymorphisms of ADH2 may not be related to the development of ALD. The two γ subunits differ at two amino acid positions, 271 and 349. The substitution of Arg_{271} in γ_1 by Gln in γ_2 may affect the rate of rate-limiting coenzyme dissociation and account for the two fold higher V_{max} for ethanol oxidation seen with γ_1 vs γ_2 (Table 2). With respect to ADH3 polymorphism, the two γ alleles appear with roughly equal frequencies in white populations, but γ_1 predominates in Japanese, Chinese, and black populations [7]. However, the relationship between ADH3 polymorphism and ALD remains unclear.

ALDH

ALDH2 contributes most to the acetaldehyde oxidizing activity in human liver [4]. About 50% of Japanese lack ALDH2 activity [5], and these ALDH2-deficient individuals suffer uncomfortable symptoms such as facial flushing, nausea and throbbing, due to elevation of the blood acetaldehyde concentration after alcohol drinking [5]. Recently, the ALDH2 genome was analyzed [12]. It has become clear that ALDH2-deficient individuals are either a homozygote of the mutant (atypical or inactive) ALDH2 genes (ALDH2[2]/ALDH2[2]) or a heterozygote of the normal and mutant ALDH2 genes (ALDH2[1]/ALDH2[2]). On the other hand, the ALDH2 genotype with no ALDH2 deficiency is a homozygote of the normal ALDH2 genes (ALDH2[1]/ALDH2[1]). In the mutant ALDH2 gene (ALDH2[2]), the normal GAA codon for glutamic acid is replaced by an AAA codon for lysin (codon 487), a single point mutaion [12]. As ALDH2 is the isotetramer enzyme, all four subunits of ALDH2 are needed to maintain its full activity. As shown in Fig. 1, in the homozygote of mutant ALDH2 genes, hepatic ALDH2 activity was completely absent, because normal ALDH2 tetramers are absent. In the heterozygote, however, small amounts of the tetramer exist and low

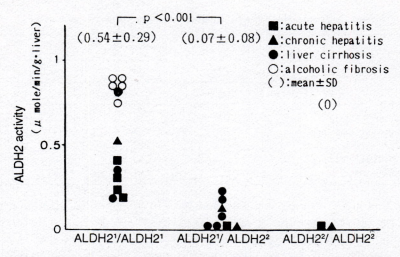

Fig. 1.   Hepatic ALDH2 activity. ALDH activity was not detected in the homozygotes of the mutant ALDH2 gene.

ALDH2 activity was detectable. We [13] have demonstrated that blood acetaldehyde levels after small amounts of ethanol (0.1 g/kg of body weight) intake in the heterozygote were significantly higher than those in the mutant homozygote (Fig. 2). These results suggest that only the mutant homozygote cannot tolerate small amounts of alcohol intake and that heterozygous subjects may be drinkers. In fact, 7 cases (14.9%) heterozygous for the ALDH2

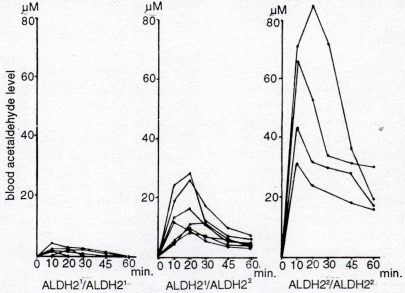

Fig. 2.   Serial changes of blood acetaldehyde levels after drinking a small amount of ethanol. Levels at the 60-min period were clearly higher in the mutant homozygoutes than in the heterozygotes without overlapping of the values.

gene were found among 47 patients with ALD, while no subject was homozygous for the mutant ALDH2 gene (Table 3). To clarify the clinical features of ALD among heterozygotes of the ALDH2 genes, alcohol intake

Table 3. **Mean alcohol intake and the incidence of each type of ALD in the different ALDH2 genotypes.**

Characteristics	Normal homozygote	Heterozygote
Alcohol intake		
No. of cases	39	7
Daily intake (gm)	136 ± 34.4*	88 ± 9.0
Total intake (kg)	$1,335 \pm 504$*	758 ± 223
ALD		
Fibrosis	21 (52.5%)	1 (14.2%)
Chronic hepatitis	1 (2.5%)	0 (0%)
Alcoholic heapatitis	6 (15.0%)	3 (42.9%)
Cirrhosis	12 (30.0%)	3 (4.9%)
Total	40 (100%)	7 (100%)

*$p < 0.01$ vs heterozygote.

and the incidence of each type of ALD in the heterozygotes was compared to those of the normal homozygotes (Table 3). The mean daily alcohol intake and total alcohol consumption in the heterozygotes were significantly lower than those in the normal homozygotes. The incidence of alcoholic fibrosis in the heterozygotes was lower than that in normal homozygotes. On the other hand, the incidence of the more severe types of ALD (alcholic hepatitis and cirrhosis) in the heterozygotes tended to be higher than that in normal homozygotes. These results indicate that a high concentration of acetaldehyde in livers is very important for the development of ALD, and that ALD develops even with moderate amounts of alcohol intake in heterozygotes of ALDH2 genes. In the heterozygotes whose liver acetaldehyde metabolism is impaired, liver damage is more severe than in normal homozygotes. Therefore, it is suggested that habitual drinkers who are heterozygotes of ALDH2 genes may be at high risk for ALD.

CYP2E1

Although the genotypes of ALDH2 are related to the development of ALD, the prevalence of ALDH2 deficiency in ALD is relatively low [5]. Therefore, in the group homozygous for the normal ALDH2 genes, other genetic factors leading to the development of ALD should be considered. CYP2E1 is the main enzyme that oxidizes ethanol in the non-ADH pathway [3]. We [14] have reported that degradationof acetaldehyde produced by the non-ADH pathway was slower than that produced by the ADH pathway. This may be related to the subcelluar localization of ALDH isozymes. In the microsomes of the human liver, only high K_m ALDH1 is present and low

K_m ALDH2 is absent [15]. Therefore, the acetaldehyde level in the hepatocytes may be high, when ethanol metabolism through the non-ADH pathway in microsomes is increased. These facts may be relevant to the degelopment of ALD.

Recently, the presence of genetic polymorphism of CYP2E1 was confirmed by Hayashi et al [7]. They classified CYP2E1 genotypes into three types: A, B, and C. Type A is homozygous for the c1 genes and type C is homozygous for the c2 genes. Type B is heterozygous for the c1 and c2 genes. High transcriptional activity of the c2 gene was confirmed by Hayashi et al (7) in studies with the choloramphenicol acetyltransferase (CAT) assay using the human hepatoma cell line Hep G2, which expresses the albumin gene. We [16] also measured the content of CYP2E1 mRNA and protein in liver biopsy samples obtained from non-alcoholic patients without liver disease. As shown in Table 4, the hepatic CYP2E1 mRNA content in type

Table 4. **Contents of CYP2E1 mRNA and protein and PNP hydroxylase activity in livers of each CYP2E1 genotype**

Genotype	mRNA[a]	Protein[b]	Activity[c]
A	2.9 ± 0.45	4.2 ± 1.0	1.25 ± 0.03
B	$9.1 \pm 0.32*$	$24.3 \pm 2.8*$	$3.85 \pm 1.54*$

[a] Arbitray densitometric unit/μg total RNA
[b] Arbitray densitometric unit/mg microsomal protein
[c] n mole 4-NC formed/ min/mg mircosomal protein
*$P < 0.00$-5 vs type A

B (c1/c2) was 3 times higher than in type A (c1/c1). The content of CYP2E1 protein in type B was also significantly higher than in type A. There was good correlation between CYP2E1 mRNA and protein contents and also between CYP2E1 protein content and activity (Fig. 3). These results indicate that the CYP2E1 genotype influences markedly not only the transcription of the human CYP2E1 gene but also the level at which the corresponding enzyme is expressed in liver, suggesting that polymorphisms of the CYP2E1 gene may be linked to the development of ALD through enhancement of ethanol metabolism in the non-ADH pathway.

To evaluate the possibility mentioned above, we [17] analyzed the genotypes of CYP2E1 in patients with or without ALD. Table 5 shows that most patients with ALD had the c2 gene but few had c1 gene. The gene frequencies of CYP2E1 in patients with ALD were significantly different from those in patients with hepatobiliary disease but not from those in ALD and in healthy controls. On the other hand, all heavy drinkers without liver disease had the c1 gene but not the c2 gene. Gene frequencies of c1 and c2 were quite different from that in ALD. These results indicate that polymorphism of CYP2E1 gene are related to the development of ALD and suggest that the c2 gene may be one of the most important determinants of ALD.

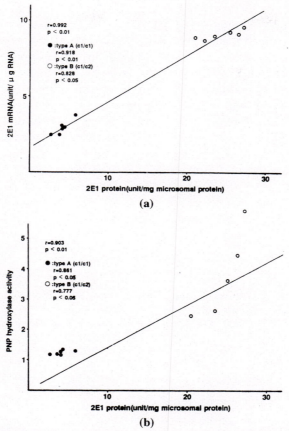

Fig. 3. Relationship among the hepatic contents of CYP2E1 mRNA and protein, and its activity. There is a good correlation between the hepatic contents of CYP2E1 mRNA and protein, and also berween CYP2E1 protein contents and its activities.

Table 5. Prevalence of the genotypes of CYP2E1

Groups	n	Sex (M/F)	A (c1/c1) (%)	B (c1/c2) (%)	C(c2/c2) (%)	Gene frequency	
				Genotypes			
ALD	50	45/5	8 (16.0)*	39 (78.0)	3 (6.0)	c1: 0.550,	c2: 0.450*
Non-ALD	34	24/10	22 (64.7)	12 (35.3)	0 (0)	c1: 0.824,	c2: 0.176
Non-hepatobiliary disease	88	62/26	62 (70.5)	25 (28.4)	1 (1.1)	c1: 0.844,	c2: 0.153
Hevy drinkers without ALD	10	10/0	10(100)	0(0)	0(0)	c1: 1.00,	c2: 0.00
Healthy controls	66	36/30	45 (68.2)	19 (28.8)	2 (3.0)	c1: 0.808,	c2: 0.192

*$p < 0.002$ vs other groups.

Summary

For a long time, the question of why heavy drinkers do not always develop ALD has remained unanswered. Still, there is no clear answer. In the last 10 years, the catalytic properties and structure of the molecular forms of ADH, ALDH and CYP2E1 and their genes have been studied. Studies of the relationship of these genotypes to the alcohol elimination rate, alcohol drinking behavior and ALD have been performed. Some of them appear definitive, whereas others will require confirmation. Overall, the studies have highlighted the importance of acetaldehyde concentration in the hepatocyte as an etiologic factor in liver injury. Consequently, it is also suggested that habitual drinkers who are heterozygotes of ALDH2 genes may be at high risk for ALD and that the c2 gene of CYP2E1 may be one of the most important determinants of the development of ALD in the group homozygous for normal ALDH2 genes.

References

1. Takada, A., Takase, S. and Tsutsumi, M. (1993). Characteristic features of alcoholic liver disease in Japan: A review. Gastroenterol Jpn, 28, 137–148.
2. Lieber, C.S. (Ed.) (1992). Medical and Nutritional Complications of Alcoholism. Plenum Medical Company, New York and London.
3. Koop, D.R. and Coon, M.J. (1986). Ethanol oxidation and toxicity: Roles of alcohol-P450 oxygenase. Alcohol Clin Exp Res, 10, 44–49.
4. Bosron, W.F., Ehrig, T. and Li, T.K. (1993). Genetic factors in alcohol metabolism and alcoholism. Semin Liver Dis, 13, 126–135.
5. Harada, S., Misawa, S., Agarwal, D.P. and Goedde H.W. (1980). Liver alcohol dehydrognease and aldehyde dehydrogenase in Japanese: Isoenzyme variation and its possible role in alcohol intoxication. Am J Hum Genet, 32, 8–15.
6. Bosron, W.F. and Li, T.K. (1986). Genetic polymorphism of human liver alcohol and aldehyde dehydrogenase, and their relationship to alcohol metabolism and alcoholism. Hepatology, 6, 502–510.
7. Hayashi, S., Watanabe, J. and Kawajiri, K. (1991). Genetic polymorohisms in the 5-franking region change transcriptional regulation of the human cytochrome P450IIE1. J Biochem 110, 559–565.
8. Xu, Y., Carr, L.G., Borson, W.F. et al (1988). Genotyping of human alcohol dehydrogenase at the ADH2 and ADH3 loci following DNA sequence amplification. Genetics, 2, 2019–214.
9. Bosron, W.F. and Li. T.K. (1988). Catalytic and structural properties of the human liver *b* alcohol dehydrogenase isozymes. Biochemical and Social Aspects of Alcohol and Alcoholism (Eds: Kuriyama, K., Takada, A. and Ishii, H.) pp. 31–34, Excepta Medica, Amsterdam.
10. Yamamoto, K., Ueno, Y., Mozoi, Y. et al (1993). Genetic polymorphism of alcohol and aldehyde dehydrogenase and the effects on alcohol Metabolism. Jpn J Alcohol Dron alcoholic liver disease. Jpn J Alcohol Drug Dependece, 28, 13–25.
11. Harada, S., Takase, S., Horiike, N. et al (1993). Genetic and epidemiologic studies on alcoholic liver disease. Jpn J Alcohol Drug Dependence, 28, 400–413.

12. Enomoto, N., Takada, A. and Date, T. (1991). Genotyping of the aldehyde dehydrogenase 2 (ALDH2) gene using the polymerase chain reaction: Evidence for single point mutation in the ALDH2 gene of ALDH2-deficiency. Gastroenterol Jpn, 26, 440–447.
13. Enomoto, N., Takase, S., Yasuhara, M. and Takada, A. (1991). Acetaldehyde metabolism in different aldehyde dehydrogenase-2 genotypes. Alcohol Clin Exp Res, 15, 141–144.
14. Yasuhara, M., Matsuda, Y. and Takada, A. (1986). Degradation of acetaldehyde produced by the nonalcohol dehydrogenase pathway. Alcohol Clin Exp Res, 10, 545–549.
15. Takase, S., Tsutsumi, M. and Takada, A. (1989). Subcellular localization of aldehyde dehydrogenase isozymes in human liver. Gastroenterol Jpn. 24, 31–39.
16. Tsutsumi. M., Wang, S.J., Takase, S. and Takada, A. (1994). Hepatic messenger RNA contents of cytochrome P4502E1 in patients with different P4502E1 genotypes. Alcohol Alcohol, 29, 29–32.
17. Tsutsumi. M., Wang, S.J., Takada, A. (1994). Genetic polymorphisms of cytochrome P4502E1 related to the development of alcoholic liver disease. Gastroenterology, 107, 1430–1435.

Liver and Environmental Xenobiotics
S.V.S. Rana and K. Taketa (Eds)

4. An Enhanced Liver Injury Induced by Carbon Tetrachloride in Acatalasemic Mice

**Kunihiko Ishii, Da-Hong Wang, Li-Xue Zhen,
Masaki Satho and Kazuhisa Taketa**

Department of Public Health, Okayama University Medical School,
2-5-1 Shikata-cho, Okayama 700, Japan

Carbon tetrachloride (CCl_4) had been widely used as a lolvent to some organic compounds, such as oil, resin or tar. CCl_4 had also been used as a raw material of halo-fluorocarbon for coolant or as an extinguish agent of fire. Since some cases of acute toxic injury caused by CCl_4 used as a solvent have been reported, the above-mentioned use of CCl_4 is now uncommon. However, it is still widely used in animal models to induce acute and chronic liver injuries for investingating the mechanisms of CCl_4-induced liver injury.

Cameron [1] first studied in 1936 the hepatotoxicity of CCl_4 to rats followed by Slater [2–9], Recknagel [10–16] and others, who studied the mechanisms of CCl_4 hepatotoxicity during 1960–1989. Recent studies on the mechanisms of CCl_4-induced liver injury have shown the involvement of Kupffer cells [17–21], cytokines [17, 22–25] and neutrophilic leukocytes [17]. It appears likely that CCl_4 hepatotoxicity is caused not only by free radicals produced directly from CCl_4 but also by other free radicals, such as superoxide anion ($O_2^- \cdot$) or hydroxyl radical ($\cdot OH$) produced by Kupffer cells or neutrophil infiltrates.

Hydroxyl radical is now considered to play an important role in cell damage [26–33], and its major source is hydrogen peroxide (H_2O_2). The intracellular level of H_2O_2 in biological systems is regulated by two enzymes, catalase in the peroxisome and glutathione peroxidase in both the cytosol and the mitochondria. The former is considered to play a major role in H_2O_2 degradation in liver, especially when H_2O_2 is overproduced [34, 35].

In order to test the hypothesis that $\cdot OH$ is directly involved in the liver injury caused by CCl_4, we studied CCl_4-induced liver injuries of acatalasemic mice in comparison with those of normal mice. Catalase activities in blood and liver of acatalasemic mice are one-sixteenth and one-third those of normal mice, respectively, as shown in Table 1.

Table 1. Catalase activities of liver and blood in normal and acatalasemic mice

Mouse	Catalase activity	
	Liver (PU/mg protein)	Blood (PU/g Hb)
Normal	4.6 ± 1.2* (n = 5)	844 ± 128** (n = 8)
Acatalasemic	1.4 ± 0.4* (n = 5)	52.3 ± 7.4** (n = 8)

*$P < 0.05$; **$P < 0.01$

In our study [36], the degree of CCl_4-induced liver injury was increased in acatalasemic mouse as compared with normal mouse. In this paper, we will briefly review the literatures of CCl_4-induced liver injuries from the aspect of their mechanisms, including our recent findings [36] of enhanced CCl_4 hepatotoxicity in acatalasemic mice.

Morphological Studies of CCl_4-Induced Liver Injuries in Acatalasemic and Normal Mice

Male normal (C3H/AnLCs^{a}Cs^a) and acatalasemic (C3H/AnLCs^{b}Cs^b) mice of 5–10 weeks of age were given intraperitoneally each 0.0125 ml CCl_4 (20% in olive oil)/g body weight. Blood samples were collected from the femoral artery at 12, 18, 24 and 48 hr following CCl_4 treatment, and each group consisted of 7 to 10 animals. Sera were separated for determination of activities of GOT and GPT. Livers were excised and stained for hematoxylin-eosin (H-E) and also used for biochemical determinations.

Pictures of a low magnification of liver histology examined under light microscope are shown in Fig. 1. Untreated mouse livers showed normal histology (Figs. 1, N1 and A1). At 12 hr of CCl_4 treatment, small areas of centrilobular necrosis appeared in normal mice, while the central areas were relatively uninvolved and periportal areas were slightly necrotic in acatalasemic mice (Figs. 1, N2 and A2). At 18 hr, necrotic areas in the central zone became more apparent in acatalasemic mice than in normal ones (Figs. 1, N3 and A3). The difference in the necrotic area between normal and acatalasemic mice became marked at 24 hr (Figs. 1 N4 and A4). It may be also noted that the necrotic area was more clearly demarcated in acatalasemic mouse liver. The difference in necrotic area was the most obvious at 48 hr with extended necrosis in liver of actalasemic mice (Figs. 1, N5 and A5). At a higher magnification (Figs. 2, N and A), neutrophils and mononuclear cells infiltrated in the necrotic area and Kupffer cells were activated and mobilized in the same area without marked difference in their extent between normal and acatalasemic mice at 12 hr after treatment. However, the number of infiltrated cells were less in acatalasemic mice than in normal mice at 48 hr, and regenerative changes of perinecrotic area were not seen in acatalasemic mice (Figs. 3, N and A). These results confirm

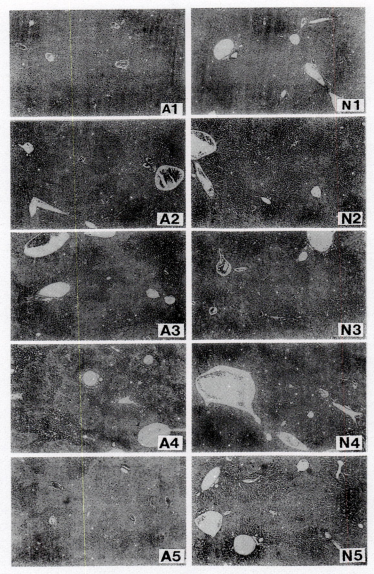

Fig. 1.   Liver histology of mice after CCl$_4$ treatment. H-E, × 30. N1 and A1, 0 hr; N2 and A2, 12 hr; N3 and A3, 18 hr; N4 and A4, 24 hr; N5 and A5, 48 hr after the treatment. N series, normal; and A series, acatalasemic mice.

our previous biochemical observations shown in Fig. 4; namely similar elevations of serum GOT and GPT in normal and acatalasemic mice at 12 hr and higher serum levels of GOT and GPT in acatalasemic mice than in normal mice at 18–24 hr of CCl$_4$ treatment.

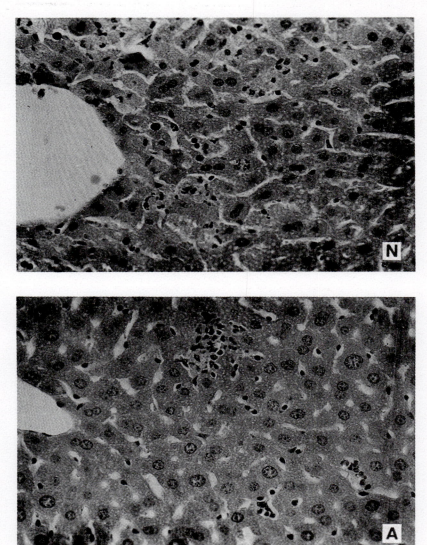

Fig. 2. Liver histology at higher magnification at 12 hr showing neutrophils and Kupffer cells infiltration into the centrilobular area of CCl_4 treatment. H-E staining × 320. N, normal; and A, acatalasemic mice.

Mechanisms of an Enhanced CCl_4 Liver Injury in Acatalasemic Mouse

1. Biochemical Events in Earlier Stages of CCl_4 Intoxication before 12 hr

Carbon tetrachloride in blood enters the hepatocytes along the blood flow from the portal tracts via the sinusoids to the central veins, where the hepatocytes have active microsomal cytochrome P-450 predominantly

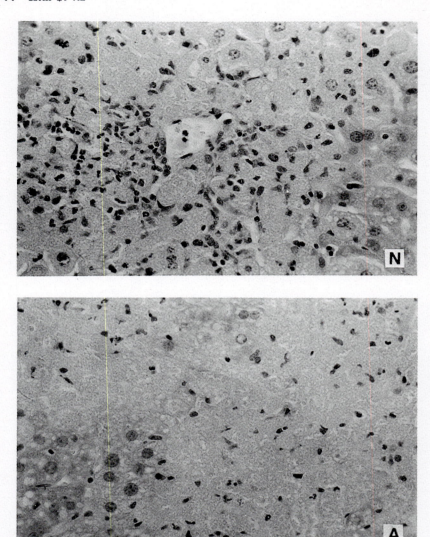

Fig. 3. **Liver histology at higher magnification at 48 hr of CCl₄ treatment showing the decreased number of infiltrated cells in necrotic area of acatalasemic mouse liver. H-E staining × 320. N, normal; and A, acatalasemic mice.**

[37, 38]. Fig. 5 schematically illustrates the initial event of CCl_4 metabolism; namely, a one-electron reductive dehalogenation catalyzed by cytochrome P-450 to produce $CCl_3 \cdot$ [39]. In this event, a complex of CCl_4 and ferric cytochrome P-450 is formed [40]. The rate of reductive dehalogenation of CCl_4 is influenced by the oxygen (O_2) concentration. The reaction rate is the highest at 2–5 v/v% of atmospheric O_2 tension, partially inhibited under excessive O_2, and completely inhibited under anaerobic conditions [39].

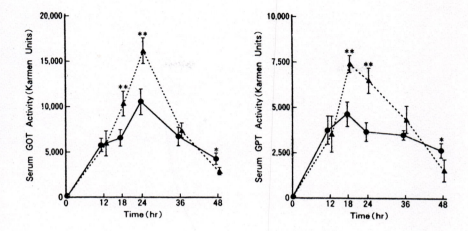

Fig. 4. Time courses of serum GOT and GPT activities in normal and acatalasemic mice after CCl4 treatment. •, normal; ▲, acatalasemic mice. Symbols represent mean values and vertical lines represent SD's in a group of more than seven mice. *P < 0.05; and **P < 0.01, with respect to normal. Reproduced with permission from Wang et al (see [36]).

The maximal rates of lipid peroxidation proceed at partial pressures of oxygene between 0.5 and 10 mmHg [41]. Since the O_2 concentrations around the central vein of the liver lobule are 2–5% and cytochrome P-450 is localized in the centrilobular area, the reductive metabolism of CCl_4 by cytochrome P-450 occurs readily in this area. The $\cdot CCl_3$ radical thus produced reacts more rapidly with O_2 to yield $CCl_3O_2\cdot$ than with amino acids, nucleotides and fatty acids [42, 43]. $CCl_3O_2\cdot$ is likely to be related to the initiation of lipid peroxidation in cell membranes, because $CCl_3O_2\cdot$ reacts faster with polyunsaturated fatty acids than $\cdot CCl_3$ [43] does. The $CCl_3O_2\cdot$ peroxidizes membrane phospholipids of the endoplasmic reticulum leading to a structural disorganization [44–46] of the membranes. However, the functions of mitochondria of hepatocytes are only minimally affected by $CCl_3O_2\cdot$ [47] in the stage of early CCl_4 intoxication as is shown in Fig. 6 with increased serum levels of microsomal glucose-6-phosphatase (G 6 Pase) and cytosol GOT and GPT but not the mitochondrial enzymes.

In the initial stage of CCl_4 intoxication, there are marked decreases in hepatic microsomal enzyme activities, including Ca^{2+}-adenosine triphosphatase (Ca^{2+}-ATPase), G-6-Pase and the cytochrome P-450 monooxygenase system in 3 to 6 hr after CCl_4 treatment [47, 48]. Since the activity of Ca^{2+}-ATPase in microsome is decreased, a high concentration of cytosolic Ca^{2+} may result from the release of Ca^{2+} from the microsome [49–52], and the increased Ca^{2+} leads to the alteration of membrane structure, ultimately causing the final break down of plasma membranes. Further, the free radicals of lipids formed in the liver microsomal membranes by $CCl_3O_2\cdot$ are likely to diffuse

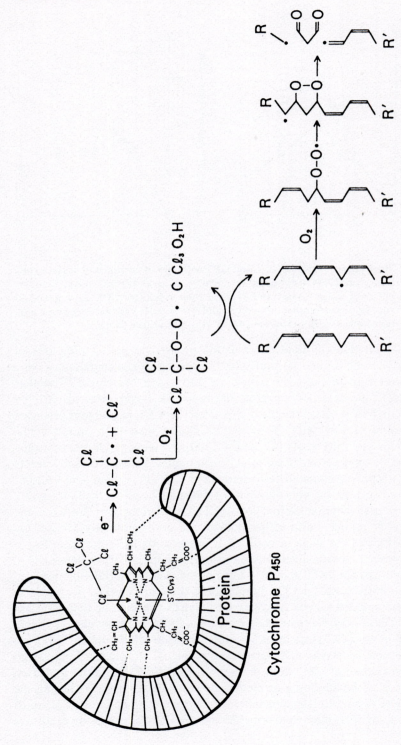

Fig. 5. Metabolic activation of CCl₄ by cytochrome P-450 and formation of free radicals, lipid peroxides and low molecular aldehydes.

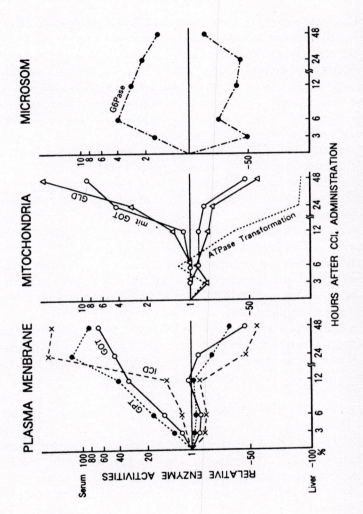

Fig. 6. Plasma levels of cytoplasmic, mitochondrial and microsomal enzymes in rats treated with CCl₄. Reproduced with permissin (see [47]).

out the plasma membrane, causing a continuing chain reactions at the membrane. However, the direct evidence of plasma membrane damage caused by $CCl_3O_2\cdot$ is not available yet. The cytosol GOT and GPT, therefore, are released to the blood stream in the early stage because of the plasma membrane damage shown in Fig 6.

2. Biochemical Events in Later Stages of CCl_4 Intoxication after 12 hr

In our studies on acatlasemic mice, the increases of serum GOT and GPT levels in acatalasemic mouse became greater than in normal mouse in 18-24 hr of CCl_4 treatment [36] as shown in Fig. 4. Results are compatible with morphological findings that the necrotic areas in acatalasemic mouse liver are more extensive than those in normal mouse liver (see Figs. 1, N4–N5 and A–A5). The enhanced CCl_4-induced liver injury in later stages of acatalasemic mice is difficult to explain by $\cdot CCl_3$ or $CCl_3O_2\cdot$ produced directly by reduction of CCl_4. The more extensive injury was probably caused by an overproduction of $\cdot OH$ radical from an undecomposed excess H_2O_2 as a result of low catalase activity. The $\cdot OH$ thus produced might have acted as an initiator of the chain reaction of lipid peroxidation leading to extensive cell destruction.

Slater [5] has pointed out that CCl_4-induced liver necrosis develops explosively in histological examination of liver tissues in 12–18 hr after CCl_4 administration. He assumed that in the later stages, either CCl_4 itself was metabolized to a deleterious free radical or more potent free radicals produced in the presence of CCl_4 may play an important role in the final centrilobular necrosis of liver.

Since Kupffer cells and neutrophilic leukocytes were found around necrotic area both in normal and acatalasemic mice at 12 hr after CCl_4 treatment, it seems possible to speculate that $O_2^-\cdot$ is also released from the Kupffer cells or neutrophils. The superoxide anion is a negatively charged radical ion and unable to pass through the cell membranes and is less reactive than $\cdot OH$; therefore, the peroxidative effects of $O_2^-\cdot$ is limited in a smaller area. On the other hand the hydrogene peroxide formed from $O_2^-\cdot$ by dismutation can readily cross cell membranes and diffuse out to a larger extent than $O_2^-\cdot$. Hydrogene peroxide further reacts with ferrous ion to produce $\cdot OH$, which is a highly reactive free radical and probably trigger the lipid peroxidation and its chain reaction with nearest membrane lipids to form lipid radicals (Fig. 7). Therefore, $\cdot OH$ could be the free radical that has direct cytotoxic effect on hepatocytes in the later stages of CCl_4 intoxication. This mechanism is compatible with the present findings that the hepatic injury caused by CCl_4 in acatalasemic mouse was severer than in normal mouse in later stages of CCl_4 intoxication. Direct demonstration of increased $\cdot OH$ in acatalasemic mouse liver by means of an ESR trapping in future studies will prove the present hypothesis.

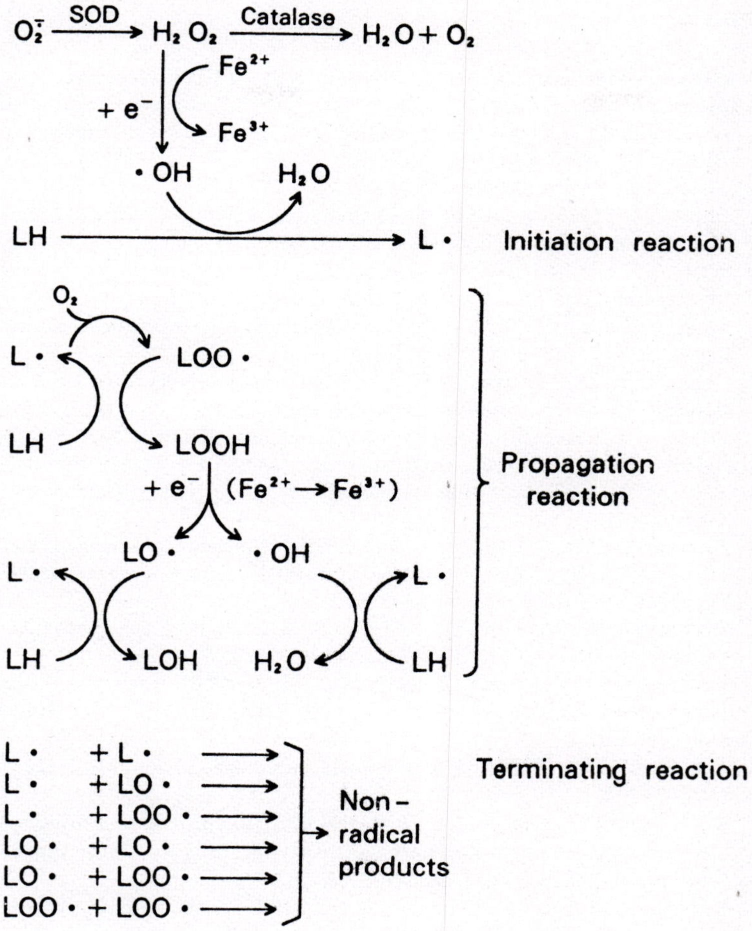

Fig. 7. Lipid peroxidation and its chain reaction initiated by hydroxyl radical.

Summary

The toxic effect of CCl_4 on the liver involves two stages. This was observed not only in biochemical but also in pathological findings as enhanced hepatocyte necrosis in later stages of CCl_4-treated acatalasemic mice. It was inferred that $CCl_3 \cdot$ and $CCl_3O_2 \cdot$ play an initiating or triggering role in the early stages of CCl_4 hepatotoxicity before 12 hr, while the $\cdot OH$ derived from H_2O_2 and originally coming from $O_2^- \cdot$ released from Kupffer cells or neutrophils probably caused an enhanced additional cell necrosis after 12 hr of CCl_4 treatment in acatalasemic liver.

References

1. Cameron, G.R. and Karunaratne, W.A.E (1936). J. Path. Bact., 42, 1.
2. Slater, T.F. Strauli, U.D. and Sawyer, B.C. (1964). Changes in liver nucleotide concentrations in experimental liver injury I. Carbon tetrachloride poisoning. Biochem. J., 93, 260–266.
3. Slater, T.F. (1965). Biochem. J., 97, 22C.
4. Slater, T.F. (1965). A note on the relative toxic activities of tetrachloromethane and trichloro-1-fluoro-methane on the rat. Biochem. Pharm., 14, 178–181.
5. Slater, T.F. (1966). Necrogenic action of carbon tetrachloride in rat: a speculative mechanism based on activation. Nature (London) 209, 36–40.
6. Slater, T.F. and Riley, P.A. (1970). Free-radical damage in retrolental fibroplasia. Lancet ii, 467, 805–814.
7. Slater, T.F. and Sawyer, B.C. (1971). The stimulatory effects of carbon tetrachloride on peroxidative reactions in rat liver fractions in vitro. Inhibitory effects of free radical scavengers and other agents. Biochem. J., 123, 823–828.
8. Slater, T.F. (1982). Lipid peroxidation. Biochem. Soc . Trans., 10, 70–71.
9. Slater, T.F. (1982). Free radical mechanisms in tissue injury. Biochem. J., 222, 1–15.
10. Recknagel, R.O. and Anthony, D.D. (1959). Biochemical changes in carbon tetrachloride fatty liver: Separation of fatty changes from mitochondria degeneration. J. Biol. Chem., 234, 1052–1059.
11. Recknagel, R.O. and Litteria, M. (1959). Activation of acid phosphatase in carbon tetrachloride fatty liver. Fedn. Proc., 18, 125.
12. Recknagel, R.O. Lombardi, B. and Schotz, M.C. (1960). A new insight into the pathogenesis of carbon tetrachloride fatt infiltration. Proc. Soc. exp. Biol. Med., 104, 608–610.
13. Recknagel, R.O. (1967). Carbon tetrachloride hepatotoxicity. Pharmac. Rev., 19, 145–208.
14. Recknagel, R.O., Glende, E.A. Jr, Ugazio, G., Koch, R.R. and Srinivasan, S. (1974). New data in support of the lipoperoxidation theory for Carbon tetrachloride liver injury. Israel. J. Med. Sci., 10, 301–311.
15. Recknagel, R.O. and Glende, E.A. Jr. (1988) Free radicals involved in hepatotoxicity of carbon tetrachloride. In: Handbook of Free Radicals and Antioxidants in Biomedicine, Vol. III, pp 3–16, Miquel, J., Quintanilha, A. and Weber, H. (eds) CRC Press, Florida.
16. Recknagel, R.O., Glende, E.A., Dolak, J.A. and Waller, R.E. (1989). Mechanisms of carbon tetrachloride toxicity. Pharmacol. Ther., 43, 39–54.
17. Edwards, M.J., Keller, B.J., Kauffman, F.C. and Thurman, R.C. (1993). The involvement of Kupffer cells in carbontetrachloride toxicity. Toxicol. Appl. Pharmacol. 119, 275–279.
18. Gunawardhana, L., Mobley, S.A. and Sipes, I.G. (1993). Modulation of 1,2-dichlorobenzene hepatotoxicity in the Fischer-334 rat by a scavenger of superoxide anions and an inhibitor of Kupffer cells. Toxicol. Appl. Pharmacol., 119, 205–213.
19. Johnson, S.J., Hines, J.E, and Burt. A.D. (1992). Macrophage and perisinusoidal cell kinetics in acute liver injury. J. Pathol., 166 (4), 351–358.
20. elSisi, A.E., Earnest, D.L. and Sipes, I.G. (1993). Vitamin A potentiation of carbon tetrachloride hepatotoxicity: Role of liver macrophages and active oxygen species. Toxicol. Appl. Pharmacol., 119(2), 295–301.
21. Raiford, D.S. and Thigpen, M.C. (1994). Kupffer cell stimulation with

Corynebacterium parvum reduces some cytochrome P450-dependent activities and diminishes acetaminophen and carbon tetrachloride-induced liver injury in the rat. Toxicol. Appl. Pharmacol., 129(1), 36-45.

22. Rockey, D.C., Housset, C.N. and Friedman, S.L. (1993). Activation-dependent contractility of rat hepatic lipocytes in culture and in vivo. J. Clin. Invest., 92(4), 1795–1804.

23. Wang, L., Yamasaki, G., Johnson, R.J. and Friedman, S.L. (1994). Induction of beta-platelet-derived growth factor receptor in rat hepatic lipocytes during cellular activation in vivo and in culture. J. Clin. Invest., 94(4), 1563–1569.

24. Laskin, D.L. and Pendino, K.J. (1995). Macrophages and inflammatory mediators in tissue injury. Annu. Rev. Pharmacol. Toxicol., 35, 655–677.

25. Liu, S.L., DEgli Esposti, S., Yao, T., Diehl, A.M. and Zern, M.A. (1995). Vitamin E therapy of acute CCl_4-induced hepatic injury in mice is associated with inhibition of nuclear factor kappa B binding. Hepatology, 22(5), 1474–1781.

26. Willson, R.L., (979). Hydroxyl radicals and biological damage in vivtro: What relevance in vivo?. Ciba Foundation Symposium No. 202, 65, 19–35.

27. Makino, K., Imaishi, H., Morinishi, S. Takeuchi, T. and Fujita, Y. (1986). An ESR study on lipid peroxidation process. Formation of hydrogen atoms and hydroxyl radicals. Biochem. Biophys. Res. Commun., 141, 381–386.

28. Kim, T., Kuzuya, T., Hoshida., S., Nisida, M., Fuji, H. and Tada, M. (1988). Endothelial cells as a source of free radical generation during myocardial reperfusion. Circulation, 78(4), II-371.

29. Sugiyama, M., Ando, A. and Ogura, R. (1989). Vitamin B2-enhancement of sodium chromate(VI) - - Induced DNA single strand breaks: ESR study of the action of Vitamin B2. Biochem. Biophys. Res. Commun., 159, 1080–1085.

30. Kuzuya, T., Hoshida, S., Kim, Y., Nishida, M., Fuji, H., Kitabatake, A., Tada, M. and Kamada, T. (1990). Detection of oxygen-derived free radical generation in the canine post-ischemic heart during late phase of reperfusion. Circ. Res., 66, 1160–1165.

31. Halliwell, B. and Aruoma, O.I. (1991). DNA damage by oxygen-derived species. Its mechanism and measurement in mammalian system. FEBS letter, 281, 9–19.

32. Yagi, K., Komura, S., Ishida, N., Nagata, N., Kohono, M. and Ohishi, N. (1993). Generation hydroxyl radical from lipid hydroxides contained in oxidatively modified low-density lipoprotein. Biochem. Biophys. Res. Commun., 190, 386–390.

33. Togashi, H., Shinzawa, H., Hung, Y., Takahashi, T., Noda, H., Oikawa, K. and Kamada, H. (1994). Ascorbic acid radical, superoxide, and hydroxyl radical are detected in reperfusion injury of rat liver using electron spin resonance spectroscopy. Magnetic Resonance in Madicine, 5, 27–30. (in Japanese).

34. Cohen, G. and Hochstein, P. (1963). Glutathione peroxide: the primary agent for the elimination of hydrogen peroxide in erythrocytes. Biochemistry, 2, 1420.

35. Boveris, A. and Chance B. (1973). The mitochondrial generation hydrogen peroxide. Biochem. J., 134, 707–716.

36. Wang, D.H., Ishii, K., Zhen, L.X. and Taketa, K. (1996). Enhanced liver injury in acatalasemic mice following exposure to carbon tetrachloride. Arch. Toxicol., 70, 189–194.

37. Baron, J., Redick, J.A. and Guengerich, F.P. (1981). An imunohistochemical study on the localizations and distributions of phenobarbital and 3-methyl-cholanthrene-inducible cytochromes P-450 within the livers of untreated rats. J. Biol. Chem., 256, 5931–5937.

38. Zimmerman, H.J. (1978). Hepatotoxicity: The adverse effects of drugs and other chemicals on the liver. New York, Appleton-Century-Crofts.
39. Mico, B.A. and Pohl, L.R. (1983). Reductive oxygenation of carbon tetrachloride: Trichloromethylperoxy radical as a possible intermediate in the conversion of carbon tetrachloride to electrophilic chlorine. Arch. Biochem. Biophys., 225, 596–609.
40. Ohomura, T. (1973). Biochemical process of chemical substances: Drug metabolization, pp. 57–97, Khodansha Sientific, Tokyo.
41. De Groot, H. and Noll, T. (1986). The crucial role of low steady state oxygen partial pressures in haloalkane free-radical mediated lipid peroxidation: possible implications in haloalkane liver injury. Biochem. Pharmacol., 35, 15–19.
42. Albano, E, Lott, K.A.K., Slater, T.F., et al. (1982). Spin-trapping studies on the free-radical products formed by metabolic activation of carbon tetrachloride in rat liver microsomal fractions isolated hepatocytes and in vivo in the rat. Biochem. J., 204, 593–603.
43. Slater, T.F. (1984). Free-radical mechanisms in tissue injury. Biochem. J., 222, 1–15.
44. Reynolds, E.S. and Ree, H.J. (1971). Liver parenchymal cell injury. VII. Membrane denaturation following carbon tetrachloride. Lab. Invest., 25, 269–278.
45. Torielli, M.V.: in Biochemical Mechanism of Liver Injury (ed. Slater T.F.), pp. 622–668, Academic Press, London.
46. Farber, J.L. and El-Mofty, S.K. (1975). The biochemical pathology of liver cell necrosis. Am. J. Pathol., 81, 237–250.
47. Kawaguchi, K., Taketa, K., Hayashi, S. et al (1968). Plasma levels of cytoplasmic, mitochondrial and microsomal enzymes in the animals administered with carbon tetrachloride and in the patients with various liver diseases. J. Jpn. Intern. Med., 57, 70–79. (in Japanese).
48. Colby, H.D., Brogan, W.D. and Miles, P.R. (1981). Carbon tetrachloride-induced changes in adrenal, microsomal mixed-function oxidases and lipid peroxidation. Toxicol. Appl. Pharmacol., 60, 492–499.
49. Younes, M., Albrechit, M. and Siegers, C.P. (1983). Interrelationship between in vivo lipid peroxidation, microsomal Ca^{2+}-sequestration activity and hepatotoxicity in rats treated with carbon tetrachloride, cumene hydroperoxide or thioacetamide. Res. Commun. Pathol. Pharmacol., 40, 405–415.
50. Fulceri, R., Benedetti, A. and Comporti, M. (1984). On the mechanisms of inhibition of calcium sequestering activity of liver microsomes in bromotrichloromethane intoxication. Res. Commun. Pathol. Pharmacol., 46, 235–243.
51. Long, R.M. and Moore, L. (1986). Elevated cytosolic calcium in rat hepatocytes exposed to carbon tetrachloride. J. Pharmacol. Exp. Ther., 238, 186–191.
52. Long, R.M., Moore, L. (1986). Inhibition of liver endopalsmic reticulum calcium pump by CCl_4 and release of a sequestered calcium pool. Biochem. Pharmacol., 35, 4131–4137.

Liver and Environmental Xenobiotics
S.V.S. Rana and K. Taketa (Eds)
Copyright © 1997, Narosa Publishing House, New Delhi, India

5. Liver Injury in Ischemia and Reperfusion

Koji Ito, Junichi Uchino, Yasuaki Nakajima and Jun Kimura

First Department of Surgery, Hokkaido University School of Medicine,
Sapporo, Japan

In recent years it has been widely accepted that oxygen-derived free radicals played an important role in causing cellular damage in postischemic organs, including the liver [1–6]. Interruption of blood flow to the liver is often necessary during extensive hepatectomy, and is an unavoidable process in liver transplantation. Thus, prevention against ischemia and reperfusion injury is an important matter.

Although many investigators have reported the relationship between postischemic liver injury and free radicals, the mechanism concerned with the injury is not clear yet. The process of free radicals generation should be discussed separately in organ and cell levels, and the contribution of infiltrating cells also has to be taken into account. This chapter summarizes current review and our recent achievements.

Organ Level Study

Direct detection of free radicals in the whole liver is rather difficult because their half-life is short and the liver contains large amounts of antioxidant substances. So the effect of radical scavengers or the decrease of antioxidant substances are usually observed.

During ischemia, adenine nucleotides are rapidly broken down to form hypoxanthine. Concomitantly, the enzyme, xanthine dehydrogenase, is converted to xanthine oxidase. When blood flow is resumed to the ischemic organ, hypoxanthine is oxidized to xanthine and during this reaction oxygen free radicals are formed. Oxygen radicals damage cell membranes by peroxidation of fatty acids in the phospholipid structure of the membranes. During this process, lipid peroxide radicals, lipid hydroxy-peroxides and other lipid fragmentation products, which are themselves active oxidizing agents, are formed [7]. Thus, the free radical reactivity has a tendency to generate a chain of reaction to produce radical species resulting in an enhancement of the ultimate destructive effect.

Allopurinol, a xanthine oxidase inhibitor, was reported to protect the liver from postischemic injury. When it was administered to rats prior to ischemia of the liver, restitution of protein synthesis and removal of cellular edema during reperfusion was faster and more complete than those in the control animals [8]. As adenine nucleotide levels and energy charge in hepatic tissue during reperfusion were not affected by allopurinol, inhibition of free radical production could have taken place. On the other hand, Kooij et al reported that conversion of xanthine dehydrogenase into xanthine oxidase did not occur to any significant extent in the *in vivo* rat livers with ischemia for 2 hrs and after reperfusion [9]. As a result, the sources of the radicals are still unclear and further studies will be needed to define the mechanism of the effect of allopurinol.

Pretreatment of rats with coenzyme $Q_{10}(C_0Q_{10})$ before hepatic ischemia improved mitochondrial respiratory rate and tissue energy level in the postischemic liver. Since preservation of mitochondrial function by C_0Q_{10} was observed only during reperfusion, and the postischemic increase in the formation of lipid peroxides was prevented with the substance, it was concluded that the beneficial effect of C_0Q_{10} was due to its action as a free radical scavenger [10].

Glutathione (GSH) is one of the important radical scavenger in the liver. When hepatic content was reduced, either by administration of diethylmaleate or by fasting, cell death during reperfusion after ischemia in rats was more extensive than that in the livers with high GSH content [11]. Injured cells were predominantly located in the vicinity of periportal fields, this being most obvious in GSH-depleted animals, further supported the concept of oxygen-induced damage. In the same study, treatment of fasted animals with cobalt chloride increased hepatic content of GSH and the extent of postischemic cell death was reduced. GSH was also reported to accelerate the resynthesis of adenosine triphosphate and to suppress the increase of lipid peroxide after ischemia and reperfusion in rat liver [12].

Superoxide dismutase (SOD) and catalase (CAT) are well known as free radical scavengers. Pretreatment of SOD and/or CAT before ischemia showed less edema and weight gain, and improvement of the liver function was apparent from the laboratory, physical, and histological comparisons in isolated perfused dog livers [13].

The use of allopurinol, or of SOD or CAT lead to significant protection of the hepatocytes when the rat liver was subjected to 90 min of warm ischemia. Allopurinol had the best protective effect, followed by CAT and SOD. It was suggested that hydrogen peroxide (H_2O_2) was more toxic than superoxide anion O_2^- with respect to the hepatic parenchyma [14].

Chemiluminescence spectrometry is a sensitive and precise method to measure the reactive oxygens unless identification of reactive oxygen species is required. Luminol-enhanced chemiluminescence (LEC) technique was applied to the isolated perfused rat liver model. The livers under perfusion with Luminol-containing buffer were subjected to 30 min of ischemia followed by 60 min of reperfusion. Transient bursts of oxygen radical production were observed on reperfusion. SOD treatment diminished reperfusion-induced chemiluminescence transient by more than 80% [15]. In an isolated perfused organ study, after making the median and left lateral lobes of rat liver ischemic in situ for 30 min, the livers were removed 1, 3, 6, 24, or 48 hr after reinstitution of blood flow. LEC was recorded before and for 90 min following phorbol myristate acetate (PMA, stimulater of Kupffer cells and neutrophils) perfusion. An increase in PMA-induced LEC was evident at 1 hr and continued to increase up to 6 hr. By 24 hr the magnitude of the PMA response had returned to control levels. This indicated that a large influx of inflammatory cells had occurred in the liver following *in vivo* ischemia-reperfusion and that these cells were well fixed in the tissue and capable of mounting a large and sustained burst of radical production on stimulation with PMA [16].

Myeloperoxidase (MPO) activity, which was increased after ischemia and reperfusion, was proportional to the number of neutrophils in the liver tissue. Pretreatment with long-acting SOD significantly attenuated the elevated MPO activity and the number of neutrophils [17]. These results indicated that reperfusion after ischemia induced an accumulation of neutrophils in the liver, and oxygen free radicals were important mediators of this neutrophil accumulation.

We demonstrated that pretreatment with antibody to neutrophil adhesion molecules attenuated ischemia-reperfusion injury in mice liver [18]. Sixteen hours before ischemia, antibody was given intravenously. Blood supply to the left lateral and the median lobes of the liver was occluded for 70 min. Plasma ALT, percentage of necrotic area and MPO-positive cell counts in the postischemic liver lobe were estimated 24 hr after reperfusion. Those three parameters were significantly decreased in antibody-pretreated group compared to the control group.

Consequently, there have been many pieces of evidence that free radicals participated in the ischemia-reperfusion liver injury. But the source of free radicals remains still unclear. One reason is that these radicals are strongly affected by the surrounding scavengers or reductive substances and the other is that their half-life is very short. Furthermore, infiltrating cells in the liver are considered to affect them. Thus, analysis of the source of free radicals in the cell level is required.

Cell Level Study

In the liver, the endothelial cells, Kupffer cells, fixed neutrophils and hepatocytes could act as the sources of free radicals. So far, electron spin resonance (ESR) is the only method that is able to directly identify the species of reactive oxygens.

Concentrated suspensions of cultured fetal bovine aortic endothelial cells were made anoxic by incubation at 37°C for 45 min. The cells were reoxygenated by addition of an aerobic solution of the spin trap 5,5'-dimethyl-

1-pyrroline-N-oxide (DMPO), and ESR spectra were obtained. The spectra of these reoxygenated cells exhibited DMPO-OH (trapped hydroxy radical). Both SOD and CAT totally abolished this radical signal, suggesting that O_2 was sequentially reduced from O_2^- to H_2O_2 and to hydroxy radical. Endothelial cells subjected to anoxia and reoxygenation, the conditions observed in the ischemic and reperfused tissues, were considered to generated a burst of superoxide-derived hydroxy free radicals, which in turn caused cell injury and cell death [19].

Kupffer cells, isolated from rat livers and cultured for 24 hr, were exposed to anoxia for 2 hr and reoxygeneted. Immediately upon reoxygenation, O_2^- formation was observed spectrometrically. At the time when the relase of O_2^- decreased, i.e., 2 hr after reoxygenation, the great majority of the cells were dead. Despite the time shift existing between O_2^- liberation and cell injury, the two events were closely linked together [20].

Neutrophils are well known to generate reactive oxygen species and accumulate in postischemic liver. Neutrophils from calves were isolated from peripheral blood. Aliquots of HBSSs-containing DMPO and the metal-chelating reagent were added to HBSS-containing neutrophils. The solution was incubated for 2 min and stimulated by PMA. Immediately after stimulation, ESR measurements were performed. DMPO-OOH adduct (trapped O_2^-) was consistently observed. [21]. Additionally, activated neutrophils caused conversion of xanthine dehydrogenase to xanthine oxidase in endothelial cells, the mechanism of which might be related to the cytotoxic effect of activated neutrophils [22].

Although it was considered that extracellular reactive oxygen species formed by nonparenchymal and/or infiltrating cells were responsible for the hepatocytes injury that occurred during reperfusion, isolated hepatocytes themselves were reported to produce oxygen free radicals. Hepatocytes were prepared from rats and incubated. After anoxic period of 1–2.5 hrs, the cells were reoxygenated. On reoxygenation reactive oxygen species could be detected by enhanced chemiluminescence [23].

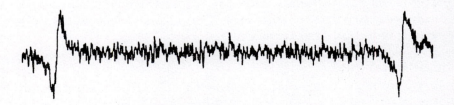

Fig. 1.   ESR spectrum of reoxygenated hepatocytes subjected to anoxia and reoxygenation.

We examined to determine whether hepatocytes could release free radicals to the outer environment. Hepatocytes were isolated by a collagenase perfusion

3. Lindberg, B. (1977). Liver circulation and metabolism in hemorrhagic shock. Acta Chir. Scand., Suppl. **476:** 1–8.
4. Farber, J.L. and Young E.E. (1981). Accelerated phospholipid degradation in anoxic rat hepatocytes. Arch. Biophys., **211:** 312–320.
5. Fornander, J., Bergmark, J., Jagenburg, R. and Hasselgren, P.O. (1985). Evaluation of an *in vivo* method for the study of hepatic protein synthesis in liver ischemia. Eur. Surg. Res., **17:** 91–100.
6. Kayawake, S., Narbaitz, R. and Kako, K.J. (1982). Effects of chlorquine and Nifedipine on the phospholipid content and enzyme activity in the subcellular fraction of ischemic rat liver. Basic Res. Cardiol., **77:** 140–157.
7. Del Maestro, R.F. (1980). An approach to free radicals in medicine and biology. Acta Physiol. Scand., Suppl., **492:** 153–168.
8. Nordstrom, G., Seeman, T. and Hasselgren, P.O. (1985). Beneficial effect of allopurinol in liver ischemia. Surgery, **97:** 679–684.
9. Kooij, A., Schiller, H.J., Schijns, M., Van Noorden, C.J.F. and Fredekiks, W.M. (1994). Conversion of xanthine dehydrogenase into xanthine oxidase in rat liver and plasma at the onset of reperfusion after ischemia. Hepatology **19:** 488–1495.
10. Marubayashi, S., Dohi, K., Ezaki, H., Hayashi, K. and Kawasaki, T. (1982). Preservation of ischemic rat liver mitochondrial functions and liver viability with C^0Q^{10}. Surgery. **91:** 631–637.
11. Jennische, E. (1984). Possible influences of glutathione on postishemic liver injury. Acta Pathol. Microbiol. Scand. **92:** 55–64.
12. Marubayashi, S., Dohi, K. and Kawasaki, T. (1985). Role of freeradicals in ischemic rat liver cell injury. Prevention of damages by vitamin E, coenzyme Q^{10}, or reduced glutathione administration. Surg. Forum. **36:** 136–138.
13. Atalla, S.L., Toledo-Pereyra. L.H., MacKenzie, G.H. and Cederna, J.P. (1985). Influence of oxygen-derived free radical scavengers on ischemic livers. Transplantation **40:** 584–590.
14. Nauta, R.J., Tsimoyiannis, E., Uribe, M., Walsh, D.B., Miller, D. and Butterfield, A. (1990) Oxygen derived free radicals in hepatic ischemia and reperfusion injury in the rat. Surg. Gynecol. Obstet. **171:** 120–125.
15. Okuda, M., Ikai, I., Chance, B. and Kumar, C. (1991). Oxygen radical production during ischemia-reperfusion in the isolated perfused rat liver as monitored by luminol enhanced chemiluminescence. Biochem. Biophys. Res. Comm. **174:** 217–221.
16. Iwata, S., Jamison, D.D. and Chance, B. (1993). Chemiluminescent response to PMA in isolated rat liver after in situ ischemia-reperfusion. Free Radic. Biol. Med. **15:** 575–580.
17. Komatsu, H., Koo, A., Ghadishah, E., Zeng, H., Kuhlenkamp, J.F., Inoue, M., Guth, P.H. and Kaplowitz, N. (1992). Nutrophil accumulation in ischemic reperfused rat liver: evidence for a role for superoxide free radicals. Am. J. Physiol. **262:** G669–676.
18. Tamura, M., Nakajima, Y., Omura, T. Ito, K., Kimura, J., Kusumoto, K., Isai, H., Uchino, J., Nakane, A. and Minagawa, T., (1995). Can anti-Mac-1 and anti-TNF monoclonal antibody protect the liver from warm ischemia-reperfusion injury in mice? Transplant/ Proc. **27:** 768–770.
19. Zweier, J.L., Kuppusamy, P. and Lutty, G.A. (1988). Measurement if endothelial cell free radical generation: evidence for a central mechanism of free radical injury in postischemic tissues. Proc. Natl. Acad. Sci/ **85:** 4046–4050.
20. Rymsa, B., Wang, J.F. and Groot, H.D. (1991). O_2^- release by activated Kupffer cells upon hypoxia-reoxygenation. Am. J. Physiol. **261:** G602–G607.

21. Kuwabara, M., Nishimura, Y., Sato, F., Takahashi, T. Tajima, M., Takahashi, K. and Nagahata, H. (1993). Spin-trpping and chemilumiicescence studies of neutrophils from a Holstein-Friesian calf with boving leukocyte adhedion deficiency, Free Rad. Res. Comms. **18:** 309–318.

22. Phan, S.H., Gannnon, D.E., Ward, P.A., and Karmiol S. (1992). Mechanism of neutrophil induced zanthine dehydrogense to xanthine oxidase conversion in endothelial cells: evidence of a role for elasetase Am. J. Respir. Cell Mol. Bio. **6:** 279–278.

23. Caraceni, P., Rosenblum, E.R., Van Thiel. D.H., adn Borle, A.B. (1994). Reoxygenation injury in isolated rat hepatocytes relation to oxygen free radicals and lipid peroxidation. Am. J. Physilo. **226:** G799–806.

24. Ito, K., Kuwabara, M., Nakajima, Y., Kimura., J. and Uchino, J. (1994). Scavenging activity of superoxide anion in cultured rat hepatocytes. Transplant. Proc. **26:** 2259–2260.

Liver and Environmental Xenobiotics
S.V.S. Rana and K. Taketa (Eds)

6. Liver Injury and Serum Hyaluronan

Takato Ueno and Kyuichi Tanikawa

Second Department of Medicine, Kurume University School of Medicine,
67 Asahi-machi, Kurume 830, Japan

Introduction

Hyaluronan (HA) (hyaluronic acid, hyaluronate), a glycosaminoglycan macromolecule, is one of the major non-structural elements of the extracellular matrix. The major biological roles of HA include the maintenance of water and protein homeostasis as well as the protection of cells from potentially harmful effects. In the liver, most HA is produced by Ito cells (fat-storing cells, lipocytes, stellate cells) located in the Disse's spaces [1]. On the other hand, HA in the tissue enters the blood stream through the lymph, and is rapidly taken up via receptors into hepatic sinusoidal endothelial cells (SEC), where degradation follows [2, 3].

Commonly, the thin peripheral portions of SEC are fenestrated, presenting a sievelike appearance. Moreover, the basement membranes, which are visible in capillaries, are hardly seen on the basal side of SEC (Fig. 1a). In chronic liver diseases such as liver cirrhosis, however, continuous basement membranes are observed on the basal side of SEC, causing hepatic sinusoidal capillarization [4]. In these conditions, SEC show morphological changes resembling the characteristics of vascular endothelial cells: in addition to the formation of basement membranes, the decrease or disappearance of fenestrae and the presence of Weibel-Palade bodies (WBP), which control the production of factor VIII-related antigen (FVIIIRAg) (Fig. 1b) [5]. In hepatic sinusoidal capillarization, SEC show morphological changes and seem to decrease HA degradation. This is a detailed review of recent reports as to the relationship between serum HA levels and liver injury, as well as a summary of our own research regarding HA in liver diseases. We determined serum HA levels in our studies using a previously reported sandwich enzyme-binding assay (Chugai Seiyaku, Tokyo Japan) [6].

Serum Hyaluronan Levels in Various Liver Diseases

The first study of the serum HA levels of patients with liver disease was made in 1985 [7]. In our study, all disease groups showed mean serum HA level higher than that of the normal subjects, and the level increased with progression of the disease (Fig. 2). In previous reports marked elevation in

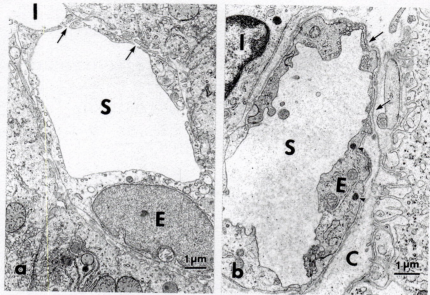

Fig. 1. Transmission electron micrographs showing the sinusoidal area of human livers. (a) Normal liver. An area of SEC shows many fenestrae (arrows) without WPB in the cytoplasm, but there are no basement membranes on the basal side of the cell. (b) Alcoholic liver cirrhosis. SEC show no fenestrae but contain many WPB (arrowheads) in the cytoplasm and continuous basement membranes (arrows) to the side. Disse's space is filled with collagen fibers. Typical hepatic sinusoidal capillarization is shown. S—sinusoid. E—sinusoidal endothelial cell. I—Ito cell. C—collagen.

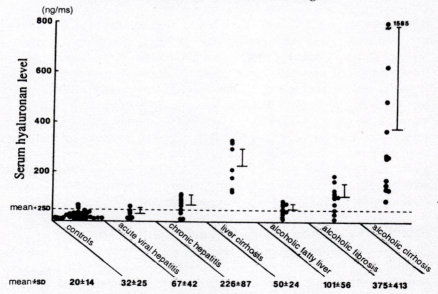

Fig. 2. Serum HA levels in patients with various liver diseases.

serum HA is seen in patients with alcoholic cirrhosis, virus induced cirrhosis, primary biliary cirrhosis and primary sclerosing cholangitis, but not in those with non-cirrhotic, liver diseases [7–13]. Turnover studies with labeled HA in patients with liver cirrhosis have disclosed that clearance rate was slower in the patients, but that the total amount of HA turnover was approximately the same as in healthy persons [9]. The results indicate that the high HA level in liver cirrhosis was due to defective clearance of circulating HA in the liver. Engström-Laurent et al [7] suggested that serum HA was a predictive marker for cirrhosis and might be a useful test for the changes of SEC.

Serum Hyaluronan Level and Morphological and Functional Changes of SEC

Serum Hyaluronan Level and Morphological Changes of SEC

In 1963, Schaffner and Popper reported that hepatic sinusodial capillarization appeared during the progression of hepatic fibrosis [4]. A reduction or disapperance of fenestrae in SEC with basement membrane formation on the basal side of the cells, and WPB in the cells are seen in this hepatic sinusoidal capillarization.

We investigated the relationship between serum HA level and the morphological changes of SEC as part of our study of the HA metabolism in the liver and the changes of the hepatic sinusoids occurring in chronic liver diseases. In our observation of liver biopsy specimens by electron microscopy, the patients were classified according to the presence or absence of basement membranes on the basal side of SEC and WPB, in the cytoplasm of SEC into the following three groups: Group A, who showed neither feature; Group B, who showed basement membranes, and Group C, who showed both. The three groups were compared as to the relationship between each feature and the serum HA levels. Group A showed the lowest mean serum HA level, the mean being lower than the cut-off value (130ng/ml). In Group B, all patients had levels < 200 ng/ml but higher than the cut-off value. The level in Group C was the highest among the three groups (A < B, $P < 0.05$. B < C, $P < 0.01$) (Fig. 3). Furthermore, the level in all patients in Groups B and C, who showed the basement membranes on the basal side of the SEC, were higher than the cut-off value. It is thus suggested that the serum HA level is related to the morphological changes of SEC, and that hepatic sinusoidal capillarization is frequently recognized in the liver of the patients showing serum HA level higher than the cut-off value. In addition, hepatic sinusoidal capillarization is invariably recognized in patients with liver cirrhosis.

Serum Hyaluronan Level and Functional Changes of SEC

Hepatic sinusoidal capillarization not only causes morphological changes

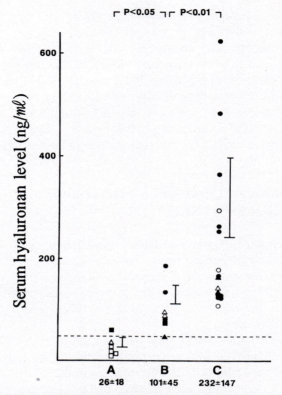

Fig. 3. Relationship between serum HA level and localization of basement membrace and WBP in SEC. □—acute viral hepatitis. △—chronic hepatitis. ○—liver cirrhosis. ■—alcoholic fatty liver. ▲—alcoholic fibrosis. ●—alcoholic cirrhosis. A—neither basement membrane nor WPB in cytoplasm. B—basement membrane without WPB. C—both basement membrane and WPB.

of the SEC, but is also likely to induce functional changes in these cells. For example, the production of FVIIIRAg, which is contained in WPB, is reported to appear in SEC when hepatic sinusoidal capillarization is present [14].

In an examination of the relationship between serum HA level and the immunolocalization of FVIIIRAg in SEC, the mean serum HA level in the patients showing FVIIIRAg in the SEC was found to be significantly higher than that of patients without FVIIIRAg. All the patients showing FVIIIRAg had liver cirrhosis, and in most of these patients the HA level was markedly elevated, i.e. > 200 ng/ml (Fig. 4). Thus, the measurement of serum HA level is useful for evaluating the morphological and functional changes of the SEC when hepatic sinusoidal capillarization is present. These morphological changes of the SEC may result in the functional transformation of the SEC to vascular endothelial cells, causing a gradual reduction in

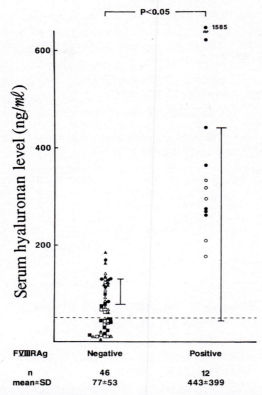

Fig. 4. Relationship between serum HA level and the immuno-localization of FVIII RAg in SEC. □—acute viral hepatitis. △—chronic hepatitis. ○—liver cirrhosis. ■—alcoholic fatty liver. ▲—alcoholic fibrosis. ●—alcoholic cirrhosis.

their function of degrading HA in the blood, resulting in an increase in the blood HA level.

Usefulness of Serum Hyaluronan Measurement in Diagnosis of Liver Cirrhosis

In a few reports, the measurement of serum HA concentration is suggested to be useful for the diagnosis of liver cirrhosis [5, 7–13], which is associated with various complications such as esophageal and gastric varices, encephalopathy, ascites and hepatocellular carcinoma.

To perform the differential diagnosis between liver cirrhosis and non-cirrhosis, cut-off levels of HA, type IV collagen, laminin and type III procollagen-N-peptide (PIIIP), indocyanine green 15 min retention rate (ICGR15) and the platelet count in blood were established based on receiver operating characteristic curves according to various liver pathological diagnoses. The respective cut-off levels for HA, type IV collagen, laminin, PIIIP, ICGR 15 and platelet count are each 130 ng/ml, 250 ng/ml, 2.5 U/ml,

18 ng/ml, 18% and $14 \times 10^4/mm^3$. The diagnostic efficiencies at these levels are 91% for laminin, 90% for HA, 83% for type IV collagen, 74% for platelet count, 64% for ICGR15 and 58% for PIIIP. Moreover, the diagnostic efficiency for liver cirrhosis is 96% in patients showing HA level of more than 130 ng/ml and type IV collagen level of exceeding 250 ng/ml (Table 1). The measurement of serum HA or serum HA and type IV collagen concentration is therefore useful for the diagnosis of liver cirrhosis.

Table 1. Diagnosis of liver cirrhosis using serum hepatic fibrotic markers, ICGR 15, and platelet count

	HA	Type IV collagen	HA and type IV collagen	Laminin	PIIIP	Platelet count	ICGR15
Cut-off value	130 ng/ml	250 ng/ml		2.5 U/ml	18 ng/ml	$14 \times 10^4/$ mm^3	18%
Sensitivity (%)	87	77	68	56	60	67	64
Specificity (%)	90	86	95	96	57	72	63
Efficiency (%)	90	83	96	91	58	74	64

Interferon Therapy in Patients with Chronic Hepatitis C and Serum Hyaluronan

Serum Hyaluronan as a Predictor of Response to Interferon-α Therapy in Chronic Hepatitis C

The agent most widely studied for the treatment of chronic hepatitis C has been interferon-α (IFN-α), the application of which has now been approved throughout the world for this indication. The predictive factors that have been tentatively identified for the response of IFN-α are the degree of liver fibrosis as well as hepatitis C virus genotype, the titer of hepatitis C virus, and the term and dose for IFN-α therapy [15, 16].

The extent of liver fibrosis seems to show little change during IFN-α therapy, although portal inflammation, piecemeal necrosis, and lobular injury are decreased [17].

We investigated the relationship between the serum HA level and liver histology before therapy and the responsiveness to IFN-α therapy for at least 6 months. The serum HA level was significantly elevated in the nonresponders compared to the responders. Most of the patients having serum HA level of more than 100 ng/ml were nonresponders who had chronic active hepatitis with bridging necrosis demonstrated at liver biopsy (Fig. 5). The extent of hepatic fibrosis was significantly greater in the nonresponders than in the responders ($P < 0.001$). These results suggest that patients having a serum HA level above 100 ng/ml and chronic active hepatitis with bridging necrosis are unlikely to respond to IFN-α.

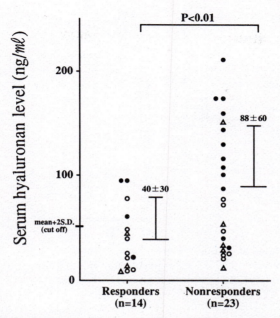

Fig. 5. Serum HA level before IFN-α therapy in patients with chronic hepatitis C. $\triangle$—chronic persistent hepatitis. $\bigcirc$—chronic active hepatitis. $\bullet$—chronic active hepatitis with bridging necrosis.

Serum HA Level for the Assessment of Liver Fibrosis in Chronic Hepatitis C Treated with IFN-α

The levels of serum markers of liver fibrosis such as PIIIP, type IV collagen and laminin are known to decrease in the responders after IFN-α therapy [18–22]. However, since the change of these markers exceeds the limits of normality in some patients with chronic hepatitis C, it is difficult to assess whether liver fibrosis is improved through IFN-α therapy or not. We calculated the ratio for serum HA level before treatment to that after treatment. In most of the groups of patients without improvement of liver fibrosis, the ratio was less than 1.5. It is therefore suggested that liver fibrosis is improved in the patients showing ratio of more than 1.5 for serum HA (Fig. 6). Thus, serum HA level is useful for the evaluation of the improvement in liver fibrosis after IFN-α therapy in chronic hepatitis C.

Serum Hyaluronan Level in Acute Liver Damage and Liver Transplantation

Serum Hyaluronan Level in Acute Liver Damage

In acute viral hepatitis, the serum HA level is slightly increased compared with that in normal subjects. Moreover, during the postoperative course after liver surgery, the serum HA level is invariably higher in patients with complication than in those without complication [23]. These phenomena

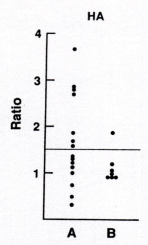

Fig. 6. Ratio of serum HA level before and after IFN-α therapy. A—group with improvement after IFN-α therapy. B—group without improvement after IFN-α therapy.

suggest that the HA receptor dysfunction of SEC occurs in acute liver damage [24].

Serum Hyaluronan Level in Liver Transplantation

Measurement of serum HA level has been suggested to be useful for the monitoring graft function after liver transplantation. Both acute and chronic rejection are associated with increase of serum HA level [25]. These results suggest that the critical target of liver injury is the hepatic microvasculature, particularly with the damage to the SEC. In experimental models, it has been demonstrated that the HA elimination rate is a sensitive marker for SEC function in the viable liver following brief ischemia [26, 27].

Serum Hyaluronan Level as a Hemodynamic Predictor

Gibson et al. examined the ralationship between serum HA level and sinusoidal blood flow in patients with alcoholic liver diseases, and found that serum HA is a predictor of deranged hepatic sinusoidal hemodynamics [28]. They also indicated that serum HA reflects short-term drug-induced changes in sinusoidal perfusion in patients with alcoholic liver disease and portal hypertension [29].

Conclusions

HA is an unbranched polysaccharide. Commonly, most HA is degraded via HA receptors of the SEC. The serum HA level is increased in various liver disorders, and serum HA determination is useful in the diagnosis of liver disorders. At present the pathophysiological mechanisms of the increased serum level are not satisfactorily understood. Decrease of the egress from the liver as well as increase of HA production are both very important factors. SEC injury and the hepatic sinusoidal capillarization may also contribute to the decrease of serum HA uptake or degradation. This review, therefore, has focused on the role of measurement of serum HA level in the diagnosis of liver cirrhosis, which is usually accompanied by the typical hepatic sinusoidal capillarization, in prediction of the response to IFN-α therapy for chronic hepatitis C, in the evaluations of the improvement in liver fibrosis after IFN-α therapy, in the monitoring of the acute or chronic rejection after liver transplantation, and in the prediction of the hepatic sinusoidal hemodynamics. Overall, it seems to be important to clearify the mechanism of high circulating HA concentration in liver disorders, and the clinical value of monitoring the serum HA level in various liver disorders may consequently mount.

References

1. Gressner, A.M. and Harrmann, R. (1988). Hyaluronic acid synthesis and secretion by rat liver fat storing cells in culture, Biochem Biophys Res Commun, Vol. 151, pp. 222–228.
2. Eriksson, S., Fraser, J.R.E., Laurent, T.C., Pertoft, H. and Smedsrød, B. (1983). Endothelial cells are a site of uptake and degradation of hyaluronic acid in the liver, Exp Cell Res, Vol. 144, pp. 223–228.
3. Forsberg, N. and Gustafson, S. (1991). Characterization and purification of the hyaluronan-receptor on liver endothelial cells, Biochem Biophys Acta, Vol. 1078, pp. 12–18.
4. Schaffner, F. and Popper, H. (1963). Capillarization of hepatic sinusoids in man, Gastroenterology, Vol. 44, pp. 239–242.
5. Ueno, T., Inuzuka, S., Torimura, T., Tamaki, S. Koh, H., Kin, M. Minetoma, T., Kimura, Y., Ohira, H., Sata, M., Yoshida, H. and Tanikawa, K. (1993). Serum hyaluronate reflects hepatic sinusoidal capillarization, Gastroenterology, Vol. 105, pp. 475–481.
6. Chichibu, K., Matsuura, T., Shichijo, S. and Yokoyama, M. (1989). Assay of serum hyaluronic acid in clinical application, Clin Chim Acta, Vol. 181, pp. 317–324.
7. Engström-Laurent, A., Lööf, L., Nyberg, A. and Schröder, T., (1985). Increased serum levels of hyaluronate in liver disease, Hepatology, Vol. 5, pp. 638–642.
8. Frébourg, T., Delpech, B., Bercoff, E., Senant, J., Bertrand, P., Deugnier, Y. and Bourreille, J. (1986). Serum hyaluronate in liver diseases: study by enzymoimmunological assay, Hepatology, Vol. 6, pp. 392–395.
9. Fraser, J.R.E., Engström-Laurent, A., Nyberg, A., and Laurent, T.C. (1986). Removal of hyaluronic acid from the circulation in rheumatoid disease and primary biliary cirrhosis, J Lab Clin Med, Vol. 107, pp. 79–85.
10. Nyberg, A., Engstrom-Laurent, A., Lööf, L. (1988). Serum hyaluronate in primary biliary cirrhosis—a biochemical marker for progressive liver damage, Hepatology, Vol. 8, 142–146.
11. Babbs, C., Haboubi, N.Y., Mellor, J.M., Smith, A., Rowan, B.P. and Warnes, T.W. (1990). Endothelial cell transformation in primary biliary cirrhosis : a morphological and biochemical study, Hepatology, Vol. 11, pp. 723–729.

12. Ramadori, G., Zöhrens, G., Manns, M., Rieder, H., Dienes, H.P., Hess, G. and Meyer Zum Büschenfelde, K.H. (1991). Serum hyaluronate and type III procollagen aminoteminal propeptide concentration in chronic liver disease. Relationship to cirrhosis and disease activity, Eur J Clin Invest, Vol. 21, pp. 323–330.

13. Nyberg, A., Lindqvist, U. and Engström-Laurent, A. (1992). Serum hyaluronan and aminoterminal propeptide of type III procollagen in primary biliary cirrhosis: relation to clinical symptoms, liver histopathology and outcome, J Inter Med, Vol. 231, PP. 485–491.

14. Taguchi, K. and Asano, G. (1988) Neovascularization of pericellular fibrosis in alcoholic liver disease, Acta Pathol Jpn, Vol. 38, pp. 615–626.

15. Fried, M.W. and Hoofnagle, J. H. (1995). Therapy of hepatitis C, Semin Liver Dis, Vol. 15, pp. 82–91.

16. Pagliaro, L., Craxi, A., Cammaá, C., Tiné, F., Marco, V.D., Iacono, O.L. and Almasio, P. (1994). Interferon-a for chronic hepatitis C: an analysis of pretreatment clinical predictors of response, Hepatology, Vol. 19, pp. 820–828.

17. Castilla, A., Prieto, J. and Fausto, N. (1991). Transforming growth factors $\beta 1$ and a in chronic liver disease: effects of interferon alfa therapy, N Engl J Med, Vol. 324, pp. 933–940.

18. Camps, J., Castilla, A., Ruiz, J., Civeira. M.P. and Prieto, J. (1993) Randomsed trial of lymphoblastoid a -interferon in chronic hepatitis C: effects on inflammation, fibrogenesis and viremia, J Hepatol, Vol. 17, pp. 390–396.

19. Capra, F., Casaril, M., Gabrielli, G.B., Tognella, P., Rizzi, A., Dolci, L., Colombari, R., Mezzelani, P., Corrocher, R. and De Sandre, G. (1993). a-Interferon in the treatment of chronic viral hepatitis: effects on fibrogenesis serum markers, J Hepatol, Vol. 18, pp. 112–118.

20. Castilla, A., Bansell, J.C., Civeira, M.P. and Prieto, J. (1993). Lymphoblastoid a-interferon for chronic hepatitis C: a randomized controlled study. Am J Gastroenterol, Vol. 88, pp. 233–239.

21. Yabu, K., Kiyosawa, K., Mori, H., Matsumoto, A., Yoshizawa, K., Tanaka, E. and Furuta, S. (1994). Serum collagen type IV for the assessment of fibrosis and resistance to interferon therapy in chronic hepatitis C, Scand J Gastroenterol, Vol. 29, pp. 474–479.

22. Gallorini, A., Plebani M., Pontisso, P., Chemello, L., Masiero, M., Mantovani, G. and Alberti, A. (1994). Serum markers of hepatic fibrogenesis in chronic hepatitis type C treated with alfa-2A interferon, Liver, Vol. 14, pp. 257–264.

23. Ohdo, M. (1994). Perioperative changes of serum hyaluronic acid on hepatic resection of microwave coagulonecrotic therapy, J. Kurume Med Association, Vol. 57, pp. 1163–1170.

24. Deaciuc, I.V., Bagby, G.J. and Spitzer, J.J. (1993). Association of galactosamine-induced hepatitis in the rat with hyperhyaluronaemia and decreased hyaluronan uptake by the isolated, perfused liver, Biochem Pharmacol, Vol. 46, pp. 671–675.

25. Adams, D.H., Wang, L., Hubscher, S.G. and Neuberger, J.M. (1989). Hepatic endothelial cells: targets in liver allograft rejection? Transplantation, Vol. 47, pp. 479–482.

26. Shimizu, H., He, W., Guo, P., Dziadkoviec, I., Miyazaki, M. and Falk, R.E. (1994). Serum hyaluronate in the assessment of liver endothelial cell function after orthotopic liver transplantation in the rat. Hepatology., Vol. 20, pp. 1323–1329.

27. Sutto, F., Brault, A., Lepage, R. and Huet, P.M. (1994). Metabolism of hyaluronic

acid by liver endothelial cells: effect of ischemia-reperfusion in the isolated perfused rat liver, J Hepatol, Vol. 20, pp. 611–616.

28. Gibson, P.R., Fraser, J.R.E., Brown. T.J., Finch, C.F., Jones, P.A., Colman, J.C. and Dudley, F.J. (1992). Hemodynamic and liver function predictors of serum hyaluronan in alcoholic liver disease, Hepatology, Vol. 15, pp. 1054–1059.

29. Gibson, P.R., Fraser, J.R.E., Colman, J.C. Jones, P.A., Jennings, G. and Dudley F. J. (1993). Chage in serum, hyaluronan: a simple index of short-term drug-induced changes in hepatic sinusoidal perfusion, Gastroenterology, Vol. 105, pp. 470–474.

7. Phthalic Acid Esters and Liver

D. Parmar and P.K. Seth

Industrial Toxicology Research Centre, P.O. Box 80
M.G. Marg, Lucknow-226 001, India

Introduction

Phthalic acid esters (PAEs) are the most commonly used plasticizers which are added to provide desired flexibility and clarity to the polyvinyl chloride (PVC) plastics used in packaging, storage and delivery of food, drugs and cosmetics. Some of the PAEs are also used as the vehicle for perfumes. A finished plastic product may contain as much as 50% of the plasticizer by weight. Since these plasticizers are not polymerized to the plastic matrix, they may with time and use migrate out from the finished plastics although these plastic products are obviously designed to retain the plasticizers and thereby remain flexible. Di (2-ethylhexyl)phthalate (DEHP), one of the most widely used PAE (Fig. 1), has been shown to leach out from the finished plastic products into blood, physiological fluids, commercial solvents and food materials and subsequently enter in human beings through food chain and during transfusion, hemodialysis and use of plastic bioimplants and other biomedical devices [1–3]. Varying quantities of DEHP and other phthalate esters have been detected in water, fish and aquatic invertebrates as well as in the bovine and human tissues [1–6].

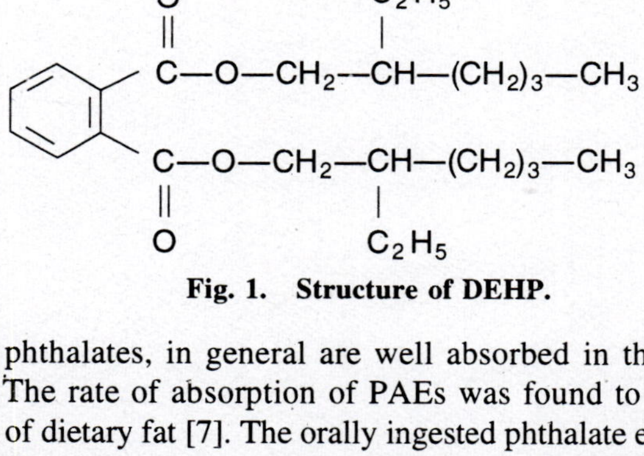

Fig. 1. Structure of DEHP.

  Dialkyl phthalates, in general are well absorbed in the gastrointestinal (GI) tract. The rate of absorption of PAEs was found to be influenced by the content of dietary fat [7]. The orally ingested phthalate esters are absorbed in the gut primarily as the corresponding monoester derivatives [8]. However, evidence for significant absorption of intact diester from the GI tract has also been demonstrated in various animal species [9–13]. Albro [11], who studied the absorption threshold of DEPH, have reported that administration of plasticizer above the threshold results in a steady increase in the amount of unhydrolyzed phthalic diester reaching the liver.

Following absorption, PAEs are known to be metabolized, and rapidly cleared out from the body. The obligatory first step in the metabolism of PAEs is hydrolysis to the monoester and corresponding alcohol by non specific lipases present in pancreatic secretion, intestinal mucosa and a number of body organs like liver, lung, kidney etc. [10–13].

Dimethyl phthalate (DMP) and to a lesser extent, dibutyl phthalate (DBP) has been shown to be eliminated in urine as monoester metabolites [15], whereas phthalate esters of longer chain lenghts, such as DEHP, undergo modifications after hydrolysis to monoester to achieve sufficient polarity for renal excretion. Studies on the metabolism of DEHP in rats and mice, suggest that mono (2-ethylhexyl) phthalate (MEHP), formed as a result of hydrolysis of DEHP, undergoes a series of oxidations in liver as shown in Fig. 2 [10, 11]. Only the side chain of MEHP was found to be oxidized as no alterations of the aromatic ring was reported in mammals.

Marked species differences have been reported in the metabolism of the PAEs (Fig. 3). Rats, in particular, differ from mice, guinea pigs and humans in the elimination of PAEs metabolites as species other than rats excrete the oxidation products of the monoester mainly in the form of glucuronide conjugates [10, 11]. Urinary analysis of the metabolites have revealed that the excreted metabolites of DEHP consist primarily of terminal oxidation products (diacids, ketoacids) in urine from rodents (rats and mice), but primarily of unoxidized or minimally oxidized (MEHP, hydroxyacid) products in urine from primates [10, 11]. Lhuguenot et al [16] studied dose-and time-dependent alterations in the metabolic profile of DEHP and MEHP in rats *in vivo* and in rat primary hepatocyte cultures. At low dose (50 mg/kg) of MEHP, the relative amounts of ω (metabolites I, V, X and XII) and ω-1 (metabolites VI and IX) oxidation products remained essentially constant while at high dose (500 mg/kg) an increase in ω-oxidation products and a decrease in ω-1 oxidation products were seen with time. Similar time and dose dependent alterations in the profile of MEHP metabolism were also observed in rat hepatocyte cultures [16]. Based on these studies, Lhuguenot et al [16] proposed metabolites I and VI as final products of MEHP metabolism.

The phthalate esters have generally been considered to be the chemicals of low order of toxicity. The LD50 values for some of the PAEs in various animal species is shown in Table 1. Although phthalates are known to be metabolized rapidly, the cumulative toxicity of PAEs has been observed on their repeated administrations. The low acute LD50 doses of both di-n-octyl phthalate (DOP) and DEHP were found to have 22 to 28 times more toxicity on repeated administrations [17, 18].

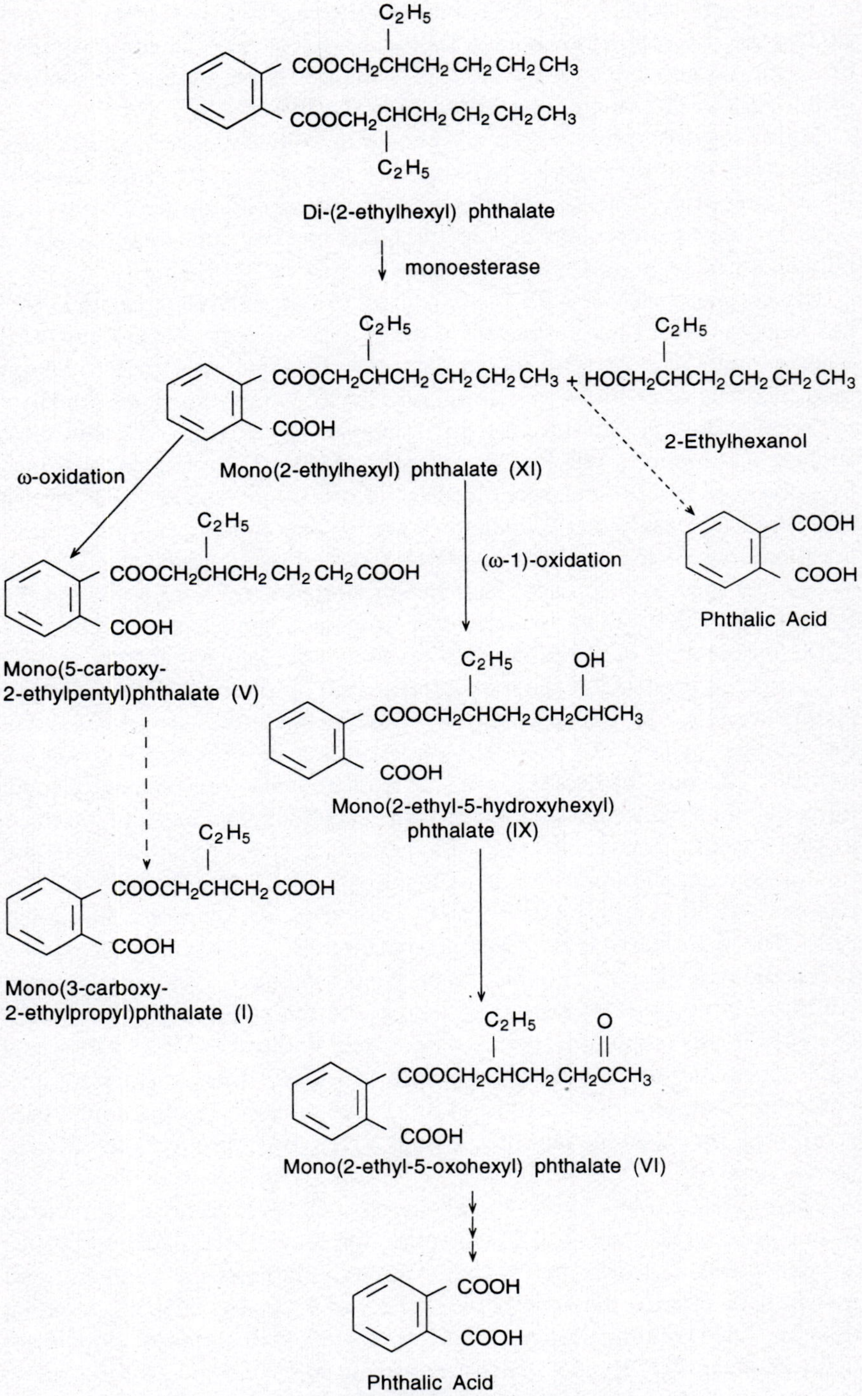

C_2H_5

$COOCH_2CHCH_2CH_2CH_2CH_3$

$COOCH_2CHCH_2CH_2CH_2CH_3$

C_2H_5

Di-(2-ethylhexyl) phthalate

↓ monoesterase

C_2H_5 C_2H_5

$COOCH_2CHCH_2CH_2CH_2CH_3$ + $HOCH_2CHCH_2CH_2CH_2CH_3$

$COOH$

Mono(2-ethylhexyl) phthalate (XI)   2-Ethylhexanol

ω-oxidation

C_2H_5

$COOCH_2CHCH_2CH_2CH_2COOH$

(ω-1)-oxidation

$COOH$

$COOH$

$COOH$

Phthalic Acid

Mono(5-carboxy-
2-ethylpentyl)phthalate (V)

C_2H_5 OH

$COOCH_2CHCH_2CH_2CHCH_3$

$COOH$

Mono(2-ethyl-5-hydroxyhexyl)
phthalate (IX)

C_2H_5

$COOCH_2CHCH_2COOH$

$COOH$

Mono(3-carboxy-
2-ethylpropyl)phthalate (I)

C_2H_5 O
               ‖

$COOCH_2CHCH_2CH_2CCH_3$

$COOH$

Mono(2-ethyl-5-oxohexyl) phthalate (VI)

$COOH$

$COOH$

Phthalic Acid

Fig. 2 Metabolism of DEHP.

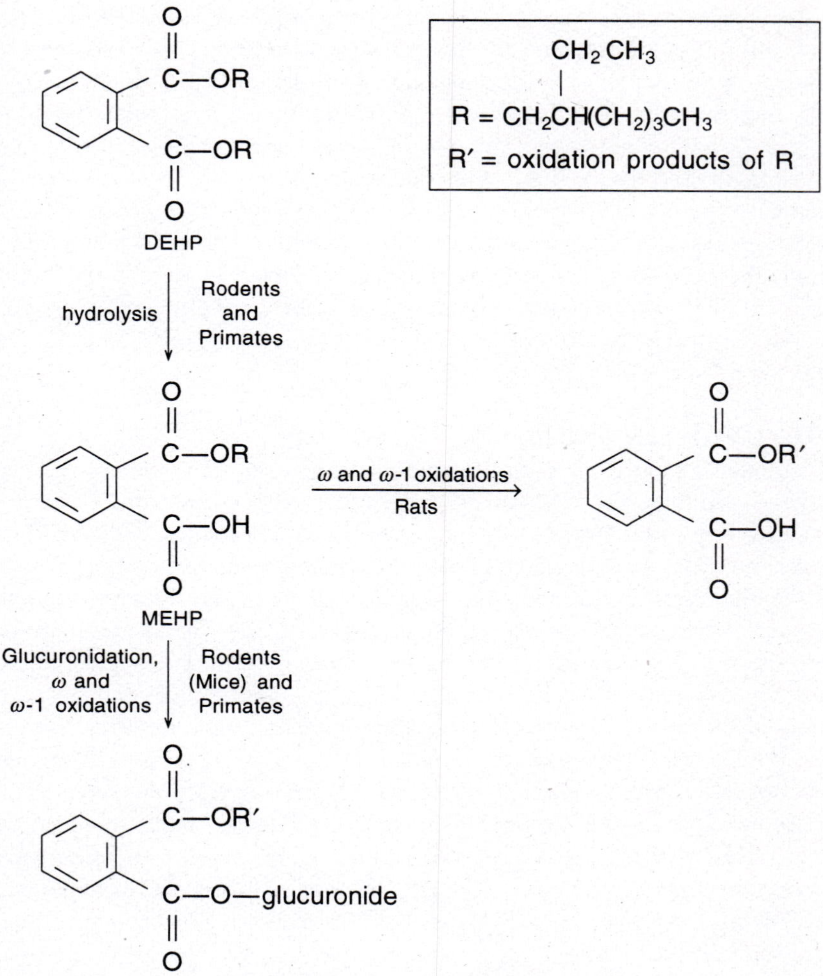

Fig. 3 Species differenecs in metabolism of DEHP.

Table 1. Acute toxicity of DEHP

Species	Route	LD50 (g/kg)
Mouse	i.p	14.2–20
Rat	i.p	50
Rat	p.o.	26
Rat	i.v.	13
Rabbit	p.o.	34
Rabbit	i.p.	31
Rabbit	Dermal	20
Guinea Pig	Dermal	10

Liver has been shown to be the target organ affected by the PAEs. Acute and chronic administration of PAEs has been reported to exert variable effects on the hepatic function depending on the animal species [6, 9–11, 19]. In general, phthalates have been found to induce liver enlargement [6, 13, 19–21]. This increase in liver weight has been attributed to rapid cell division (hyperplasia) along with the detachment of cells (hypertrophy). Hepatic hyperplasia appears to be the initial physiological response to DEHP in rats as reflected by the increase in cell division within 24 hours after a single dose of DEHP and in early stages of treatment in the chronic studies [22, 23]. The increase in the liver weight caused by phthalates has been found to reverse to normal or even below normal levels on prolonged exposure.

Effect of PAEs on Hepatic Morphology

Histopathological examination of phthalate induced enlargement of livers have shown fatty vacuolation and congestion followed by cloudy swelling, excessive pigmentation, bile duct proliferation and occasional fatty degeneration [6, 19, 20]. Microscopic examinations revealed structural changes in the bile ducts, a decline in centrilobular glycogen and fat deposits in the periportal area in the liver of rats treated with DEHP. The accumulation of lipofuscin deposits indicated the peroxidation of cellular lipids [6, 9, 24]. A definite increase in hepatic peroxisomes in the centrilobular and periportal areas of the liver and an increase in the number of mitochondria was also observed. Lipid filled lysosomes were also observed in some cases. Moreover, most of the morphological changes were seen in the male rats even at low doses but appeared in the females only at high doses, indicating a greater susceptibility of male rats than the females. Hepatic necrosis and atrophy were also reported in rats fed DBP. Histopathological studies revealed centrilobular necrosis and degeneration with distension of the capsule and proliferation of the bile ducts in mice fed DBP in the diet. Murakami et al [25] also reported increase in peroxisome, lysosome and mitochondria on ultrastructural examination of the liver cells.

Effect of Phthalates on Lipid Metabolism

Ever since Nazir et al [26] detected DEHP in association with triglycerides of bovine mitochondria, the interaction of PAEs with lipid metabolism has been a subject of active investigation (Table 2). Stein et al [7] showed an interaction of dietary fat with DEHP where presence of the phthalate in diet potentiated the growth promoting effects of lipids in rats. Exposure to phthalates, in general, has been found to be associated with the reduction in circulating cholesterol and serum triglyceride levels which accounted for the reduction in liver steroidogenesis [27–33]. Bell et al [32–34] reported reduced uptake of ^{14}C-mevalonate and ^{14}C-acetate by the liver minces of DBP exposed rats. Monooctyl phthalate (MOP), the monoesterified metabolitie of DOP, has been reported to reduce the circulating concentrations of triglycerides and total cholesterol while increase the serum concentrations of phospholipids and nonesterified fatty acids. MOP was further found to increase palmitic and oleic acid contents while decreasing stearic acid contents in serum phospholipids, increase cholesteryl ester and triglycerides, decrease linoleic acids contents in serum triglycerides and arachidonic acid contents in serum phospholipids thus suggesting alterations in the hepatic metabolism of fatty acid and cholesterol [34]. Nair and Kurup [35] further showed that DEHP when given in diet increased the cellular ubiquinone levels, which acts as inhibitor in cholesterol synthesis.

Effect of PAEs on Carbohydrate Metabolism

PAEs have been found to effect the carbohydrate metabolism in liver (Table 2). DEHP is reported to deplete the hepatic glycogen deposits in the rodents. A decrease in glycogen in livers of mice and rats [6, 19, 24, 36–39] and ferrets [37] receiving DEHP has been reported. Sakurai et al [38] showed marked depression of glucose and glycogen in livers of rats receiving diet containing DEHP. This depletion in hepatic glycogen appears to be due to the increase in hepatic glucose utilization in DEHP treated rats as a result

Table 2.   Effect of phthalates on lipid, energy and carbohydrate metabolism

Phthalate	Species	Principal findings	References
DEHP	Rat	Interaction with dietary fat	[7]
DBP, DEHP and DOP	Rat	Reduction in circulating cholesterol and serum triglycerides	[27–33]
DBP	Rat	Reduced uptake of ^{14}C-mevalonate	[32, 34]
DOP	Rat	Increased concentrations of phospholipids & nonesterified fatty acids	
DEHP	Rat, mouse, ferret	Depletion of hepatic glycogen deposits	[6, 9, 36–39]
DEHP	Rat	Increased glyceraldehyde 3-phosphate dehydrogenase, malic dehydrogenase and lactic dehydrogenase	[40]
DEHP	Rat	Retardation of gluconeogenesis	[39]
DEHP, DOP	Rat	Inhibition of glycogenesis and glycogenolysis	[40]
DBP, DEHP and DOP	Rat	Electron transfer inhibitors, depression of mitochondrial respiration	[42–44]
DBP, DEHP	Rat, mouse	Uncoupling of oxidative phosphorylation	[44]
DEHP	Rat	Inhibition of SDH, ATPase, diaphorase	[34, 45]

of the decrease in the activity of hepatic glucose 6-phosphatase. The activities of glyceraldehyde 3-phosphate dehydrogenase, malic dehydrogenase and lactic dehydrogenase were also found to be increased after DEHP exposure [40].

Studies on the rates of incorporation of labelled pyruvate into blood glucose and liver glycogen and alterations in the levels of intermediates of carbohydrate metabolism indicated retardation of gluconeogenesis [39]. Mushtaq et al [40], have shown that DEHP inhibits glycogenesis and glycogenolysis in rat liver. They observed a significant decrease in the activity of glucose 6-phosphate dehydrogenase, phosphorylase and glucose 6-phosphatase in livers of DEHP exposed rats. Similar alteration, but to a lesser extent were observed after exposure to DOP in rodents [41].

Interaction of PAEs with Mitochondrial Membrane

Mitochondria appear to be the target of phthalates (Table 2). Adverse effects of PAEs on mitochondrial function have been reported by several investigators. PAEs, in general, were found to inhibit the mitochondrial respiration in rat liver [6, 9, 41–43]. Takahashi [42] suggested that PAEs act as energy transfer inhibitors to depress the mitochondrial respiration. The studies of Ohyama [43] have indicated that PAEs are electron and energy transport inhibitors, while Inouye et al [44] have suggested that phthalates induce uncoupling of oxidative phosphorylation. Phthalates were found to produce aberrations in mitochondrial function, e.g. DBP enhanced K^+ efflux from isolated mitochondria, usually not produced by standard uncoupling agents [44]. Srivastava et al [36, 45] reported sensitivity of various components of electron transport chain towards DEHP as indicated by decrease in the activities of succinate dehydrogenase (SDH), cytochrome c-oxidase, malic dehydrogenase and diaphorase and an increase in the alkaline phosphate activity in liver of DEHP treated rats. DEHP was also found to inhibit the activity of total and Mg^+ stimulated adenosine triphosphatase (ATPase) activity of rat liver [36, 45]. These effects of DEHP were present even after 11 days of final treatment with the diester, suggesting that the enzymatic alteration observed after treatment with PAEs were perhaps not related to the presence of DEHP, as by this time all the plasticizer is expected to be excreted [6, 9, 10, 13].

Effect of PAEs on Peroxisome Proliferation

The earlier reports that PAEs can cause proliferation of hepatic peroxisomes [6, 19, 38, 46, 47] have aroused a great concern as this phenomenon is believed to be associated with the production of hepatic tumours and induction of hepatocellular carcinomas in rats and mice [48, 49]. Studies have shown that an increase in hepatic peroxisomes is a marker of DEHP exposure in rodents. The induction in the number of peroxisomes has been shown to be accompanied with a several fold increase in the activity of H_2O_2 generating peroxisomal fatty acid β-oxidation system and a two fold increase in the activity of catalase [6, 19, 49–52]. DEHP induced peroxisome proliferation is also found to be associated with a remarkable increase in the content of PPA-80 (peroxisome proliferation associated 80,000 molecular weight polypeptide), identified as bifunctional protein of the peroxisomal fatty acid β-oxidation system [53, 54]. Further, this increase in the amounts of peroxisomal fatty acid β-oxidation enzymes following PAEs exposure has been shown to be due to specific increases in messenger RNA in the liver suggesting the transcriptional activation of the genes of peroxisomal β-oxidation enzymes [55].

Using primary rat hepatocyte cultures, Gray et al [56] reported that monoesters as compared to intact diester were more effective in producing peroxisome proliferation and that straight chain monoesters from methyl to n-octyl have little effect on rat hepatic peroxisomes compared with the branched chain monoester, MEHP. Mitchell et al (57) further identified the different metabolites of DEHP which could be responsible for the proliferation of peroxisomes induced by the diester. 2-ethylhexanol and ω-carbon oxidation products, mono (5-carboxy-2-ethylpentyl) phthalate (metabolite V) and mono (3-carboxyethylpropyl) phthalate (metabolite I) produced little or no increase in CN insensitive palmitoyl-CoA oxidation whereas ω-1 carbon oxidation products , mono(2-ethyl-5-oxohexyl)phthalate (metabolite VI) and mono (2-ethyl-5-hydroxyhexyl) phthalate (metabolic IX) produced a large (7- to 11-fold) induction of peroxisomal enzyme activity mirroring that produced by MEHP itself. Although MEHP is known to be biotransformed to the ω-1 oxidation products, the peroxisome proliferation due to MEHP per se cannot be ruled out.

Marked difference have been reported amongst different animal species to induce peroxisomal proliferation [6, 51, 58, 59]. Amongst various species tested, rats and mice were found to be most sensitive, hamster intermediate and guinea pigs, primates and man insensitive or non-responsive to DEHP [51, 58, 59]. *In vitro* studies with cultured hepatocytes, too show a similar species difference in response to DEHP. Little or no effect of MEHP and metabolite VI, the active peroxisome proliferators, on palmitoyl CoA oxidation in marmoset, guinea pig or human hepatocytes have further suggested intrinsic differences in the response of liver cells to DEHP [58–62].

Studies aimed to elucidate the mechanism(s) of peroxisome proliferation have suggested that alterations in lipid metabolism may be an important factor in the genesis of the peroxisome proliferation. It has been shown that DEHP induces a diverse number of effects upon enzymes, organelles and cofactors involve in lipid metabolism. An increase in ω and β oxidation of fatty acids, acyl CoA hydrolases, CoA and carnitine has been reported following administration of DEHP and other peroxisome proliferators to the rodents [48, 57–65]. Lock et al [62] who observed that lipids which accumulate in liver on administration of DEHP, disappear when the peroxisomes are induced, suggested the mechanism for the induction peroxisomes via perturbation of lipid metabolism. Studies in their laboratory have shown that mono (2-ethyl-5-oxohexyl) phthalate (metabolite VI), the active proliferator derived from DEHP, causes a concentration dependent decrease in the oxidation of fatty acids in isolated cells and selectively inhibits medium chain fatty acids (octanoyl), but not palmitoyl and carnitine in isolated mitochondrial by inhibiting mitochondrial β-oxidation enzymes and depleting essential CoA. This inhibition of mitochondrial β-oxidation due to sequestration of CoA thus leads to the accumulation of medium and long chain fatty acid or their CoA esters in the cell and these in turn lead to the increased synthesis of peroxisomes and enzyme and enzymes involved in fatty acid oxidation in an attempt to maintain lipid homeostasis.

Interaction of Phthalates with Other Xenobiotics

Alterations in barbiturate sleeping time and ethanol sleeping time following exposure to phthalates suggest that phthalate esters could interact with other drugs and chemicals and modify their biological response. A single administration of DEHP was found to increae the hexobarbital or pentobarbital sleeping time in rats or mice while repeated administration of a number of phthalates caused singnificant and dose dependent decrease in hexobarbital sleeping time in rats [19, 66–68]. Likewise, single exposure of DEHP increased the ethanol-induced sleeping time while repeated administration decreased the same [19]. DEHP has also been shown to modify the biological response of parathion, an organophosphorus insecticide by lowering the inhibitory activity of parathion in DEHP-treated animals [19, 69]. Alterations in the response of carbon tetrachloride was also observed following DEHP exposure [19, 70]. Studies in our laboratory have shown that DEHP produces such changes by acting at the pharmacokinetic phase since it modifies the activity of the enzymes responsible for their metabolic dispositions. Tomaszweski et al [71] suggested that DEHP may act as an antagonist for the hepatic damage caused by other chemicals such as 2,3,7,8-tetra-chlorodibenzo-p-dioxin (TCDD). Pretreatment with DEHP mitigated many of the toxic effects of TCDD. Sager and Little [72] showed that DEHP affected the binding of propyl-2,3-dihydroalprenol (DHA), a β-adrenergic blocking agent on the mononuclear leukocytes thereby suggesting that DEHP could potentially affect the mode of action of β-adrenergic class of pharmaceuticals. Perera et al [73] reported that DEHP induced effects on the peroxisomal system of the liver appeared to be increased in rats kept on a choline deficient diet.

Interaction of PAEs with Cytochrome P450 Monooxygenases

Exposure to phthalate esters have been shown to be associated with the proliferation of smooth endoplasmic reticulum [19, 62, 63] which results in a concomitant increase in certain microsomal enzyme, in particular the cytochrome P450s [19, 61–65, 74]. This increase in microsomal P450 enzymes has been attributed to both an increase in the rate of *de novo* protein synthesis as demonstrated by the elevated rate of incorporation of amino acids into microsomal proteins and decrease in protein degradation as indicated by the increase in half lives of total microsomal proteins [75].

Studies in our laboratory have indicated that alterations in the P450 enzymes could be correlated with the amount of the intact diester and its hydrolytic products reaching the liver. Depending on route and duration of exposure both P450 enzyme induction and inhibition has been observed [16, 76–78]. The inhibitory effect observed after single oral or i.p. or repeated i.p. administrations of DEHP has been attributed to the direct effect of the plasticizer or its metabolites while the induction in the P450 monooxygenases after repeated oral administrations for 7 days has been shown to be due to the self induction of the P450 monooxygenases as MEHP and its further metabolites are known to be metabolized by the same P450 enzymes (Fig. 4). Pharmacokinetic studies have also shown an increase in the circulating concentrations of MEHP and 2-ethylhexanol after single oral or i.p. exposure as compared to that after repeated oral administration of the plasticizer [78, 79]. Moreover, a lesser degree of induction in the levels of P450 contents and the activity of P450 dependent aniline hydroxylase and ethylmorphine

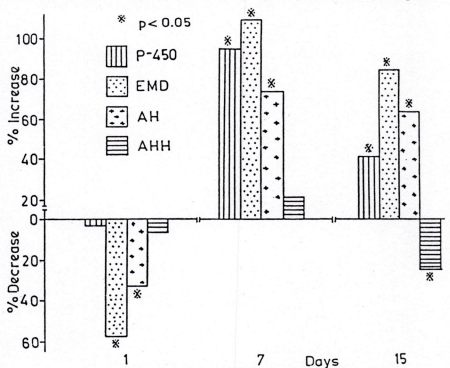

Fig. 4 Time dependent effects of DEHP on P450 enzymes.

Table 3:   Age related effects of DEHP on hepatic cytochrome P450 monooxygenases

	3 Week		6 Week		10 Week	
	Control	Treated	Control	Treated	Control	Treated
Cytochrome P450*						
1 day	0.41 ± 0.02	0.21 ± 0.03[a]	0.51 ± 0.03	0.38 ± 0.05	0.58 ± 0.05	0.53 ± 0.10
7 days	0.47 ± 0.04	1.05 ± 0.08[a]	0.52 ± 0.04	0.97 ± 0.09[a]	0.55 ± 0.06	0.88 ± 0.08[a]
15 days	0.50 ± 0.04	0.33 ± 0.02[a]	0.54 ± 0.03	0.81 ± 0.05[a]	0.54 ± 0.06	0.78 ± 0.06[a]
Aniline hydroxylase**						
1 day	47.9 ± 5.3	13.4 ± 1.8[a]	46.4 ± 5.0	23.2 ± 1.6[a]	50.4 ± 4.6	33.5 ± 3.4[c]
7 days	45.9 ± 4.0	105.7 ± 1.0[a]	44.2 ± 3.4	90.8 ± 7.0[a]	53.5 ± 8.5	89.8 ± 7.8[c]
15 days	45.8 ± 2.5	27.5 ± 2.0[a]	46.2 ± 2.4	84.0 ± 4.8[a]	51.9 ± 4.0	76.7 ± 5.0[a]
Ethylmorphine N-demethylase**						
1 day	0.23 ± 0.02	0.10 ± 0.02[a]	0.29 ± 0.04	0.17 ± 0.03[c]	0.31 ± 0.04	0.21 ± 0.08
7 days	0.25 ± 0.05	0.77 ± 0.09[a]	0.29 ± 0.04	0.60 ± 0.03[b]	0.31 ± 0.06	0.54 ± 0.08[a]
15 days	0.28 ± 0.05	0.18 ± 0.03	0.31 ± 0.05	0.51 ± 0.09[c]	0.30 ± 0.02	0.43 ± 0.02[d]
Arylhydrocarbon hydroxylase***						
1 day	19.4 ± 2.3	9.7 ± 1.3[a]	27.9 ± 3.7	18.4 ± 2.5[b]	30.3 ± 4.0	28.5 ± 1.6
7 days	24.3 ± 3.9	45.3 ± 3.2[a]	27.7 ± 3.7	50.3 ± 3.5[b]	29.9 ± 2.9	34.9 ± 3.1
15 days	26.5 ± 1.4	10.6 ± 0.7	26.7 ± 1.8	13.8 ± 0.9a	28.4 ± 2.5	21.4 ± 0.4[d]

All values are mean ± S.E. of five animals.

[a]$P < 0.001$; [b]$P < 0.01$; [c]$P < 0.05$; *nmoles mg/protein; **pmoles p-aminophenol formed/min/mg protein; ***nmoles HCHO formed/min/mg protein; ****pmoles 3-OH-benzo (a) pyrene formed/min/mg/protein.

Table 4.   Species specific effects of DEHP on hepatic cytochrome P450 monooxygenases

	Ethylmorphine N-demethylase[a]		Aniline hydroxylase[b]		Arylhydrocarbon hydroxylase[c]	
	Control	Treated	Control	Treated	Control	Treated
			7 days			
Rat	0.305 ± 0.05	0.638 ± 0.08*	53.5 ± 8.5	89.8 ± 7.8*	28.9 ± 2.9	34.9 ± 3.1
Mouse	0.387 ± 0.04	0.562 ± 0.03*	60.2 ± 4.6	78.0 ± 3.9*	28.1 ± 1.5	29.7 ± 0.7
G.pig	0.183 ± 0.01	0.278 ± 0.01	51.5 ± 2.0	63.0 ± 2.0*	19.7 ± 0.4	23.6 ± 0.4*
Rabbit	0.111 ± 0.01	0.055 ± 0.01*	49.6 ± 1.5	20.2 ± 1.9*	21.2 ± 3.4	7.9 ± 1.1*
			15 days			
Rat	0.326 ± 0.02	0.537 ± 0.37*	55.8 ± 4.0	81.9 ± 9.0*	25.8 ± 2.3	19.3 ± 0.4*
Mouse	0.405 ± 0.03	0.528 ± 0.04*	61.1 ± 1.5	68.6 ± 1.8*	26.5 ± 2.6	17.9 ± 2.3*
G. pig	0.138 ± 0.02	0.060 ± 0.01*	51.9 ± 2.6	30.1 ± 1.8*	26.1 ± 1.8	20.3 ± 0.5*
Rabbit	—	—	—	—	—	—

*$p < 0.05$ when compared with control.
None of the rabbits survived 15 days treatment.
[a]nmole HCHO formed/min/mg protein; [b]pmole p-aminophenol formed/min/mg protein; [c]pmole 3-OH benzo (a) pyrene formed/min/mg protein.

or aminopyrine N-demethylase while a derease in that of arylhydrocarbon hydroxylase when the DEPH exposure was continued for 15 days suggests not only the involvement of multiple forms of P450 in the metabolism of DEHP but also the differences in the sensitivity of these different forms of P450 towards DEHP [77, 80, 81].

Significant differences in the interaction of DEHP with the hepatic P450 monooxygenases in different age group of animals (Table 3) and amongst different animal species (Table 4) further provides evidence for the involvement of multiple forms of P450s in the metabolism of DEHP [77, 80, 81, 83]. Our studies have indicated that the age related differences in the intraction of DEHP with P450 monooxygenases could be related to the varying contents and form (s) of P450s present in different age group of animals and their relative sensitivity towards the diester and its metabolites [77]. Likewise the inability of some of the animal species (rabbits, guinea pigs and primates) to metabolize DEHP has been attributed to the differences in the interaction of DEHP with P450 monooxynases, which are known to exist in different isoenzymic forms amongst the different animal species [80]. Our studies exhibiting species specific effect of DEHP on P450 monooxygenases in rats, mice guinea pigs and rabbits suggested differences in the sensitivity of these P450s towards DEHP and its metabolites [80].

Studies aimed to identify the specific P450 isozymes involved in the metabolism of DEHP have shown that P450 4A1 isoenzyme, associated with ω-and ω-1 hydroxylation of fatty acids, preferentially catalyzes the hydroxylation of MEHP, the hydrolytic product of DEHP [62–65, 82–84]. Immunochemical studies with specific antibodies have shown that P450 4A1 is elevated 5–10 fold in the liver of rats treated with DEHP [62, 82–84]. Transcriptional activation of the P450 4A1 gene has also been reported which closely parallels the increases in P450 4A1 protein and enzymatic activity for the ω-hydroxylation of lauric acid. *In vitro* studies utilizing rat hepatocytes cultures have shown that both MEHP and ω-1 oxidation product, mono(2-ethyl-5-oxohexyl) phthalate (metabolite VI) produced a dose related increase in the activity of lauric acid hydroxylase (LAH). Whereas the ω-carbon oxidation products, mono(5-carboxy-2-ethylpentyl)phthalate (metabolite V) and mono (3-carboxy-2-ethylpropyl) phthalate (metabolite I) failed to produce such effects except at very high concentrations [16]. Similar structure-activity relationship has been observed with peroxisome proliferation as well. Interestingly, the inability of DEHP to interact with P450 4A1 in animal species which do not show any evidence of peroxisome proliferation such as guinea pigs, marmosets and humans suggest that P450 enzyme system maybe involved in the process of peroxisome proliferation [16, 62]. Studies by Albro [10, 11] have suggested that MEHP, the hydrolytic product of DEHP is treated as a fatty acid, which initially cannot be oxidized by peroxisomes, so is subjected to ω and ω-1 oxidation by P450 4A1, followed by β-oxidation in liver peroxisomes. Recent studies have infact shown that the induction of P450 4A1 by peroxisome proliferators is the primary hepatic response resulting in an increase of cellular ω-hydroxy fatty acids, which undergo further ω-oxidation in liver peroxisomes [16, 61, 62].

Hepatocarcinogenicity of PAEs

Long term exposure of DEHP to rodents has been shown to cause cancer of the liver in both rats and mice [6, 85–88]. The plasticizer was found to produce increased incidence of hepatocellular neoplasms in both sexes of Fischer 344 (F344) rats and B6C3F1 mice [6, 85–88]. Porliferation of the preneoplastic nodules was also observed in the liver of the rats even when no carcinomas were present. As a result of these studies, DEHP has been classified in EPA Group B2 (probable human carcinogen) for male and female mice and rats [88]. The U.S. Department of Health and Human Services suggests that it is reasonable to consider DEHP as a carcinogen [88] and IARC classifies this compound as a 2B, a possible carcinogen [88].

Even though the exact mechanism by which DEHP acts as a carcinogen are not fully understood, the current available evidences have hypothesized that peroxisome proliferation and hyperplasia as the two main events related to carcinogenicity of DEHP [61, 88]. Though there are indirect evidence relating peroxisome proliferation to carcinogenesis, absence of a clear increase in hepatic peroxide concentrations and its interaction with cellular biomolecules and because hyperplasia consistently accompanies peroxisome proliferation, it has been proposed that carcinogenesis induced by DEHP is result of the initiation of cell division by exposure to DEHP [22, 87, 88]. Exposure to DEHP is known to cause almost immediate increase in cell division in rats and mice as indicated by a significant increase in DNA synthesis in rat and mice liver [88].

Conclusion

Phthalic acid esters (PAEs), commonly used as plasticizers to impart flexibility to polyvinyl chloride (PVC) plastics are known to leach out from the finished plastic products into the materials stored in them and subsequently enter in human beings. Acute and chronic exposure to di(2-ethylhexyl) phthalate (DEHP), one of the most widely used plasticizer, produces marked changes in the hepatic function as judged by an increase in liver weight, and morphological and biochemical changes. PAEs, in general are found to inhibit mitochondrial respiration in rodent liver. A decrease in circulating cholesterol and triglycerides is also associated with DEHP exposure. DEHP has also been shown to inhibit both glycogenesis and glycogenolysis. These changes in lipid and carbohydrate metabolism following DEHP exposure are found to be associated with the proliferation of peroxisomes in rodent liver. An increase in hepatic peroxisomes is considered to be a marker of

DEHP exposure in rodents. DEHP has been further shown to modify the biological response of drugs and other xenobiotics. Such interactions appear to occur at the pharmacokinetic phase as DEHP is shown to alter the activity of the microsomal cytochrome P450 (P450) enzymes in liver. Not all the animal species and animals of different ages were equally susceptible to DEHP. The inability of DEHP to interact with P450 in animal species which do not show any evidence of peroxisome proliferation suggests that P450 enzyme induction and peroxisome proliferation maybe closely linked which may determine the hepatic response to DEHP.

References

1. Jaeger, R.J. and Rubin, R.J. Migration of a phthalate ester plasticizer from polyvinyl chloride blood bags into stored human blood and its localization in human tissues. N. Engl. J. Med. **287**, 1114, 1972.
2. Jaeger, R.J. and Rubin, R.J. Di(2-ethylhexyl) phthalate, a plasticizer contaminant of platelet concentrates. Transfusion **13**, 107, 1973.
3. Pollack, G.K., Buchanan, J.F., Kohli, R.K. and Shen, D.D. Circulating concentrations of di(2-ethyhexyl)phthalate and its deesterified phthalic acid products following exposure in patients receiving hemodialysis. Toxicol. Appl. Pharmacol. **79**, 257, 1985.
4. Peakall, D.B. Phthalate esters: Occurence and biological effects. Residue Rev. **54**, 1, 1975.
5. Metcalf, R.L., Booth, G.M., Schuth, C.K., Hansen, J.J. and Lu, P.Y. Uptake and fate of DEHP in aquatic organisms and in a model ecosystem. Environ. Health Perspect. **4**, 27, 1973.
6. Thomas, J.A. and Thomas, M.J. Biological effects of DEHP and other phthalic acid esters. CRC Crit. Rev. Toxicol. **13**, 283, 1984.
7. Stein, M.S., Cassi, P.I. and Nair, P.P. Influence of dietary lipids in rats. J. Nutr. **104**, 187, 1973.
8. Lake, B.G., Phillips, J.C., Linnell, J.C and Gangolli, S.D. The *in vitro* hydrolysis of some phthalate diesters by hepatic and intestinal preparations from various species. Toxicol. Appl. Pharmacol. **39**, 239, 1977.
9. Carpenter, D., Weil, C.S. and Smyth, H.F. Jr. Chronic oral toxicity of DEHP for rats, guinea pigs and dogs. AMA Arch. Ind. Hyg. Occup. Med. **8**, 219, 1953.
10. Albro, P.W., Hass, J.R., Peack, C.C., Odam, D.G., Corbett, J.T., Bailey, F.J., Blatt, H.E. and Barrett, B.B. Identification of the metabolites of DEHP in urine from the African green monkey. Drug Metab. Dispos. **9**, 23, 1981.
11. Albro, P.W. Absorption, metabolism and excretion of DEHP by rats and mice. Environ. Health Perspect. **65**, 293, 1986.
12. William, D.T. and Blanchfield, B.J. Retention, excretion metabolism of DEHP administered orally to the rat. Bull. Environ. Contam. Toxicol. **11**, 371, 1974.
13. Daniel, J.W. and Bratt, H. The absorption, metabolism and tissue distribution of DEHP in rats. Toxicol. **2**, 51, 1974.
14. Albro, P.W and Thomas, R.O. Enzymatic hydrolysis of DEHP by lipases. Biochem. Biophys. Acta **206**, 308, 1973.
15. Albro, P.W and Moore, B. Identification of the metabolites of simple phthalate diesters in rat urine. J. Chromatogr. **94**, 209, 1974.

16. Lhuguenot, J.C., Mitchell, A.M, Milner, G, Lock, E.A and Elcombe, C.R. The metabolism of DEHP and MEHP in rats: *in vivo* and *in vitro* dose and time dependency of metabolism. Toxicol. Appl. Pharmacol. **80**, 11, 1985.

17. Autian, J. Toxicity and health threats of phthalate esters: review of the literature. Environ. Health Perspect. **4**, 3, 1973.

18. Autian, J. Antifertility and dominant lethal assays for mutagenic effects of DEHP. Environ. Helth Perspect. **45**, 115, 1982.

19. Seth, P.K. Hepatic effects of phthalate esters. Environ. Helath Perspect. **45**, 27, 1982.

20. Gray, T.J.B., Butterworth, K.R., Gaunt, I.F., Grasso, P and Gangolli, S.D. Short term toxicity study of DEHP in rats. Fd. Cosmetic Toxicol. **15**. 389, 1977.

21. Nikonorow, M., Mazur, H and Peikacz, H. Effect of orally administered plasticizers and polyvinyl chloride stabilizers in the rat. Toxicol. Appl. Pharmacol. **26**, 253, 1973.

22. Smith-Oliver, T and Butterworth, B.E. Corelation of the carcinogenic potential of DEHP with induced hyperplasia rather than with genotoxic activity. Mutat. Res. **188**, 21, 1987.

23. Busser, M.T and Lutz, W.K. Stimulation of DNA synthesis in rat and mouse liver by various tumor promoters. Carcinogenesis **8**, 1433,1987.

24. Mitchell, F.E., Price, S.C., Hinton, R.H., Grasso, P and Bridges, J.W. Time and dose response study of the effect on rats of the plasticizer, DEHP. Toxicol. Appl. Pharmacol. **81**, 371, 1985.

25. Murakami, K., Nichiyama, K and Higuti, T. Mitochondrial effect of orally administered dibutyl phthalate in rats. Jap. J. Hyg. **41**, 796, 1986.

26. Nazir, D.J., Alcarza, A.P., Bierl, B.A., Beroza, M and Nair, P.O. Isolation, identification and specific localization of DEHP in bovine heart muscle mitochondria. Biochem. **10**, 4428, 1971.

27. Dostal, L.A., Jenkins, W.L and Schwetz, B.A. Hepatic peroxisome proliferation and hypolipidemic effects of DEHP in neonatal and adult rats. Toxicol Appl. Pharmacol. **87**, 81, 1987.

28. Reddy, J.K., Mody, D.E., Azarnoff, D.L and Rao, M.S. DEHP, an industrial plasticizer induces hypolipidemia and enhances hepatic catalase and carnitine acetyltransferase activities in rats and mice. Life Sciences **18**, 94, 1976.

29. Yangita, T., Kobayashi, K. and Enomoto, N. Accumulation of hepatic phospholipids in rats fed DEHP. Biochem. Pharmacol. **27**, 2283, 1978.

30. Yangita, Y., Kuzuhara, S., Enomoto, N., Shimada, T and Sugano, M. Effects of DEHP on the content and composition of hepatic mitochondrial and microsomal phospholipids in the rat. Biochem. Pharmacol. **28**, 3115, 1979.

31. Rhodes, C., Orton, T.C., Pratt, I.S., Batten, P.L., Bratt, H., Jackson, S.J and Elcombe, C.R. Comparative pharmacokinetics and subacute toxicity of DEHP in rats and marmosets: Extrapolation of effects in rodents to man. Environ. Health Perspect. **65**, 299, 1986.

32. Bell, F.P., Makowski, M., Schneider, D and Patt, C.S. Inhibition of steroidogenesis in brain and liver of fetal and suckling rats from dams fed DEHP, plasticizer. Lipids **14**, 372, 1979.

33. Bell, F.P. Effects of phthalate esters on lipid metabolism in various tissues, cells and organelles in mammals. Environ. Health Perspect. **45**, 41, 1982.

34. Bell, F.P., Patt, C.S., Brundage, B., Gillies, P.J. and Phillips, W.A. Studies on lipid biosynthesis and cholesterol content of liver and serum lipoproteins in rats fed various phthalate esters. Lipids **13**, 66, 1978.

35. Nai, N and Kurup, C.K. Increase in hepatic ubiquinone on administration of DEHP to the rat. J. Biosc. **11**, 391, 1987.

36. Srivastava, S.P., Agrawal, D.K. and Seth, P.K. Effect of DEHP on activity of succinic dehydrogenase and adenosine triphosphatase of some vital organs of rat. Toxicology, **7**, 163, 1977.

37. Lake, B.G., Branton, P.G., Gangolli, S.D. Butterworth, K.R. and Grasso, P. Studies on hepatic effects of orally administered DEHP in the ferret. Toxicology, **6**, 314, 1976.

38. Sakurai, T., Miyazawa, S. and Hashimoto, T. Effects of DEHP administration on carbohydrate and fatty acid metabolism in rat liver. J. Biochem. (Tokyo), **83**, 313, 1978.

39. Gebracht, U., Eining. C., Oesterle, D., Deml, E., Schlatterer, B and Eigenbrodt, E. DEHP alters carbohydrate enzyme activities and incidence in rat liver. Carcinogenesis, **11**, 2111, 1990.

40. Mushtaq, M., Srivastava, S.P. and Seth, P.K. Effect of DEHP on glycogen metabolism in rat liver. Toxicology, **16**, 153, 1980.

41. Mann, A.H., Price, S.C., Mitchell, F.E., Grasso, P., Hinton, R.H. and Bridges, J.W. Comparison of the short term effects of DEHP, DHP and di-n-octyl phthalate in rats. Toxicol. Appl. Pharmacol., **77**, 116, 1985.

42. Takahashi, T. Biochemical studies on phthalate esters. II. Effects of phthalate esters on mitochondrial respiration of rat liver. Biochem. Pharmacol., **26**, 19, 1977.

43. Ohyama, T. Effects of phthalate esters on respiration of rat liver mitochondria. J. Biochem., 79, 153, 1976.

44. Inouye, B., Ogino, Y., Ishida, T., Ogata, M. and Utsumi, K. Effects of phthalate esters on mitochondrial oxidative phosphorylation in the rat. Toxicol. Appl. Pharmacol., **43**, 189, 1978.

45. Srivastava, S.P., Agrawal, D.K., Mushtaq, M. and Seth, P.K. Effect of DEHP on chemical constituents and enzymatic activity of rat liver. Toxicology, **11**, 271, 1978.

46. Reddy, J.K., Azarnoff, D.L. and Hignete, C.E. Hypolipidemic hepatic proliferators form a novel class of chemical carcinogens. Nature (London), **283**, 397, 1980.

47. Moody, D.E. and Reddy, J.K. Hepatic peroxisome (microbody) proliferation in rats fed plasticizers and related compounds Toxicol. Appl. Pharmacol., **45**, 497, 1978.

48. Reddy, J.K. and Rao, M.S. Peroxisome proliferators and cancer mechanisms and implications. Trends Pharmacol. Sci., **7**, 438, 1986.

49. Reddy J.K. and Lalwani, N.D. Carcinogenesis by hepatic peroxisome proliferators: evalution of the risk of hypolipidaemic drugs and industrial plasticizers to humans. CRC Crit. Rev. Toxicol., **12**, 1, 1983.

50. Warren, J.R., Simmon, V.F. and Reddy, J.K. Properties of peroxisome proliferators in the lymphocyte 3H-thymidine and salmonella mutagenesis assay. Cancer Res., **40**, 36, 1980.

51. Inestrosa, N.C., Bronfman, M. and Leighton, F. Detection of peroxisomal fatty acyl-coenzyme A oxidase activity. Biochem. J., **182**, 779, 1979.

52. Osumi, T. and Hashimoto, T. Enhancement of fatty acyl-CoA oxidising activity in rat liver peroxisomes by DEHP. J. Biochem., **83**, 1361, 1978.

53. Lalwani, N.D., Reddy, M.K. M-Mark. M. and Reddy, J.K. Induction, immunochemical identity and immunofluorescence localization of peroxisome proliferation associated polypeptide (PPA-80) and peroxisomal enoyl CoA hydratase of mouse liver and renal cortex. Biochem . J., **198**, 177, 1981.

54. Reddy, J.K., Reddy, M.K., Usman, M.I., Lalwani, N.D. and Rao, M.S. Comparison of hepatic peroxisome proliferative effect and its implication for hepatocarcinogenicity of phthalate esters, DEHP and DEHA with a hypolipidaemic drug. Environ. Health. Prespect., **65**, 315, 1986.

55. Reddy, J.K., Goel, S.K., Nemali, M.R., Carcino, J.J., Laffler, T.G., Reddy, M.K., Serbeck, S.J., Osumi, T., Hashimoto, T., Lalwani, N.D and Rao, M.S. Transcriptional regulations of peroxisomal fatty acyl-CoA oxidase and enoyl-CoA hydratase/3-hydroxyacyl CoA dehydrogenase in rat liver by peroxisome proliferators. Proc. Natl. Acad. Sci., USA, **83**, 1747, 1986.

56. Gray, T.J.B., Beamand, J.A., Lake, B.G., Foster, J.R. and Gangolli, S.D. Peroxisome proliferation in cultured rat hepatocytes produced by clofilorate and phthalate ester metabolites. Toxicol. Lett., **10**, 273. 1982.

57. Mitchell, A.M., Lhuguenot, J.C., Bridges, J.W. and Elcombe, C.R. Indentification of the proximate peroxisome proliferators(s) derived from DEHP. Toxicol. Appl. Pharmacol., **80**, 23, 1985.

58. Elcombe C.R and Mitchell, A.M. Peroxisome proliferation due to DEHP: Species differences and possible mechanisms. Environ. Health Persect. **70**, 211, 1986.

59. Lake, B.G., Gry, T.J.B., Foster, J.R., Stubberfield, C.R and Gangolli, S.D. Comparative studies on DEHP induced hepatic peroxisome proliferation in rat and hamster. Toxicol. Appl. Pharmacol. **72**, 46, 1984.

60. Gray, T.J.B., Lake, B.G., Beamand, J.A., Foster, J.R and Gangolli, S.D. Peroxisome proliferation in primary cultures of rat hepatocytes. Toxicol. Appl. Pharmacol. **67**, 15, 1983.

61. Mitchell, A.M., Bridges, J.W and Elcombe C.R Factors influencing peroxisome proliferation in cultured rat hepatocytes. Arch. Toxicol. **55**. 239, 1986.

62. Loke, E.A., Mitchell A.M and Elcombe, C.R. Biochemical mechanisms of induction of hepatic peroxisome proliferation. Ann. Rev. Pharmacol. Toxicol. **29**, 145, 1989.

63. Lake, B.G., Gray, T.J.B., Pels Rijcken, W.R., Beamand, J.A and Gangolli, S.D. The effect of hypolipidaemic agents on peroxisomal β-oxidation and mixed function oxidase activities in primary cultures of rat hepatocytes. Relationship between inducion of palmitoyl-CoA oxidation and lauric acid hydroxylation. Xenobiotica **14**, 269, 1984.

64. Halvorsen, O. Effects of hypolipidaemic drugs on hepatic CoA. Biochem. Pharmacol. **32**, 1126, 1983.

65. Miyazawa, F.S., Furuta, S and Hashimoto, T. Induction of a novel long chain acyl-CoA hydrolase in liver by administration of peroxisome proliferators. Eur. J. Biochem. **117**, 425, 1981.

66. Rubin, R.J. and Jaeger, R.J. Some pharmacologic and toxicologic effects of di(2-ethylhexyl) phthlate and other plasticizers. Enviran. Health Perspect. **3**, 53, 1973.

67. Seth, P.K., Srivastava, S.P., Agrawal, D.K and Mushtaq, M. Interaction of di(2-ethylhexyl)phthalate with pentobarbitone and methaqualone. Bull. Environ. Contam. Toxicol. **6**, 723, 1977.

68. Lawrence, W.H., Malik, M., Turner, J.E., Singh, A.R and Autian, J.A. A toxicological investigation of some acute short term and chronic effects of administering di(2-ethylhexyl) phthalate and other phthalates. Environ. Res. **9**, 1, 1975.

69. Srivastava, S.P., Agrawal, D.K., Mushtaq, M. and Seth, P.K. Interaction of di(2-ethylhexyl) phthalate with parathion in rats. Chemosphere **5**, 177, 1979.

70. Seth, P.K., Srivastava, S.P., Mushtaq, M., Agrawal, D.K and Chandra, S.V. Effect of di(2-ethylhexyl)phthalate on rat liver injured by chronic carbon tetrachloride treatment. Acta Pharmacol. Toxicol. **44**, 161, 1979.

71. Tomaszweski, K.E., Montogomery, C.A and Melnick, R.L. Modulation of 2, 3, 7, 8-tetrachlorodibenzo-p-dioxin toxicity in F344 rats by DEHP. Chem. Biol. Interact. **65**, 205, 1988.

72. Sager, G and Little, C. The effect of the plasticizers, TBEP, tris 2-butoxyethylphosphate and DEHP on beta-adrenergic ligand binding to alpha-1-acid glycoprotein and mononuclear leukocytes. Biochem. Pharmacol. **38**, 2551, 1989.

73. Perera, M.I., Katyal, S.L and Shinozuka, H. Suppression of choline deficient diet induced hepatocyte membrane lipid peroxidation in rats by the peroxisome proliferators 4-chloro-6-(2,3-xylidino)-2-pyrimidinylthio (N-betahydroxyethyl) acetamide and DEHP. Cancer Res. **46**, 3304, 1986.

74. Okita, R and Chance, C. Induction of laurate w-hydroxylase by DEHP in rat liver microsomes. Biochem. Biophys. Res. Commun. **121**, 304, 1984.

75. Ganning, A.E., Olsson, M.J., Elhammer, A and Dallner, G. The influence of DEHP on protein turnover in rat liver. Toxico. Lett. **48**, 185, 1989.

76. Agrawal, D.K., Agrawal, S and Seth, P.K. Effects of DEHP on drug metabolism, lipid peroxidation and sulphydryl content of rat liver. Drug Metab. Dispos. **10**, 77, 1982.

77. Parmar, D., Srivastava, S.P and Seth, P.K. Age related effects of DEHP on hepatic cytochrome P450 monooxygenases in wistar rat. J. Pharmacol. Toxicol. **75**, 177, 1994.

78. Pollack, G.M., Shen, D.D and Door, M.B. Contribution of metabolites to the route and time dependent hepatic effects of DEHP in the rats. J. Pharmacol. Exp. Ther. **248**, 176, 1989.

79. Pollack, G.M., Li, R.C.K., Ermer, J.C and Shen, D.D. Effect of route of administration and repetitive dosing on the disposition kinetics of DEHP and is mono-de-esterified metabolite in rats. Toxicol. Appl. Pharmacol. **79**, 246, 1985.

80. Parmar, D., Srivastava, S.P and Seth, P.K. Effect of DEHP on hepatic mixed function oxidases in different animal species. Toxicol. Lett. **40**, 209, 1988.

81. Parmar, D., Srivastava, S.P., Srivastava, Sri, P and Seth, P.K. Hepatic mixed function oxidases and cytochrome P450 contents in rat pups exposed to DEHP through mother's milk. Drug Metab. Dispose. **13**, 368, 1985.

82. Sharma, R., Lake, B.G., Foster, J. and Gibson, G.G. Microsomal cytochrome P450 induction and peroxisomal proliferation by hypolipidaemic agents in rat liver. Biochem. Pharmacol. **37**, 1193, 1988.

83. Sharma, R., Lake, B.G and Gibson, G.G. Co-induction of microsomal cytochrome P450 and peroxisomal fatty acid β-oxidation pathway in the rat by clofibrate and DEHP. Biochem. Pharmacol. **37**, 1203, 1988.

84. Bains, S.K., Gardiner, S.M., Mannweler, K., Gillette, D and Gibson, G.G. Immunochemical study on the contribution of hypolipidaemic induced cytochrome P450 to the metabolism of lauric acid and arachidonic acid. Biochem. Pharmacol. **34**, 3221, 1985.

85. Kluwe, W.M., Haseman, J.K., Douglas, J.F and Huff, J.E. The carcinogenicity of dietary DEHP in Fischer 344 rats and B6C3F1 mice. J. Toxicol. Environ. Health **10**, 797, 1982.

86. Melnick, R.L., Morrissey, R.E and Tomaszewki, K.E. Studies by the National Toxicology Program on DEHP. Toxicol. Indust. Health **3**, 99, 1987.

87. Ward, J.M., Hagiwara, A., Anderson, L.M, Lindsey, K and Diwan, B.A. The chronic hepatic and renal toxicity of DEHP, acetaminophen, sodium barbital and PB in male B6C3F1 mice: Autoradiographic, immunohistochemical and biochemical evidence for levels of DNA synthesis not associated with carcinogenesis or tumor promotion. Toxicol. Appl. Pharmacol. **96**, 494, 1988.
88. Toxicological profile for di(2-ethylhexyl) phthalate (DEHP): An update. U.S Department of Health and Human Service, 1992.

Liver and Environmental Xenobiotics
S.V.S. Rana and K. Taketa (Eds)

8. Role of Nitric Oxide (NO) in the D-Galactosamine-Induced Liver Injury

Hironori Sakai, Hidehiko Isobe and Hajime Nawata

Third Department of Internal Medicine Faculty of Medicine,
Kyushu University Fukuoka, 812–82 Japan

Introduction

Nitric oxide (NO), a highly reactive free radical gas, was recently identified as a metabolite of L-arginine formed by the enzyme nitric oxide synthase [1–4]. Due to its lipophilicity, NO can pass easily into the intracellular area and affect cell metabolism. Thus, NO has a number of important biological functions as an intercellular and intracellular messenger [5]. Within the cell, NO activates soluble guanylate cyclase, which leads to an increase in cGMP levels [6]. Through this mechanism, endothelial-derived NO induces relaxation of vascular smooth muscle, vasodilation , and inhibits platelet aggregation and adherence [7–9]. As a vasodilator, it may play an important role in regulating the systemic and regional circulation [10–13]. No also plays a role in signal transduction within the central nervous system [14]. Furthermore, NO has been shown to exert various effects on hepatocytes such as the inhibition of both protein synthesis [15, 16] and mitochondrial respiration [17, 18], and an alteration of cytochrome P-450 enzyme activity [19–21].

While NO is constitutively produced by endothelial cells and cerebellum, hapatocytes and Kupffer cells can produce larger amounts of NO when exposed to endotoxin or cytokines, such as tumor necrosis factor-α (TNF-α) and interleukin-1 (IL-1) [4]. In liver, sinusoidal endothelial cells also release less NO during endotoxin induced inflammation [22]. Many substances, including cytokines, prostaglandins, and vasoactive and procoagulant factors have been shown to be stimulated by endotoxin *in vitro* and *in vivo* and may contribute to the clinical effects of endotoxin. However, the secondary mediator responsible for the pathological effects of endotoxin has not been identified. A number of recent studies have led to the possibility that NO could be one of important secondary mediators of endotoxemia. Therefore, it is important to elucidate the pathophysiological role of NO in liver injury associated with endotoxemia or other systemic inflammatory diseases. On the one hand, recent studies have demonstrated a protective role of NO in experimental models of liver inflammation [23, 24]. On the other, its deleterious effects have also been reported [15–21, 25].

The D-galactosamine is known to be a specific hepatotoxic agent. Administration of GalN in experimental animals leads to liver injury, of which the morphological aspects closely resemble those of human acute viral hepatitis [26]. The early biochemical changes induced by GalN in hepatocytes are characterized by a marked decrease in the uridine phosphate's level. This decrease impairs biosynthesis of RNA and macro–molecular cell constituents, resulting in damage to, and ultimately in the death of, hepatocytes [27]. Recently, several reports have shown that endotoxin and cytokines such as TNF-α play an important role in the development of liver injury in this model [28–32]. Naturally, GalN administration should accelerate the production of NO in the liver.

We designed the experments to deterimine whether inhibition of NO synthesis modulates the GalN-induced liver injury.

Experimental Procedures
Male Wistar WKA strain viral antigen- and pathogen-free rats (body weight 200–250 g) were used. They were allowed rodent laboratory chow and water *ad libitum.*

Measurement of hepatic tissue blood flow: The liver was exposed by laparotomy under sodium pentabarbital (60 mg/kg ip) anesthesia and a platinum electrode (diameter: 80 μm) was inserted into the median lobe. The animal was then ventilated with hydrogen gas. Hepatic tissue blood flow was measured by the hydrogen gas clearance method using MHG-D1 (Unique Medical, Tokyo, Japan) [33].

Measurement of total serum NO_2/NO_3: The serum samples were assayed for the stable and products of NO, NO_2 and NO_3. After the precipitation of protein with sulfosalicylic acid, NO_3 in the sample was reduced to NO_2 with copper-coated cadmium, and then the total NO_2 concentration in the sample was measured using a colorimetric method based on the Griess reaction (1% sulfanilamide, 0.1% naphthylethylenediamine dihydrochloride and 2.5% H_3PO_4) [34].

Effects of arginine derivatives on D-galactosamine induced liver injury: Rats were divided into six groups: (a) saline-treated rats, (b) N^G-nitro-D-arginine methyl ester HCl (D-NAME)-treated rats, (c) N^G-nitro-L-arginine methyl ester HCl (L-NAME)-treated rats, (d) D-galactosamine and saline-treated rats, (e) D-galactosamine and D-NAME-treated rats and (f) D-galactosamine and L-NAME-treated rats. GalN was adjusted to pH 7.4 with NaOH and was injected intraperitoneally at a dose of 1000mg/kg at time 0. Each arginine derivative was injected intraperitoneally at a dose of

40 mg/kg at time 0 and then again every 8 hours for 48 hours. Serum samples were collected before and at 48 hours after the injection of GalN. Hepatic tissue blood flow was also measured at 48 hours after the injection. We determined serum levels of aspartate aminotransferase (AST), alanine aminotrans-ferase (ALT) and total bilirubin. The liver was excised, fixed in 10% formalin and stained with hematoxylin and eosin for routine light microscopic examination.

Results

Effects of arginine derivatives on D-galactosamine-induced liver injury (Fig. 1): Without administration of GalN, there were no significant hepatotoxicites of L-NAME, a specific NO synthesis inhibitor, and D-NAME, an inactive isomer of L-NAME, compared with saline in rats. Administration of GalN (1000 mg/kg) in rats induced liver injury to such an extent that there were significant increases of serum aminotransferase (ALT and AST) levels but no change in serum level of total bilirubin. In rats treated with GalN and L-NAME, serum levels of AST, ALT and total bilirubin were enormously elevated compared with those treated with GalN only or GalN and D-NAME. Histopathologically, necrosis was observed around the central veins and in the subcapsular area of the liver in all groups treated with GalN. Among these three groups, the group treated with GalN and L-NAME showed the most severe hepatic necrosis. Weak portal and parenchymal inflammatory infiltration were observed that were similar in all groups treated with GalN. No arginine derivatives cause significant histological changes by themselves.

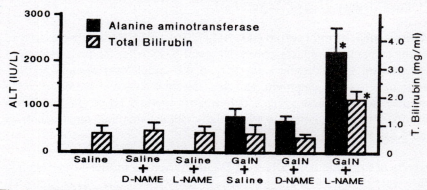

Fig. 1.   Effects of arginine derivatives on D-galactosamine-induced liver injury in rats. Values are the mean ± SD. *$P < 0.05$, significantly different from rats treated with GalN + saline and those with GalN + D -NAME.

Effects of arginine derivatives on hepatic tissue blood flow (Fig. 2): Hepatic tissue blood flow of six groups treated with or without GalN and/ or arginine derivatives are shown in Fig.2. There was no difference in

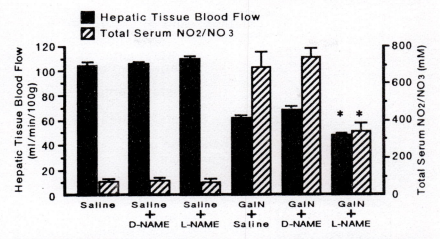

Fig. 2. Effects of galactosamine derivatives on hepatic tissue blood flow and serum NO2/ NO3 level in D-galactosamine-treated rats. Values are the mean ± SD. *$P < 0.05$, significantly different from rats treated with GalN + saline and those with GalN + D–NAME.

hepatic tissue blood flow among three groups without GalN treatment. GalN treatment significantly decreased this flow. Among these groups treated with GalN, hepatic tissue blood flow was significantly reduced in rats treated with L-NAME compared with those treated with D-NAME or saline.

Effects of D-galactosamine and arginine derivatives on No production (Fig. 2):   L-NAME or D-NAME treatment showed no significant changes in serum NO_2/NO_3 level in rats treated without GalN. However, administration of GalN markedly increased serum NO_2/NO_3 concentration at 48 hours after injection. Thought L-NAME administration significantly reduced serum level of NO_2/NO_3 in GalN-treated rats, D-NAME did not.

Discussion

Though the precise mechanism of GalN-induced liver injury has not been completely described, the participation of endotoxin and cytokines such as TNF-α has been shown in this liver injury model [28–32]. The supposed mechanism of this liver injury is shown in Fig. 3. GalN induces some biochemical changes such as depletion of uridine phosphate in hepatocytes and impairment of RNA biosynthesis, and these changes are also considered to play an important role in development of endotoxin hyperreactivity. Moreover, GalN administration causes endotoxemia derived from the gut. In this model, involvement of gut-derived endotoxin may develop the hepatocyte damage because of GalN-induced sensitization to endotoxin [29, 30, 32]. Endotoxin induces Kupffer cells to release a number of mediators including cytokines such as TNF-α and IL-1β, eicosanoids and reactive oxygen intermediates [36]. Endotoxin also increases expression of an inducible

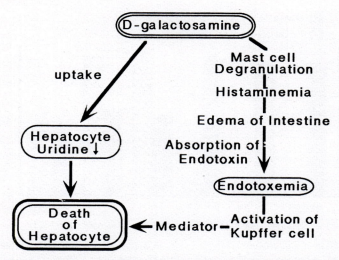

Fig. 3.   Mechanism of D-galactosamine induced liver injury [35].

form of nitric oxide synthase mRNA and protein [4, 37–40]. In the liver, a large amount of NO is produced by Kupffer cells, hepatocytes and sinusoidal endothelial cells during endotoxemia [4, 22, 41]. In the present study, we observed a marked increase of the circulating NO_2/NO_3 level in the GalN-treated rats, which was inhibited by the adminsstration of L-NAME, as expected.

There have been many studies on the vasodilatory effects of NO [10–13]

Among these, several reports showed that NO mediates the vasodilatory effects induced by ATP in the hepatic arterial and portal venous vascular beds of the healthy rabbits [42, 43]. On the other hand, in the pathological state such as liver cirrhosis, there were some reports on the relationship between NO and the systemic circulation, but not the hepatic circulation [44–47]. However, the effect of endogenous NO on hepatic tissue blood flow has not been observed in a model of liver injury. We observed in this study that hepatic tissue blood flow markedly decreased to 60% of control by the treatment with GalN and that the administration of L-NAME, a NO synthesis inhibitor, added the significant reduction of hepatic tissue blood flow in GalN-treated rats. We also found that the intravenous continuous infusion of L-NAME significantly resuced hepatic tissue blood flow in the GalN-treated rats, but not D-NAME, an inactive isomer of L-NAME. Blood flow fell to 78.6% of the base line during the infusion of L-NAME at a dose of 1000µg/kg/min. No significant changes were observed during the infusion of L-NAME in rats treated without GalN (data not shown). These results suggest that endogenous NO regulates the hepatic tissue blood flow in this model.

We demonstrated here an enhancement of GalN-induced hepatotoxicity caused by the additional treatment of L-NAME, probably due to a disturbance in hepatic tissue blood flow. Nishida et al. also reported that NO played a significant role in stabilizing the hepatic microcirculation during endotoxemia [48]. So, we suggest that NO may play an important role in protecting the liver from ischemia and leukocyte-induced oxidative injury by means of keeping hepatic tissue blood flow in GalN -induced liver injury model. However, other mechanisms may also be involved. As NO possesses anti-aggregatory and anti-platelet adhesion properties [7], the inhibition of NO production may promote intravascular coagulation [24, 49], leading to a disturbance of hepatic microcirculation. We have also reported the protective role of NO in dimethylnitrosamine (DMN)-induced liver injury in rats in which DMN destroyed hepatic sinusoidal endothelial cells causing intrasinusoidal coagulation and hepatocyte damage [50]. Since NO may alter the activity of the cytochrome P-450 enzyme system [19–21] and modulate the immune system [51–56], it would also influence the liver injury in this model.

Furthermore, NO reacts with superoxide anion radical and forms peroxynitrite anion, a powerful oxidant, which can be rapidly protonated to yield two highly toxic radicals, hydroxyl radical and nitrogen dioxide[57]. Because of the formation of peroxynitrite, coexistance of NO with superoxide may have the cytotoxic potential. However, Harbrecht et al. reported that NO reduced oxygen radical-mediated liver injury and protected liver damage [24]. There has been some controversy as to whether NO has cytoprotective [58–61] or cytotoxic properties [57, 62, 63] in radical-mediated cellular injury. Further studies should be done to establish the role of NO in various liver injury models.

Acknowledgements
We are grateful to Mr. Philip Stewart for his advice on the manuscript.

References

1. Hibbs, J.B., Jr, Taintor, R.R. and Vavrin, Z. (1987). Macrophage cytotoxicity: Role for L-arginine deiminase and imino nitrogen oxidation to nitrite. Scince 235, 473–476.
2. Sakuma, I., Stuehr, D.J., Gross, S.S., Nathan, C. and Levi, R. (1988). Indentification of arginine as a precursor of endothelium-derived relaxing factor. Proc. Natl. Acad. Sci. USA 85, 8664–8667.
3. Palmer, R.M.J., Ashton, D.S. and Moncada, S. (1988). Vascular endothelial cells synthesize nitric oxide from L-arginine. Nature 333, 664–666.
4. Stuehr, D.J. and Griffith, O.W. (1992). Mammalian nitric oxide synthases, *in Advances in Enzymology, Meister,* F.F., ed. an Interscience Publication, New York, pp. 287–346.
5. Lowenstein, C.J. and Snyder, S.H. (1992). Nitric oxide, a novel biologic messenger. Cell 70, 705–707.
6. Ignarro, L.J. (1991). Signal transduction mechanisms involving nitric oxide. Biochem. Pharmacol. 41, 485-490.

7. Moncada, S., Palmer, R.M.J. and Higgs, A. (1991). Nitric oxide: Physiology, pathophysiology and pharmacology. Pharmacol. Rev. 43, 109–142.

8. Snyder, S.H. and Bredt, D.S. (1992). Biological roles of nitric oxide. Sci. Amer. 266, 28–35.

9. Stark, M.E. and Szurszewski, J.H. (1992). Role of nitric oxide in gastrointestinal and hepatic function and disease. Gastroenterology 103, 1928–1949).

10. Rees, D.D., Palmer, R.M.J. and Moncada, S. (1989). Role of endothelium-derived nitric oxide in the regulation of blood pressure. Proc. Natl. Acad. SCI. USA 86, 3375–3378.

11 Tolins, J.P., Palmer, R.M.J., Moncada, S. and Raij, L. (1990). Role of endothelium-derived relaxing factor in regulation of renal hemodynamic responses. Am. J. Physiol. 258, H655–H662.

12. Kelm, M. and Schrader, J. (1990). Control of coronary vascular tone by nitric oxide. Circ. Res. 66, 1561–1575.

13. Rosenblum, W.I., Nishimura, H. and Nelson, G.H. (1990). Endothelium-dependent L- arg-and L-NMMA-sensitive mechanisms regulate tone of brain microvessels. Am. J. Physiol. 259, H1396–H1401.

14. Garthwaite, J., Charles, S.L. and Chess-Williams, R. (1988). Endothelium-derived relaxing factor release on activation of NMDA receptors suggests role as intercellular messenger in the brain. Nature 336, 385–388.

15. Billiar, T.R., Curran. R.D., Stuehr, F.J., West, M.A., Bentz, B.G. and Simmons, R.L. (1989). An L-arginine-dependent mechanism mediates Kupffer cell inhibition of hepatocyte protein synthesis in vitro. J. Exp. Med. 169, 1467–1472.

16. Curran, R.D., Ferrari, F.K., Kispert, P.H., Stadler, J., Stuehr, D.J., Simmons, R.L. and Billiar, T.R. (1991). Nitric oxide and nitric oxide-generating compounds inhibit hepatocyte protein synthesis. FASEB J. 5, 2085–2092.

17. Stadler, J., Curran, R.D., Ochoa, J.B., Harbrecht, B.G., Hoffman, R. A., Simmons, R.L. and Billiar, T.R. (1991). Effect of endogenous nitric oxide on mitochondrial respiration of rat hepatocytes in vitro and in vivo. Arch. Surg. 126, 186–191.

18. Stadler, J., Billiar, T.R., Curran, R.D., Stuehr,. D.J., Ochoa, J.B. and Simmons, R.L. (1991). Effect of exogenous and endogenous notric oxide on mitochondrial respiration of rat hepatocytes. Am. J. Physiol. 260, C910–916.

19. Tsubaki, M., Hiwatashi, A., Ichikawa, Y., Fujimoto, Y., Ikekawa, N. and Hori. H. (1988). Electron paramagnetic resonance study of ferrous cytochrome P-450_{scc}-nitric oxide complexes: effects of 20 (R), 22 (R)-dihydroxycholesterol and reduced adrenodoxin. Biochemistry 27, 4856–4862.

20. Stadler, J., Trockfeld, J., Schmalix, W.A., Brill, T. and Doehmer, J. (1994). Inhibition of cytochromes P4501A by nitric oxide. Proc. Natl. Acad. Sci. USA 91, 3559–3563.

21. Chamulitrat, W., Jordan, S.J., Mason, R.P., Litton, A.L., Wilson, J. G., Wood, E.R., Wolberg, G. and Vedia, L.M. (1995). Targets of nitric oxide in a mouse model of liver inflammation by corynebacte-rium parvum. Arch. Biochem. Biophy. 316, 30–37.

22. Laskin, D.L., Heck. D.E., Gardner, C.R., Feder, L.S. and Laskin, J.D. (1994). Distinct patterns of nitric oxide production in hepatic macrophages and endothelial cells following acute exposure of rats to endotoxin. J. Leukoc. Biol. 56, 751–758.

23. Billiar, T.R., Curran, R.D., Harbrecht, B.G., Stuehr, D.J., Demetris, A.J. and Simmons, R.L. (1990). Modulation of nitrogen oxide synthesis in vivo: N^G-monomethyl-L-arginine inhibits endo-toxin-induced nitrite/nitrate biosynthesis while promoting hepatic damage. J. Leukoc. Biol. 48, 565–569.

24. Harbrecht, B.G., Billiar, T.R., Stadler, J., Demetris, A.J., Ochoa, J., Curran, R.D. and simmons, R.L. (1992). Inhibition of nitric oxide synthesis during endotoxemia promotes intrahepatic thromobosis and an oxygen radical -mediated hepatic injury. J. Leukoc. Biol. 52, 390–394.

25. Hogg, N., Darley-Usmar, V., Wilson, M. and Moncada, S. (1992). Production of hydroxylradicals from the simultaneous generation of superoxide and nitric oxide. Biochem. J. 281, 419–424.

26. Keppler, D., Lesch, R.W. and Decker, K. (1968). Experimental hepatitis induced by D-galactosamine. Exp. Mol. Pathol. 9, 279–290.

27. Decher, K. and Keppler, D. (1974). Galactosamine hepatitis: Key role of the nucleotide deficiency period in the pathogenesis of cell injury and cell death. Rev. Physiol. Biochem. Pharmacol. 71, 77–106.

28. Grün, M., Liehr, H. and Rasenack, U. (1976). Significance of endo-toxaemia in experimental "galactosamine-hepatitis" in the rat. Acta Hepato-Gastroenterol. 23, 64–81.

29. Freudenberg, M.A., Keppler, D. and Galanos, C. (1986). Requirement for lipopolysaccharide-responsive macrophages in galacto-samine-induced sensitization to endotoxin. Infect. Immun. 51, 891–895.

30. Hishinuma, I., Nagakawa, J., Hirota, K., Miyamoto., K., Tsukidate, K., Yamanaka, T., Katayama, K. and Yamatsu, I. (1990). Involvement of tumor necrosis factor-*a* in development of hepatic injury in galactosamine-sensitized mice. Hepatology 12, 1187–1191.

31. Decker, K. (1993). Mechanisms and mediators in hepatic necrosis. Gastroenterol. Jpn. 28, 20–25.

32. Nagaki, M., Muto, Y., Ohnishi, H., Yasuda, S., Sano K., Naito, T., Maeda, T., Yamada, T. and Moriwaki, H. (1994). Hepatic injury and lethal shock in galactosamine-sensitized mice induced by the superantigen staphylococcal enterotoxin B. Gastroenterology 106, 450–458.

33. Aukland, K., Bower, B.F. and Berliner, R.W. (1964). Measurement of local blood flow with hydrogen gas, Circ. Res. 14, 164–187.

34. Green, L.C., Wagner, D.A., Glogowaski, J., Skipper, P.L., Wishnok, J.S. and Tannenbaum, S.R. (1982). Analysis of nitrate, nitrite and (^{15}N) nitrate in biological fluids. Anal. Biochem. 126, 131–138.

35. Shiratori, Y. and Komatsu, H. (1994). Galactosamine hepatitis. Kan. Tan. Sui. 29, 917–923. (Japanese)

36. Decker, K. (1990). Biologically active products of stimulated liver macrophages (Kupffer cells). Eur. J. Biochem. 192, 245–261.

37. Luss, H., DiSilvio, M., Litton, A.L., Vedia, L. M., Nussler, A.K. and Billiar, T.R. (1994). Inhibition of nitric oxide synthesis enhances the expression of inducible nitric oxide synthesis enhances the expression of inducible nitric oxide synthase mRNA and protein in a model of chronic liver in flammation. Biochem. Biophys. Res. Commun. 204, 635–640.

38. Buttery. L.D.K., Evans, T.J., Springall, D.R., Carpenter, A., Cohen, J. and Polak, J.M. (1994). Immunochemical localization of infucible nitric oxide synthase in endotoxin-treated rats. Lab. Invest. 71, 755–764.

39. Sato, K., Miyakawa, K., Takeya, M., Hattori, R. Yui, Y., Sunanoto, M., Ichimori, Y., Ushio, Y. and Takahashi, K. (1995). Immunohistochemical expression of inducible nitric oxide synthase (iNOS) in reversible endotoxic shock studied by a novel monoclonal antibody against rat iNOS. J. Leukoc. Biol. 57, 36–44.

40. Laskin, D.L., Valle, M.R., Hech, D.E., Hwang, S., Onishi, S.T., Durham, S.K., Goller, N.L. and Laskin, J.D. (1995). Hepatic nitric oxide production following

acute endotoxemia in rats is mediated by increased inducible nitric oxide synthase gene expression. Hepatology 22, 223–234.

41. Curran, R.D., Billiar, T.R., Steuhar, D.J., Hofmann, K. and Simmons, R.L. (1989). Hepatocytes produce nitrogen oxides from L–arginine in response to inflammatory products from kupffer cells. J. Exp. Med. 170, 1769–1774.

42. Mathie. R.T., Ralevic, V., Alexander, B. and Burnstock, G. (1991). Nitric oxide is the mediator of ATP-induced dilatation of the rabbit hepatic arterial vascular bed. Br. J. Pharmacol. 103, 1602.–1602.

43. Browse, D.J., Mathie, R.T., Benjamin, I.S. and Alexander, B. (1994). The transhepatic action of ATP on the hepatic arterial and portal venous vascular beds of the rabbit: the role of nitric oxide. Br. J. Pharmacol.. 113, 987–993.

44. Vallance, P. and Moncada, S. (1991). Hyperdynamic circulation in cirrhosis: a role for nitric oxide? Lancet 337, 776–778.

45. Atucha, N.M., García-Estañ, J., Ramírez, A., Pérez, M.D.C., Quesada, T. and Romero, J.C. (1994). Renal effects of nitric oxide synthesis inhibition on cirrhotic rats. Am. J. Physiol. 267, R1454–R1460.

46. Ros. J., Jiménez, W., Lamas, S., Claria, J., Arroyo, V., Rivera, F, and Rodés, J. (1995). Nitric oxide production in arterial vessels of cirrhotic rats. Hepatology 21, 554–560.

47. Niederberger, M., Gines, P., Tsai, .P., Martin, P., Morris, K., Weigert, A., McMurtry, I. and Schrier, R.W., (1995). Increased aortic cyclic guanosine monophosphate concentration in experimental cirrhosis is rats: evidence for a role of nitric oxide in the pathogenesis of arterial vasodilation in cirrhosis. Hepatology 21, 1625–1631.

48. Nishida, J., McCuskey, R.S., McDonnell, D. and Fox, E.S. (1994). Protective role of NO in hepatic microcirculatory dysfunction during endotoxemia. Am. J. Physiol. 267, G1135–G1141.

49. Shultz, P.J. and Raij, L. (1992). Endogenously synthesized nitric oxide prevents endotoxin-induced glomerular thrombosis. J.Clin. Invest. 90, 1718–1725.

50. Nagase, S., Isobe, H., Ayukawa, K., Sakai, H. and Nawata, H. (1995). Inhibition of nitric oxide production increases dimethyl-nitrosamine-induced liver injury in rats. J. Hepatol. 23, 601–604.

51. Hibbs, J.B., Taintor, R.R., Vavrin, Z. and Rachlin, E.M. (1988). Nitric oxide: a cytotoxic activated macrophage effector molecule. Biochem. Biophys. Res. Commun. 157, 87–94.

52. Park, K.G.M., Hayes, P.D., Garlick, P.J., Sewel, H. and Eremin, O. (1991). Stimulation of lymphocyte natural cytotoxicity by L-arginine. Lancet 337, 645–646.

53. Lander, H.M., Sehajpal, P., Levine, D.M. and Novogrodsky, A. (1993). Activation of human peripheral blood mononuclear cells by nitric oxide-generating comounds. J. Immunol. 150, 1509–1516.

54. Gregory, S.H., Wing, E.J., Hoffman, R.A. and Simmons, R.L.(1993). Reactive nitrogen intermediates suppress the primary immunologic response to listeria. J. Immunol. 150, 2901–2909.

55. Holt, P.G., Oliver, J., Bilyk, N., Mcmenamin, C., McMenamin, P.G., Kraal, G. and Thepen, T. (1993). Downregulation of the antigen presenting cell function (s) of pulmonary dendritic cells in vivo by resident alveolar macrophages. J. Exp. Med. 177, 397–407.

56. Stadler , J., Harbrecht, B.G., Silvio, M.D., Curran, R.D., Jordan, M. L., Simmons, R.L. and Billiar, T.R. (1993). Endogenous nitric oxide inhibits the synthesis of cyclooxygenase products and interleukin-6 by rat Kupffer cells. J. Leukoc. Biol. 53, 165–172.

57. Beckman, J.S., Beckman, T.W., Chen, J., Marshall, P.A. and Freeman B.A. (1990). Apparent hydroxyl radical production by peroxynitrite: implications for endothelial injury from nitric oxide and superoxide. Proc. Natl. Acad. Sci. USA 87, 1620–1624.
58. Kanner, J., Harel, S. and granit, R. (1991). Nitric oxide as an antioxidant. Arch. Biochem. Biophys. 289, 130–136.
59. Wink, D.A., Hanbauer, I., Krishna, M.C., DeGraff, W., Gamson, J. and Mitchell J.B. (1993). Nitric oxide protects against cellular damage and cytotoxicity from reactive oxygen species. Proc. Natl. Acad. Sci. USA 90, 9813–9817.
60. Kuo, P.C. and Abe, K.Y. (1995). Interleukin 1-induced production of nitric oxide inhibits benzenetriol-mediated oxidative injury in rat hepatocytes. Gastroenterology, 109, 206–261.
61. Wink, D.A., Cook, J.A., Krishna, M.C., Hanbauer, I., DeGraff, W., Gamson, J. and Mitchell, J.B. (1995). Nitric oxide protects against alkyl peroxide-mediated cytotoxicity: further insights into the role nitric oxide plays in oxidative stress. Arch. Biochem. Biophys. 319, 402–407.
62. Radi, R., Beckman, J.S., Bush, K.M. and Freeman, B.A. (1991). Per-oxynitrite-induced membrane lipid peroxidation: the cytotoxic potential superoxide and nitric oxide. Arch. Biochem. Biophys. 288, 481–487.
63. Ma, T.T., Ischiropoulos, H. and Brass, C.A. (1995). Endotoxin-stimulated nitric oxide production increases injury and reduces rat liver chemiluminescence during reperfusion. Gastroenterology 108, 463, 469.

Liver and Environmental Xenobiotics
S.V.S. Rana and K. Taketa (Eds)
Copyright © 1997, Narosa Publishing House, New Delhi, India

9. Generation of Reactive Oxygen Species, DNA Damage and Lipid Peroxidation in Liver by Structurally Dissimilar Pesticides

S.J. Stohs, D. Bagchi, M. Bagchi and E.A. Hassoun

Department of Pharmaceutical and Administrative Sciences, Creighton University
2500 California Plaza, Omaha NE 68178

Introduction

The structurally dissimilar polyhalogenated cyclic hydrocarbons (PCH), chlorinated acetamide herbicides (CAH) and organophosphate insecticides (OPS) are classified as pesticides or contaminants of pesticides, and/or environmental pollutants. PCH such as endrin and chlordane, and CAH such as alachlor are halogenated and lipophilic [1–3], while OPS as fenthion and chlorpyrifos are organic triesters of phosphoric acid and phosphorothioic acid and are also lipophilic and highly toxic [3].

Exposure of animals to these structurally diverse xenobiotics elicits a number of similar effects, including the lipid mobilization, porphyria, hypothyroidism, an increased liver to body weight ratio, and progressive weight loss with hypophagia [3–6]. Another common biological property of PCH is their ability to induce microsomal drug metabolizing enzymes [7]. Alachlor-induced mutagenicity and DNA damage and development of nasal tumors are well documented [8–10].

Recent findings in our laboratories [11, 12] indicate that the toxic manifestations induced by PCH may be associated with the enhanced production of reactive oxygen species, which provides an explanation for the multiple types of toxic responses as well as the characteristic wasting syndrome. Reactive oxygen species may serve as common mediators in programmed cell death (apoptosis) in response to many toxicants and pathological conditions [13]. OPS as phosphamidon, trichlorofon and dichlorvos have been reported to induce oxidative stress, both *in vivo* and in hepatocytes, as shown by inhibition of SOD activity, enhanced malondialdehyde production, lactate dehydrogenase leakage, and a decrease in glutathione peroxidase activity [14-16]. CAH as alachlor induce enhanced excretion of urinary lipid metabolies including malondialdehyde, formaldehyde, acetaldehyde and acetone [17]. The increase in excretion of these urinary products may be due to a combination of increased lipid metabolism and peroxidation induced by alachlor [17]. Ample evidence supports the hypothesis that oxygen free radicals mediate cell injury and lead to tumor promotion and carcinogenesis [18], and most of these xenobiotics have been implicated in tumor formation [19–21].

The comparative abilities of PCH as endrin and chlordane, CAH as alachlor, and OPS as chlorpyrifos and fenthion to produce reactive oxygen species with subsequent tissue damage were assessed by chemiluminescence, lipid peroxidation and DNA-single strand breaks (DNA-SSB).

Materials and Methods

Chemicals
Endrin, chlordane, chlorpyrifos and fenthion were obtained from Supelco (Bellefonte, PA). Alachlor was a generous gift from Monsanto (St. Louis, MO). All other chemicals and solvents used in this study were obtained from Sigma Chemical Company (St. Louis, Mo) and were of analytical grade or the highest grade available.

Animals and Treatment
Female Sprague-Dawley rats (160–180 g) were purchased from Sasco, Inc. (Omaha, NE). All animals were housed two per cage and allowed to acclimate to the environment for four to five days prior to experimental use. The animals were allowed free access to tap water and food (Purina Rodent Lab Chow # 5001). The rats were maintained at a temperature of 21°C with lighting from 6 a.m. to 6 p.m. daily. Group of rats were treated orally with endrin, chlordane, alachlor, chlorpyrifos and fenthion in two equal doses (0.25 LD_{50}) of 2.25, 60, 300, 41 and 54 mg/kg body weight, respectively, in corn oil at 0 hr and 21 hr. Control animals received the vehicle. All animals were killed by decapitation at 24 hrs.

Preparation of Liver Homogenates
Livers from control and treated animals were quickly removed and placed in ice cold 50 mM Tris-KCl buffer (pH 7.4) containing 150 mM KCl, 1 mM dithiothreitol, and 10% glycerol. Portions of the livers were homogenized with 5 ml buffer/gm in a Potter Elvehjem homogenizer (Wheaton, Millville, NJ) fitted with a Teflon pestle (four 30 sec strokes). Protein content of the liver homogenates was determined by the standard method of Lowry et al. [22] using bovine serum albumin as the standard.

Portions of the liver samples were placed in an ice cold buffer of White et al. [23] for isolation of hepatic nuclei which were used for the determination of DNA-single strand breaks (SSB). The buffer consisted of 120 mM KCl, 30 mM NaCl, 0.3 mM spermine, 1.0 mM spermidine, 0.25 M sucrose, 4.0 mM ethylenediaminetetraacetic acid tetrasodium salt, 1 mM ethyleneglycol-bis-(β-aminothyl ether) N, N'-tetraacetic acid, 1 mM phenylmethylsulfonyl fluoride, 15 mM 2-mercaptoethanol and 15 mM Tris-HCl (pH 7.4). The livers were homogenized in a loose fitting, all glass Dounce homogenizer at 1 g/4 ml buffer, and centrifuged at 480 × g for 15 min. The nuclear pellets were washed once and resuspended in one-half the original volume of homogenizing buffer used for the whole homogenate.

Lipid Peroxidation

Lipid peroxidation was determined on the hepatic whole homogenates from control and treated animals according to the method of Buege and Aust [24] based on the formation of thiobarbituric acid reactive substances (TBARS). Malondialdehyde was used as the standard and prepared according to the method of Largilliere and Melancon [25]. A molar extinction coefficient of $1.56 \times 10^5 \, M^{-1} \, cm^{-1}$ was used at 535 nm.

Chemiluminescence

Chemiluminescence was measured in Chronolog Lumivette luminometer (Chronolog Corp., Philadelphia, PA). Both *in vitro* and *in vivo* effects of the pesticides were determined on liver whole homogenates. The assays were conducted in 3 ml glass mini-vials. The vials were incubated at 37°C prior to measurement. The background chemiluminescence of each vial was checked before use. Samples containing 1 mg/ml protein were preincubated at 37°C for 30 min. Liver homogenate samples were individually incubated with various concentration of pesticides for the *in vitro* experiments. Concentration of pesticides as low as 0.1 nmole/ml and a concentration as high as 10 nmoles/ml were employed for the *in vitro* experiments. Homogenates from animals that had been treated with various pesticides were also assayed for chemiluminescence. After preincubation of each homogenate, 4 μM luminol was added to enhance chemiluminescence. All additions to the vials as well as chemiluminescence counting procedures were performed under dim lighting conditions. The incubation mixtures were maintained at pH 9 according to the method so Samuni *et al.* [26] in order to obtain maximal chemiluminescence. Results are expressed as counts/unit time minus background [27].

DNA Single Strand Breaks

DNA damage in hepatic nuclei was measured as single strand breaks (SSB) by the alkaline elution method as previously described [23, 28]. Briefly, isolated nuclei (0.1 ml of nuclear homogenate) were lysed on a 5 μm membrane filter (Millipore Corp., Bedford, MA) with a solution containing 2% w/v sodium dodecyl sulfate (SDS) and 25 mM ethylenediaminetetraacetic acid tetrasodium salt (EDTA), pH 10.4, for 20 min. DNA was then eluted with an elution solution containing 0.1% SDS and 20 mM EDTA, adjusted to pH 12.3 with tetraethylammonium hydroxide, at a flow rate of 0.1 ml/

min using a monostat, cassette pump (Fisher, Pittsburgh, PA). Seven 3 ml fractions were collected using an ISCO fraction collector (ISCO Inc., Lincoln, NE). The data from these fractions were used to calculate the elution rate constant, the measure of oxidative DNA damage.

DNA was precipitated from the collected fractions by the addition of 0.1 ml bovine serum albumin solution (2 mg/ml) and 0.1 ml of 40% (w/v) trichloracetic acid. The fractions were then kept in a refrigerator for 2–3 hr, washed once with 3.0 ml ethanol-HCl (36:1 v/v) and allowed to dry overnight. DNA content was measured microfluorometrically (excitation wavelength 436 nm, emission wavelength 521 nm) in a spectrofluorometer (American Instrument Co., Silver Springs, MD) after addition of 3,5-diaminobenzoic acid dihydrochloride as the fluorogen and incubation for 45 min at 60°C. The elution constants (k) were determined by plotting the $\log_{10}$DNA remaining on the filter against the volume of eluate, where $k = -2.3 \times$ slope of this plot.

Statistical Methods

The presence of significant differences between mean groups was determined using analysis of variance (ANOVA) with Scheff's S method as the post-hoc test. Each value is the mean $\pm$ S.D. from 4-6 experiments. The level of statistical significance employed in all cases was $P < 0.05$.

Results

The results of chemiluminescence assay for the production of reactive oxygen species in liver homogenates, prepared from untreated rats, by the pesticides are presented in Fig. 1. Maximum increases in chemiluminescence response occurred within 4-7 min of incubation and persisted for over 10 min. Increases of 3.0-, 2.7-, 3.6-, 4.9- and 4.4-fold were observed in the chemiluminescence responses following incubation of the liver homogenates with 1 nmol/ml of endrin, chlordane, alachlor, chlorpyrifos and fenthion, respectively. Concentration of the pesticides as low as 0.1 nmol/ml and a concentration as high as 10 nmol/ml were also employed (data not shown), with the maximal increases in chemiluminescence responses being observed with 1 nmol/ml.

Results of chemiluminescence assay for the production of reactive oxygen species by liver homogenates from control and pesticide-treated rats are presented in Fig. 2. The chemiluminescence response produced by liver homogenates from pesticide-treated rats rapidly increased, reaching a maximum between 6 and 8 min of incubation, while liver homogenate samples from control animals reach a peak chemiluminescence at 6 min. Chemiluminescence persisted for over 10 min. Increases of 2.2-, 2.3-, 2.9-, 2.9- and 3.4-fold were observed in the chemiluminescence responses in the liver homogenates of the animals treated with endrin, chlordane, alachlor, chlorpyrifos and fenthion, respectively.

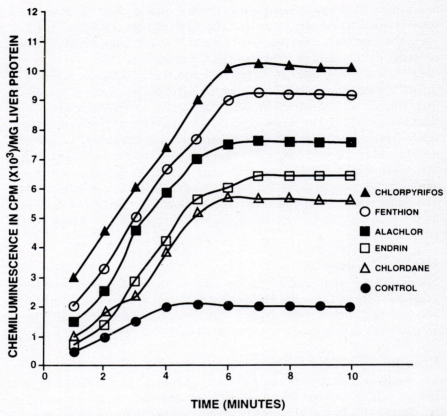

Fig. 1. Production of chemiluminescence by liver homogenate (1 mg protein/ml) incubated *in vitro* at 37°C with endrin, chlordane, alachlor, chlorpyrifos and fenthion (1 nmol/ml each). Luminol (4 μM) was added to enhance chemiluminescence. Each value is the mean of 4-6 experiments.

Effects of the pesticides on lipid peroxidation in hepatic homogenates based on the TBARS assay are summarized in Table 1. The animals were treated with two 0.25 LD_{50} doses at 0 hr and 21 hr and killed at 24 hr and lipid peroxidation assays were conducted on liver homogenates. Following treatment of the rats with endrin, chlordane, alachlor, chlorpyrifos and fenthion, increases of 2.8-, 3.0-, 4.2-, 4.3- and 4.8-fold were observed in hepatic lipid peroxidation, respectively.

DNA single strand breaks (SSB) are another index of oxidative stress and cellular damage. The effects of the five pesticides on DNA-SSB in hepatic nuclei are shown in Table 1. Rats were orally administered two 0.25 LD_{50} doses at 0 hr and 21 hr and killed at 24 hr. Nuclei were isolated from hepatic tissues as described in the methods section. Following treatment of the rats with endrin, chlordane, alachlor, chlorpyrifos and fenthion, increases of 4.4-, 3.9-, 1.6-, 3.9- and 3.5-fold were observed in hepatic DNA-SSB, respectively.

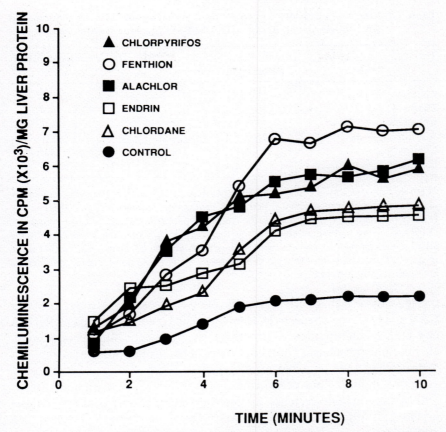

TIME (MINUTES)

Fig. 2. Production of chemiluminescence by liver homogenates (1 mg protein/ml)
following treatment of rats with pesticides in two equal doses (0.25 LD_{50})
at 0 and 21 hrs. All animals were killed 24 hr post-treatment. Each value
is the mean of 4-6 experiments.

Discussion

The polyhalogenated cyclic hydrocarbons (PCH) endrin and chlordane, the
organophosphorous pesticides (OPS) chlorpyrifos and fenthion, and the
chloroacetamide herbicide (CAH) alachlor produce toxicological problems
due to their high environmental persistence and ability to accumulate in
adipose tissues. PCH and OPS exhibit similar abilities as inducers of hepatic
drug metabolizing enzymes [7]. Alachlor is known to induce DNA damage
[8], mutagenicity [9] and nasal tumors in rats [10]. Alachlor is cytotoxic to
a wide variety of tissues [29, 30] and is extensively metabolized in rats,
mice and monkeys through several pathways [31–34]. Thus, similar
mechanisms of toxicity may be involved.

PCH as 2, 3, 7, 8-tetrachlorodibenzo-p-dioxin (TCDD) and endrin induce
an oxidative stress with the production of hepatic lipid peroxidation and
DNA-single strand breaks (SSB) [11, 12]. In order to investigate whether

Table 1. **Effects of pesticides on hepatic lipid peroxidation (TBARS content) and DNA-single strand breaks (DNA-SSB) in Sprague-Dawley rats***

Treatment	Lipid Peroxidation (nmol/mg protein)	DNA elution constants ($\times 10^{-3}$)
Control	3.9 ± 0.7^a	5.1 ± 0.13^a
Endrin	10.7 ± 1.2^b	22.2 ± 6.9^b
Chlordane	11.3 ± 0.9^b	19.6 ± 1.4^b
Alachlor	15.7 ± 1.5^c	$8.0 \pm .0.9^c$
Chlorpyrifos	15.8 ± 1.2^c	17.4 ± 3.0^b
Fenthion	18.2 ± 1.8^c	15.3 ± 1.8^b

*Female Sprague-Dawley rats were given two 0.25 LD_{50} doses of the pesticides orally at 0 and 21 hr in corn oil, and killed at 24 hr. Control animals received the vehicle. Lipid peroxidation was determined as the content of thiobarbituric acid reactive substances (TBRAS), using malondialdehyde as the standard. DNA-SSB were determined by the alkaline elution method and are expressed as DNA elution constants. Each value is the mean ± S.D. of at least 4–6 animals in each group. Values with non-identical superscripts are significantly different ($P < 0.05$).

oxidative tissue damage is characteristic of other classes of pesticides including CAH and OPS, the effects of PCH as endrin and chlordane, CAH as alachlor and OPS as chlorpyrifos and fenthion on the hepatic lipid peroxidation, chemiluminescence and DNA-single strand breaks in Sprague-Dawley rats were studied and compared.

Endrin induces lipid peroxidation in liver as well as brain and kidneys with a concomitant decrease in the glutathione (GSH) content of these organs [35, 36]. In addition, the enzyme selenium dependent glutathione peroxidase is inhibited by endrin, facilitating the accumulation of hydroperoxides [36]. Fatty changes in the foam cells with cytoplasmic vacuolation were also detected. Lipofuscin pigments, associated with lipid peroxidation, were observed in Kupffer cells and hepatocytes [37] following exposure to endrin. Degeneration and necrotic changes with inflammatory cell filtration were also observed in the liver as well as kidneys. Pretreatment of rats with butylated hydroxyanisole (BHA), vitamin E, vitamin C, vitamin E succinate, ellagic acid and cysteine significantly inhibited hepatic lipid peroxidation and glutathione depletion, as well as the enhanced excretion of urinary lipid metabolites induced by endrin [35–38]. These antioxidants also provided partial protection against lethality produced by 8 mg endrin/ kg body weight, suggesting that free radicals and reactive oxygen species are involved in the toxic manifestations of endrin [35].

Based on the above studies, endrin can serve as a basis of reference for other pesticides. The present studies clearly demonstrate that endrin produces enhanced chemiluminescence with liver tissues (Figs. 1 and 2) both *in vivo* and *in vitro*, indicative of the induced production of reactive oxygen species. Furthermore, endrin produces enhanced DNA-SSB in rat liver (Table 1)

ic of oxidative tissue damage. These results support
that endrin induces an oxidative stress and subsequent

Chlordane produces a variety of toxicologic effects associated with the
hepatic as well as gastric and nervous systems. The treatment of
leukocytes with chlordane stimulated superoxide anion
membrane potential, and increased calcium concentrations
suggested that the activation of phospholipase C might
generation of superoxide anion by chlordane. No lag
in the release of membrane-bound calcium by chlordane.
ip between stimulation of superoxide anion generation
s toxicity was suggested.

is cytotoxic to a wide variety of tissues and is extensively
metabolized, little information is available regarding its mechanism of toxicity.
Studies in our laboratories have shown that adminstration of 800 mg alachlor/
kg orally to rats results in the enhanced urinary excretion of the oxidative
lipid metabolites malondialdehyde, formaldehyde, acetaldehyde and acetone
[17]. These metabolites were identified and quantified simultaneously by
GC-MS and HPLC.

Chronic neuropsychological sequelae of occupational exposure to OPS
insecticides have been reported [40]. The incidence of non-Hodgkin's
lymphoma may be related to the use of OPS insecticides [41]. OPS as
phosphamidon, trichlorofon and dichlorvos have been reported to induce
oxidative stress, both *in vivo* and in hepatocytes, as shown by inhibition of
SOD activity, enhanced malondialdehyde production and lactate dehydrogenase leakage, and decreased glutathione peroxidase activity [14-16].

Antunes-Madeira and Madeira [42] have demonstrated that insecticides
modify basic membrane mechanisms including permeability to non-
electrolytes and transport of cations mediated by ionophores. Relatively
low concentrations of OPS and organochlorine insecticides ranging from
10^{-5} to 10^{-4} M have significant effects [42]. OPS and organochlorine
compounds have been shown to interact with membrane events including
nerve conductance [40, 43, 44], and plasma membrane [45, 46] and organelle
enzyme activities [47, 48]. OPS insecticides, besides their typical action as
inhibitors of acetylcholinesterase, interfere with the allosteric behaviour of
the enzyme through interaction with the membrane lipids [49]. The
effectiveness of the various pesticides parallels quite well their relative
degree of toxicity to mammals [12, 50, 51]. However, some insecticides
accumulate preferentially in lipid domains of cells and organisms [12, 52]
so that the local concentrations near the membranes may be rather different
than those obtained under the assumption of an homogeneous distribution
of the compounds.

Results of the present experiments clearly demonstrate that following
treatment with the pesticides, significant increases in lipid peroxidation

associated with hepatic homogenates as well as DNA damage (Table 1) were observed. Greatest hepatic lipid peroxidation was induced by the OPS chlorpyrifos and fenthion under the conditions which were employed. Alachlor induced moderate lipid peroxidation in liver, while the PCH endrin and chlordane induced the least lipid peroxidation in liver (Table 1) as compared to the other pesticides.

The CAH alachlor induced the least DNA-SSB in hepatic nuclei, which agrees with previous studies regarding the ability to produce DNA damage [8]. The PCH endrin and chlordane induced greater DNA-SSB in hepatic nuclei as compared to the OPS chlorpyrifos and fenthion.

Chemiluminescence assay is a non-specific test for the identification of reactive oxygen species. The sustained chemiluminescence produced by hepatic tissues following addition of endrin, chlordane alachlor, chlorpyrifos and fenthion is presumably due to the continued production of reactive oxygen species (Fig. 1). The incubation of luminol with these pesticides in the absence of tissue homogenates did not result in an increase in the chemiluminescence with time (data not shown). Therefore, the increase in chemiluminescence with time is not due to a direct interaction between the pesticides and luminol. The greatest chemiluminescence responses in hepatic tissues were induced by the OPS chlorpyrifos and fenthion. The CAH alachlor resulted in moderate chemiluminescence responses, while endrin and chlordane produced the lowest responses.

Hepatic chemiluminescence responses produced following *in vivo* administration of these pesticides are given in Fig. 2. The greatest chemiluminescence responses in hepatic tissues were induced by the OPS fenthion. The CAH alachlor and the OPS chlorpyrifos resulted in identical chemiluminescence responses in hepatic tissues. The PCH endrin and chlordane produced the lowest responses in the hepatic samples.

These findings clearly demonstrate that administration of structurally diverse pesticides including PCH, CAH and OPS result in the *in vitro* and *in vivo* induction of hepatic lipid peroxidation, chemiluminescence responses and DNA-SSB, suggesting that reactive oxygen species and/or free radicals may be involved in the toxic manifestations of the pesticides. Furthermore, the data indicate the tissue specificity of the pesticides with respect to these responses. The diverse responses may be due to the toxicokinetics (pharmacokinetics) of the pesticides as well as the inherent differences in reactivities with receptors. The data support the contention that reactive oxygen species may serve as common mediators associated with the toxicities of many structurally dissimilar xenobiotics.

Acknowledgements

These studies were supported in part by a grant from the Air Force Office of Scientific Research (#94–1–0048) and a Health Future Foundation Grant (#200098). The authors thank Ms. LuAnn Schwery for technical assistance.

References

1. Murphy, R. and Harvey, C. (1985). Residues and metabolites of selected persistent halogenated hydrocarbons in blood specimens from a general population survey, Environ. Hlth. Persp., Vol. 60, pp. 115–120.
2. Kimbrough, R.D. (1985). Laboratory and human studies on polychlorinated biphenyls (PCBs) and related compounds, Environ. Hlth. Persp., Vol. 59, pp. 99–106.
3. Murphy, S.D. (1986). Toxic effects of pesticides, In Toxicology: The Basic Science of Poisons, 3rd ed. (C.D. Klassen, M.V. Amdur and J. Doull, Eds.) pp. 519–581. McMillan Publishing Co., New York.
4. Shain, W., Bush, B. and Seegal, R. (1991). Neurotoxicity of polychlorinated biphenyls: Structure-activity relationship of individual congeners, Toxicol. Appl. Pharmacol., Vol. 111. pp. 33–42.
5. Bach, D. and Sela, B.A. (1984). Interaction of the chlorinated hydrocarbon insecticide lindane or DDT with lipids—a differential scanning calorimetry study, Biochem. Pharmacol., Vol. 33, pp. 2227–2230.
6. Poland, A. and Knutson, J.D. (1982). 2, 3, 7, 8-Tetrachlorodibenzo-p-dioxin and related halogenated aromatic hydrocarbons: examination of the mechanism of toxicity, Ann. Rev. Pharmacol. Toxicol., Vol. 22, pp. 517–554.
7. Viviani, A., Lutz, W.K. and Schlatter, C. (1978). Time course of the induction of aryl hydrocarbon hydroxylase in rat liver nuclei and microsomes by phenobarbital, 3-methyl cholanthrene, 2, 3, 7, 8-tetrachlorodibenzo-p-dioxin, dieldrin, and other inducers, Biochem. Pharmacol., Vol. 27, pp. 2103–2108.
8. Pinter, A., Torok, G., Surjan, A., Csik, M., Borzsonyi, M. and Kelescsenyi, Z. (1989). Genotoxicity of selected herbicides, Ann. 1st Super Sanita Vol. 25, pp.577–582.
9. Plewa, M.J., Wagner, F.D., Gentile, G.J. and Gentile, J.M. (1984). An evaluation of the genotoxic properties of herbicides following plant and animal activation, Mutat. Res., Vol. 136, pp. 233–245.
10. U.S. Environmental Protection Agency (1984). Notice of initiation of special review of regulations of pesticide products containing alachlor, Alachlor Position Document 1, pp. 1–89.
11. Stohs, S.J. (1990). Oxidative Stress induced by 2, 3, 7, 8-tetrachlorodibenzo-p-dioxin (TCDD), Free Rad. Biol. Med., Vol. 9, pp. 79–90.
12. Stohs, S.J. (1995). Synthetic Pro-oxidants: Drugs, Pesticides and other Environmental Pollutants, In Oxidative Stress and Antioxidant Defenses in Biology (S. Ahmad, Ed.), pp. 117–180. Chapman and Hall, New York.
13. Sarafian, T. A. and Bredesen, D.E. (1994). Is apoptosis mediated by reactive oxygen species? Free Rad. Res., Vol. 21, pp. 1–8.
14. Naqvi, S.M. and Hasan, M. (1992). Acetylhomocysteine thiolactone protection against phosphamidon-induced alteration of regional superoxide dismutase activity in central nervous system and its correlation with altered lipid peroxidation, Ind. J. Exp. Biol., Vol. 30, pp. 850–852.
15. Yamano, T. and Morita, S. (1992). Hepatotoxicity of trichlorfon and dichlorvos in isolated rat hepatocytes, Toxicol., Vol. 76, pp. 69–77.
16. Julka, D., Pal, R. and Gill, K.D. (1992). Neurotoxicity of dichlorvos: effect of antioxidant defense system in the rat central nervous system, Exp. Mol. Pathol., Vol. 56, pp. 144–152.
17. Akublle, P.I. and Stohs, S.J. (1991). Endrin induced production of nitric oxide by rat peritoneal macrophages, Toxicol. Lett., Vol. 62, pp. 311–316.

18. Sun, Y. (1990). Free Radicals, Antioxidant Enzymes and Carcinogenesis., Free Rad Biol. Med., Vol. 8, pp. 583–589.
19. Halliwell, B., Gutteridge, J.M.C. and Cross, C.E. (1992). Free radicals, antioxidants, and human diseases: where are we now?, J. Lab. Clin. Med., Vol. 119, pp. 598–620.
20. Klaunig, J.E. and Ruch, R.J. (1987). Strain and species effects on the inhibition of hepatocyte intercellular communication by liver tumor promoters, Cancer Lett., Vol, 36, pp. 161–168.
21. Williams, G.M. and Numoto, S. (1984). Promotion of mouse liver neoplasms by the organochlorine pesticides chlordane and hepatochlor in comparison to dichlorodiphenyl trichloroethane, Carcinogenesis, Vol. 5, pp. 1689–1696.
22. Lowry, O.H., Rosebrough, N.J., Farr, W.L. and Randall, R.J. (1951). Protein measurement with the folin phenol reagent, J. Biol. Chem., Vol. 193, pp. 265–275.
23. White, R.D., Sipes, I.G., Gandolfi, A.J. and Bowden, G.T. (1981). Characterization of the hepatic DNA damage caused by 1, 2-dibromethane using the alkaline elution technique, Carcinogenesis, Vol. 2, pp. 839–843.
24 Buege, J.A. and Aust, S.D. (1972). Microsomal lipid peroxidation, Meth. Enzymol., Vol, 51, pp. 302–310.
25. Largilliere, C. and Melancon, S.B. (1988). Free malondialdehyde determination in human plasma by high-performance liquid chromatography, Analyt. Biochem., Vol, 170, pp. 123–126.
26. Samuni, A., Krishna, M.C., Cook, J., Black, C.D.V. and Russo, A. (1991). On radical production by PMA stimulated neutrophils as monitored by luminol-amplified chemiluminescence, Free Rad. Biol. Med., Vol. 10, pp. 313–325.
27. Cederbaum, A.I. and Puntarulo, S. (1988). Comparison of the ability of ferric complexes to catalyze microsomal chemiluminescence, lipid peroxidation and hydroxyl radical generation, Arch, Biochem. Biophys., Vol. 264, pp. 482–491.
28. Bagchi, M., Hassoun, E.A., Bagchi, D. and Stohs, S.J. (1992). Endrin-induced increases in hepatic lipid peroxidation, membrace morcoviscosity, and DNA damage in rats, Arch. Environ. Contam. Toxicol., Vol. 23, pp. 1–5.
29. Rabich, H., Rosenberg, D.W. and Borenfreund, E. (1991). In vitro cytotoxicity studies with the fish hepatoma cell line, PLHC-1 (Poeciliopsis Incida), Ecotoxicol. Environ, Safety, Vol. 21, pp. 327–336.
30. Lin, M.F., Wu, C.L. and Wang, T.C. (1987). Pesticide clastogenicity in Chinese hamster ovary cells, Mutat. Res., Vol. 188, pp. 241–250.
31. Sharp, D.B. (1988). Alachlor, In Herbicides: Chemistry, Degradation and Mode of Action (P.C. Kearney and D.D. Kaufman, Eds.) pp. 1–20. Marcel Dekker, New York.
32. Feng, P.C.C. and Patanella, J.E. (1988). Identification of mercapturic acid pathway metabolities of alachlor formed by liver and kidney homogenates of rats, mice and monkeys, Pestic. Biochem. Physiol., Vol. 31, pp. 84–90.
33. Feng, P.C.C., Wilson, A.G.E., McClanahan, R.H., Patanella, J. E. and Wratten, S.J. (1990). Metabolism of alachlor by rat and mouse liver and nasal turbinate tissues, Drug Metab. Dispos., Vol. 18, pp. 373–377.
34. Kimmel, E.C., Casida, J.E. and Ruzo, L.O. (1986). Formamidine insecticides and chloroacetanilide herbicides: Disubstituted aniline and nitrosobenzenes as mammalian metabolites and bacterial mutagens, J. Agric. Food Chem., Vol. 34, pp. 157–161.
35. Numan, I.T., Hassan, M.Q. and Stohs, S.J. (1990). Protective effects of antioxidants against endrin-induced lipid peroxidation, glutathione depletion, and lethality in rats, Arch. Environ. Contam. Toxicol., Vol. 19, 302–306.

36. Numan, I.T., Hassan, M.Q. and Stohs, S.J. (1990). Endrin-induced depletion of glutathione and inhibition of glutathione peroxidase activity in rats, Gen. Pharmacol. Vol. 21, pp. 625–628.

37. Hassan, M.Q., Numan, I.T., Al-Nasiro, N. and Stohs, S.J. (1991). Endrin-induced histopathological changes and lipid peroxidation in livers and kidneys of rats, mice guinea pigs and hamsters, Toxicol. Pathol., Vol. 19, pp. 108–114.

38. Bagchi, D., Hassoun, E.A. Bagchi, M. and Stohs, S.J. (1993). Protective effects of antioxidants against endrin-induced hepatic lipid peroxidation, DNA damage, and excretion of urinary lipid metabolites, Free Rad. Biol. Med., Vol. 15, pp. 217–222.

39. Suzaki, E., Inoue, B., Okimasu, E., Ogata, M. and Utsumi, K. (1988). Stimuative effect of chlordane on the various functions of guinea pig leukocytes, toxicol. Appl. Pharmacol., Vol. 93, pp. 137–145.

40. Rosenstoch, L., Daniell, W., Barnhart, S., Schwartz, D. and Demers, P.A. (1990). Chronic neurophysiological sequelae of occupational exposure to organophosphate insecticides, Am. J. Ind. Med., Vol. 18, pp. 321–325.

41. Weisenburger, D.D. (1990). Environmental epodemiology of non-Hodgkin's lymphoma in eastern Neberaska, Am. J. Ind. Med., Vol. 18, pp. 303–305.

42. Antunes-Madeira, M.C. and Madeira, V.M.C. (1979). Interaction of insecticides with lipid membranes, Biochim. Biophys. Acta, Vol. 550, pp. 384–392.

43. Narahashi, T. and Haas, H.G. (1967). DDT: with nerve membrane conductance changes, Science, Vol. 157, pp. 1438–1440.

44. Narahashi, T. and Haas, H.G. (1968). Interaction of DDT with the components of lobster nerve membrane conductance, J. Gen. Physiol., Vol. 51, pp. 177–198.

45. Matsumura, F, and Patil, K.C. (1969). Adenosine triphosphatase-Sensitive to DDT synapses of rat brain, Science, Vol. 166, pp. 121–122.

46. Schneider, R.P. (1975). Mechanism of inhibition of rat brain (Na+K)-adenosine triphosphatase by 2, 2-bis (p-chlorophenyl)-1, 1, 1-trichloroethane (DDT), Biochem. Pharmacol., Vol. 24, pp. 939–946.

47. Bradbury, S.J. (1973). The effect of parathion on crustacean skeletal muscle. I. The mechanical threshold and dependent on Ca^{+2} ions, Comp. Biochem. Physiol., Vol. 44A, pp. 1021–1032.

48. Binder, N., Landon, E.J., Weeker, L. and Dettbarn, W.D. (1976). Effect of parathion and its metabolities on Ca^{+2} uptake activity of rat skeletal muscle sarcoplasmic reticulum *in vitro*, Biochem. Pharmacol., Vol. 25, pp. 835–839.

49. Domenech, C.E., Machado de Domenech, E.E., Balegno, H.F., de Mendoza, D. and Farias, R.N. (1977). Pesticide action and membrane fluidity, Allosteric behavior of rat erythrocyte membrane-bound acetylcholinesterase in the presence of organophosphorous compounds, FEBS Lett., 74, 243–246.

50. Metcalf, R.L. (1971) In: Pesticides in the Environment, Vol. 1, Part 1 (White-Stevens, R. Ed.), pp. 1–144. Marcel Dekker, Inc., New York.

51. Morrison, H.I., Wilkins, K., Semenciw, R., Mao, Y. and Wigle, D. (1992). Herbicides and Cancer, J. Natl. Can. Inst., Vol. 84, pp. 1866–1874.

52. Brooks, G.T. (1974). Chlorinated Insecticides: Organic and Biological Chemistry, Chapter IV, pp. 123–231. CRC Press, Cleveland.

Liver and Environmental Xenobiotics
S.V.S. Rana and K. Taketa (Eds)
Copyright © 1997, Narosa Publishing House, New Delhi, India

10. Oxidative Stress and Liver Injury by Environmental Xenobiotics

S.V.S. Rana

Department of Zoology, Ch. Charan Singh University, Meerut 250 004, India

Introduction

Oxidation processes are thought to form the basis of a number of physiological and pathophysiological phenomena that participate in diverse processes viz: ageing, inflammation, carcinogenesis, drug action, drug toxicity. defence against protozoa and many others. Moreover, oxidative damage to biological material is inflicted on compounds of all major chemical classes. It is mediated by reactive oxygen species (ROS). Oxygen radicals that are probably formed in all living organisms could be responsible for lipid peroxidation, leading to a sequence of chain of reactions. Therefore, oxidative stress so far remains to be a very attractive hypothesis for explaining many diseases and drug induced toxicity.

Lipid peroxidation has been broadly defined by A.L. Tappel (1978) as the "oxidative deterioration of polyunsaturated lipids," ie lipids that contain more than two carbon carbon double covalent bond ($>C=C<$). Unlike ground state oxygen, singlet oxygen can react rapidly with compounds containing $>C=C<$ bonds to give hydroperoxides. Membrane lipids are not only the molecules found in cells that contain many $>C=C<$ bonds. Several other molecules present can be peroxidized under appropriate conditions. Lipid peroxidation may be important in oxidative injury because: (a) it can amplify the number of free radical chain reactions; (b) some products of lipid peroxidation are toxic and (c) lipid peroxidation places a demand on reduced glutathione dependent detoxication systems and thus renders the cell less capable of detoxifying other reactive species.

In recent years, oxidative stress and its implications in diverse toxic mechanisms have attracted considerable attention. An attempt has been made here to discuss oxidant-antioxidant disturbances caused by a few environmentally significant xeno-biotics viz; industrial solvents, alcohols and heavy metals in the liver of laboratory rat. Role of calcium, cytochrome P_{450}, cytochrome P_{448}, glutathione transferase isozyme 8–8, hormones, vitamins and interactions of oxidative stress with DNA have also been discussed.

Oxidative Stress, Calcium and Cell Death

Studies over the last few years have indicated that oxidative hepatocellular injury is due to the inactivation of specific membrane transport protein such as the plasma membrane and endoplasmic reticular Ca^{++} ATPase apparently by sulphydryl oxidation [33]. Impairment of Ca transport by these systems, as well as an impaired ability of the mitochondria to retain Ca^{2+} [5, 6, 32], contribute to increased cytosolic Ca^{2+}. Sustained increases in cytosolic Ca^{2+} are thought to disrupt cytoskeletal elements and activate phospholipases and proteases leading to cell injury and finally terminating into cell death.

Recent evidence suggest that cytoplasmic ionized calcium ($[Ca^{2+}]i$) is clearly an important mediator in both accidental (necrosis) and programmed (apoptosis) cell death [81]. Increases of $(Ca^{2+})i$ occur rapidly following injury and precede other early events such as blebbing, mitochondrial swelling, and induction of immediate early genes. The latter events appear to involve Ca^{2+} dependent protein kinases and sometimes involve high concentration of Ca^{2+} in the nucleus [83]. Furthermore, several studies have implicated Ca^{2+} dependent nucleases in apoptosis and modulation of $(Ca^{2+})i$ clearly offers a protective mechanism against the development of apoptosis in thymocytes.

The low concentration of Ca^{2+} in the resting cytosol of hepatocytes is maintained by active compartmentation processes and by calcium binding proteins including calmodulin. Mitochondrial Ca^{2+} homeostasis is regulated by a cyclic mechanism, involving Ca^{2+} uptake by an energy dependent pathway and Ca release which is probably mediated by a Ca^{2+}/H^+ antiposter. The latter appears to be regulated by the redox level of intramitochondrial pyridine nucleotides [39].

Incubation of hepatocytes with various toxic agents is associated with alterations in the intracellular Ca^{2+} pools. Orrenius and Nicotera (1987) have shown that menadione, t-butyl hydroperoxide, N-acetyl-p-benzoquinone imine, carbon-tetrachloride, bromobenzene and cystamine all increase cytosolic Ca^{2+} pool. Role of calcium in carbontetrachloride toxicity was reviewed by Recknagel (1983). Calcium seqestration by the liver ER was considered one of the triumvirate of major mechanisms known so far [65], the other two being calcium sequestration by the mitochondria and calcium extrusion by the plasma membrane which maintain and regulate the calcium concentration in the cytoplasm. Relationship between calcium, oxidative stress and cell death was studied by Pavoine et al [53]. Celluar calcium intoxication can result either from a primary imbalance between the influx and efflux of calcium across the inner mitochondrial membrane. Calcium permeability of this membrane can be induced by drugs or chemicals.

Hormones can rapidly elevate the cytoplasmic concentration of Ca^{2+} by changing the properties of plasma-membrane and thereby accelerating passive uptake. However, hormones seem to specifically bring about the "opening of calcium channel," and/or facilitation of Ca-transport mechanisms.

Hormones can also promote the release of calcium from sequestration sites. The toxic potential may be greatly changed by the endocrinal status [22, 37, 38, 56, 57]. The effect of carbontetrachloride is diminished or even abolished by hypophysectomy, adrenalectomy [8, 66]. In contrast the effect of carbontetrachloride is aggravated by the administration of thyroxine [9]. We have made certain studies that show a direct co-relation of calcium, lipid-peroxidation and oxidative stress and confirm the role of calcium in lipid peroxidation and oxidative stress. Parathyroidectomy causes hypocalcemia that attributes to the diminished rat of lipid peroxidation. Removal of both the glands in carbontetrachloride treated rats resulted in increased hepatic glutathione level and simultaneously showed a greater antiper-oxidative effect (Tables 1 and 2). The fact that parathyroidectomy proved effective in inhibiting malondialdehyde production in the carbontetrachloride treated rats suggest a correlation amongst hypocalcemia, lipid peroxidation, parathyroid hormone and detoxication mechanisms. These observations suggest that endocrinal status significantly contributes in drug/chemical toxicity.

Table 1. Malondialdehyde (MDA) and glutathione (GSH) in the liver of rats treated with carbon-tetrachloride (CCl_4) after parathyroidectomy

Group No.	Treatment	Malondialdehyde (n mole/mg protein)	Glutathione (μg GSH/g fresh liver)
A	Control	0.1420 ± 0.017	1400 ± 5.63
B	CCl_4	0.4350 ± 0.025*	2800 ± 6.89*
C	UPTx	0.1710 ± 0.019*+	4600 ± 7.01*+
D	UPTx + CCL_4	0.3480 ± 0.020*+	1600 ± 5.90*+
E	BPTx	0.1840 ± 0.016*+	5000 ± 7.23*+
F	BPTx + CCl_4	0.1570 ± 0.018*+	5900 ± 7.04*+

Results are mean ± S.E of 5 observations in each group.
*$p < 0.001$ (control vs experimental rats); +$p < 0.001$ (CCl_4 vs experimental rats).
UPTx—Unilaterally parathyroidectomized; BPTx—bilaterally parathyroidectomized (from [60], reprinted with permission).

Recently, the recognition that immediate early gene expression represents a prevalent reaction to injury has been extended to consideration of the possible function of these genes in the progression of cell injury [42]. The spectrum of possible effects of these genes has been broadened to include activation of later genes as well as possibly complex interactions among their products which probably form complex signaling networks possibly with considerable redundancy. At present time, however, it is impossible to say whether the gene products (e.g. Fos, Jun, Myc) are only parallel responses or they indeed, have functions that are directly related to the mechanisms of cell injury and cell death. At present, the study of accidental and preformed cell death is revealing a number of signaling pathways including $(Ca^{2+})i$,

Table 2. Glutathione-peroxidase (GSH-px), glutathione-reductase (GR) and catalase in the liver of rats treated with CCl_4 after parathyroidectomy

Group No.	Treatment	GSH-px[a]	GR[a]	Catalase[b]
A	Control	43.4 ± 2.63	15.05 ± 2.04	43.90 ± 3.61
B	CCl_4	$17.2 \pm 1.50^*$	$26.20 \pm 1.57^{**}$	$61.15 \pm 2.16^{**}$
C	UPTx	$1.2 \pm 1.04^{***+++}$	$11.00 \pm 1.21^{n.s.+++}$	$19.47 \pm 1.07^{***+++}$
D	UPTx + CCl_4	$42.2 \pm 2.89^{n.s.+++}$	$41.60 \pm 1.04^{***+++}$	$80.69 \pm 3.02^{***+++}$
E	BPTx	$0.2 \pm 0.47^{***+++}$	$25.00 \pm 1.60^{**n.s.}$	$88.28 \pm 3.18^{***+++}$
F	BPTx + CCl_4	$9.1 \pm 3.01^{***++}$	$22.00 \pm 1.68^{*n.s.}$	$73.32 \pm 1.68^{***+++}$

Results are mean $\pm$ S.E. of 5 observations in each group.
$^*p < 0.05$; $^{**}p < 0.01$; $^{***}p < 0.001$ (control vs experimental rats); $^+p < 0.05$; $^{++}p < 0.01$; $^{+++}p < 0.001$ (CCl_4 vs experimental rats).
[a]n mples NADPH oxidised/mg protein/min in the cytosol fraction of the liver; [b]k cat/mg protein.
UPTx—Unilaterally parathyroidectomized; BPTx—bilaterally parathyroidectomized.
n.s—not significant (from [60], reprinted with permission).

a series of protein kinases and immediate early genes that appear to be involved in the mechanism(s). Elucidation of these pathways promises a lead to interventions that can prevent, ameliorate, or accelerate the cell death process.

Oxidative Stress by Industrial Solvents

The above hypothesis works well with a model hepatotoxin i.e. carbontetrachloride. In order to ascertain similar mechanisms with other xenobiotics, a study on three major industrial solvents viz: xylene, toluene and methyl alcohol was performed. A statistically significant increase in serum calcium was observed after xylene and methyl alcohol treatment. However, a non significant increase was observed after toluene and their combined treatment.

Results on malondialdehyde, showed that xylene, toluene and methyl alcohol do induce lipid peroxidation and depete GSH content in the liver. Increase in lipidperoxidation corresponded with glutathione depletion (Tables 3 and 4). Earlier studies suggest that cell injury manifested by aromatic organic compounds is principally related to the covalent binding of their reactive metabolites to macromolecules. Oxygen species thus generated cause oxidative stress finally leading to lipid peroxidation [60]. Glutathione conjugation and subsequent excretion as mercapturic acids could be the main detoxication mechanism of these solvents. Therefore, this study was followed by a study on antioxidative enzymes viz. glutathione peroxidase, glutathione reductase and catalase [61]. Inhibited activity of glutathione peroxidase suggests reduction of hydroperoxides to corresponding alcohols.

Table 3. Malondialdehyde (n mol/mg protein) in liver of rats treated individually and with a combination of xylene, toluene and methanol
(Values are mean ± of 5 observations of each group of rats)

Group No.	Treatment	Liver
A	Xylene	0.229 ± 0.031^b
B	Toluene	0.245 ± 0.060^{NS}
C	Methanol	0.318 ± 0.042^a
D	Mixture	0.306 ± 0.051^b
E	Control	0.140 ± 0.010

$^a p < 0.01$; $^b p < 0.02$.

However, activity of glutathione reductase increased so as to maintain the glutathione reserves. Catalase protected the rats by counteracting the superoxide radicals.

Table 4. Glutathione (μg/g tissue) content of liver of rats treated individually and with a combination of xylene, toluene and methanol
(Values are mean ± of 5 observations of each group of rats)

Group No.	Treatment	Liver
A	Xylene	1280 ± 3.45^a
B	Toluene	1310 ± 8.07^a
C	Methanol	930 ± 5.96^a
D	Mixture	1020 ± 10.26^a
E	Control	1400 ± 4.68

$^a p < 0.001$; $^b p < 0.01$, $c < 0.02$ (from [61], Reprinted with permission).

Earlier studies by Pathiatne et al [52] have concluded that glutathione was elevated by benzene, decreased by xylenes and not affected by toluene. Glutathione-s-transferse was induced differentially by these hydrocarbons towards various substrates.

Oxidative Stress by Alcohol(s)

Alcohol is very well known to produce hepatocellular damage. It is known to be caused by acetaldehyde or acetaldehyde altered proteins. It also brings about changes in the microsomal drug metabolising apparatus. The malondialdehyde content, hydroperoxides and conjugated dienes were increased in the liver of the acute and chronic ethanol treated rats. However, the activities of antiperoxidative enzymes decreased after ethanol treatment. Inhibition of enzymes supports increased peroxidation, increased synthesis of ecosonoids and increased damage to the tissue. It is clear that cyto-toxicity of molecular oxygen is checked by the delicate balance between the rate of generation of the partially reduced oxygen species and the rate of their removal by different defence mechanisms. Any shift in this delicate balance can lead to cellular damage. The decreased activity of these enzymes in the hepatic tissue suggests increased damage to the tissue as a result of uncontrolled generation of partially reduced oxygen species.

Table 5. Antioxidative enzymes in the liver of rat after exposure to xylene, toluene and methyl alcohol, separately and in combination

Group No.	Treatment	Glutathione peroxidase (n-mole NADPH/mg protein/min)	Glutathione reductase (n-mole NADPH/mg protein/min)	Catalase K/mg protein
A	Xylene	30.81 ± 2.12***	19.58 ± 0.85*	70.76 ± 3.65***
B	Toluene	31.66 ± 1.85***	20.64 ± 1.10**	75.16 ± 5.10***
C	Methyl alcohol	26.72 ± 2.10***	18.60 ± 0.65*	69.48 ± 3.78***
D	Mixture[+]	40.54 ± 1.46ns	14.01 ± 1.02ns	78.86 ± 6.10***

[+]Equimolar concentration of xylene, toluene, methyl alcohol.
Results are mean ± S.E. of five observations in each group of rats.
*$p < 0.05$, **$p < 0.02$, ***$p < 0.001$ (between control and experimental groups)
n.s.—Not significant (from [62], reprinted with permission).

Several possible mechanisms by which alcohol can promote oxidative stress have been suggested [11]. Alcohol and acetaldehyde decrease GSH depending on the dose. Microsomal ethanol oxidising system via cytochrome $P\text{-}_{450}$ may produce reactive free radicals which are potent oxidising species. Acetaldehyde, the metabolite of ethanol has also been shown to produce oxygen radicals as well as ethane and pentane which are peroxidized products of unsaturated fatty acids. Cytochrome $P_{450}J$ or $P_{450}II E_1$ induced by ethanol may function as an effective Fenton or Haber-Weiss catalysts of lipid peroxidation. Another possible mechanism involved in chronic ethanol-induced oxidative stress might be the increase in hepatic non-heme iron mobilised from ferritin after long term alcohol feeding. It has been recently reported by Khan et al [35] that iron induced lipid peroxidation in rat liver is accompanied by preferential induction of glutathione-S-transferase 8-8 isozyme. They suggest that induction of enzyme may be caused by increased 4 HNE (4-hydroxynonenal) levels in tissues. The specific induction of rat GST 8-8 upon exposure to iron resulting in increased lipid peroxidation and presumably due to increased 4 HNE concentrations may provide an excellent model to study the regulatory elements involved in the induction of rat GST-8-8.

Oxidative Stress by Heavy Metals

A growing body of evidence indicates that transition metals act as catalysts in the oxidative deterioration of biological macromolecules, and therefore, the toxicities associated with these metals may be due atleast in part to oxidative tissue damage. Recent studies [55, 72, 77] have shown that metals such as iron, copper, cadmium chromium, lead, mercury, nickel and vanadium exhibit the ability to produce reactive oxygen species resulting in lipid peroxidation, DNA damage, depletion of sulphydryls and altered calcium homeostasis. Specific differences in the toxicities of metal ions may be related to differences in solubilities, absorbability, transport, chemical reactivity and the complexes that are formed within the body. Inspite of these factors, the basic mechanisms involved in the production of reactive oxygen species are the same for these metal ions.

Role of iron in the initiation of lipid-peroxidation has also been reviewed by Minotti and Aust [45] and Alleman et al [2]. Recent studies have indicated that lipid peroxidation are enhanced in target tissue of rodents exposed to Cd, Co, Cu, Hg, Ni, Pb, Sn, and V compounds. Stacey et al [76] suspected that lipid peroxidation was not the primary mechanism for cell membrane damage by Cd, since anti-oxidants prevented Cd induced lipid peroxidation but did not protect against intracellular loss. Dillard and Tappel [15] observed increased TBA chromogens in liver, kidney and blood of copper sulphate treated vitamin E deficient rats. Shafiq-Ur-Rehman [69] observed two fold increase of TBA chromogen production in brain homogenates of adult rats. Sunderman et al [71] found that administration of nickel chloride to rats increased TBA chromogen concentration in liver, kidney and lung. Fukino et al [19] confirmed that administration of mercuric chloride induced TBA chromogens in rat kidney. Rana et al [62] studied mercury induced lipid peroxidation and oxidative stress in the liver, kidney, brain and gills of a fresh water fish. It has been suggested that the rate of lipid-peroxidation did not strictly correspond to oxidative stress. Time dependent effects may represent an early biochemical response, although the presence of some labile GSH-dependent factors may provide a protective mechanism. Albro et al [1] have suggested a partial mechanism given below for the production of hydrogen peroxide during trace metal catalyzed oxidation of glutathione.

$$GSH \rightleftharpoons GS^- + H^+ \tag{1}$$

$$2GS^- + Me^{+2} \rightleftharpoons\rightleftharpoons GS\text{-}Me\text{-}SG \tag{2}$$

$$GS\text{-}Me\text{-}SG + O_2 \rightarrow [?] \rightarrow GS\text{-}Me^+ + HO_2^- + GSSG$$

$$\begin{array}{cc} | & \downarrow\uparrow \\ GSH & H^+ + O_2^- \end{array} \tag{3}$$

$$FG\text{-}Me^+ + 2O_2^- \cdot + 2H^+ + GS^- \rightarrow GS\text{-}Me\text{-}SG + H_2O_2 + O_2$$

Net: $6GSH + O_2 + 2Me^{+2} \rightarrow GSSG + 2GS\text{-}Me\text{-}SG + H_2O_2 + 4H^+$ $\tag{4}$

It is suggested by this study that at high metal/GSH ratios, the species GS-Me$^+$ reacts rapidly with oxygen to form an activated precursor of hydrogen peroxide. In case of metals, autoxidation of glutathione may induce hydrogen peroxide radicals.

Chevion [12] has proposed two models for interventions in transition metal ion mediated oxidative processes, which are referred to as "pull" and "push" mechanisms. The first mechanism invokes the use of specific chelators that pull "redox active" and available metals out of binding stress, while the second mechanism invokes the use of redox inactive metals such as zinc to push redox active metals from binding sites. Evidence in support of both mechanisms and approaches to the production of oxidative tissue damage exists today [54].

Oxidative Stress and Cytochrome P-450

Recent information suggests that oxygenation of chemicals in conformationally hindered positions is known to occur by two different mechanisms, namely, (i) non enzymic hydroxylation by hydroxyl radicals generated by ionizing radiation or (ii) enzymically by the cytochrome(s) P-448 but not by the cytochrome(s) P-450 of microsomal mixed function oxidases. The cytochrome(s) P-448 are able to catalyse the oxygenation of chemicals in "conformationally hindered" or "bay-region" positions, by virtue of their unique active site which unlike the restricted active site of the cytochrome P-450, is able to accomodate molecules so as to facilitate oxygen transfer to conformationally hindered areas of the toxic chemical. Hence it is being generally realized that the cytochromes P-450 tend to detoxicate drugs, toxic chemicals and carcinogens whereas the cytochromes P_{448} generally tend to activate these chemicals. Non-oxidative metabolic activation of CCl_4 to radicals by cytochrome P_{450} is an exception to this generalization.

As the cytochrome P_{450} are generally more abundant than the cytochrome P_{448} in the adult mammalian liver, the overall function of the liver is generally of detoxication rather then activation. Furthermore, from pharmacogenetic studies, it would appear that the ratio of hapatic cytochrome P_{450} to P_{448} is genetically determined [44] and may also be affected by diet, life style and exposure to environmental chemicals [3].

This process of activation of toxic chemicals by metabolic oxygenation by cytochrome P_{448} was first recognized in the polycyclic aromatic hydrocarbons [41] but is now known to encompass a wide variety of different chemical structures ranging form paracetamol to food products. These reactive intermediates are highly eletrophilic and are more likely to react non-enzymically with critical intracellular macromolecules such as glutathione, sulphydryl enzymes, RNA mutations leading to malignancy and genotoxicity.

Antioxidant Defence

An oxidant can be defined as any substance that when present at low concentrations compared to those of an oxidisable substrate, significantly delays or prevents oxidation of that substrate.

When reactive oxygen species (ROS) are generated in living systems, a wide variety of antioxidants come into play. The relative importance of these antioxidants as protective agents depends on which ROS is generated, how it is generated, where it is generated and what target of damage is measured. If water soluble peroxyl radicals are used to impose oxidative stress, the best antioxidants will be those like ascorbate that are good at scavenging water soluble peroxyl radicals.

According to their physiological functions, cellular antioxidants can be divided into three categories: preventive antioxidants, chain breaking antioxidants and repair and *de-novo* compounds. The preventive and chain breaking antioxidants are considered as a first level of protection against oxidative damage. The second level of protection comes from a series of repair systems including enzymes [47].

Aerobic organisms have potent antioxidant defenses whose role is to neutralize and minimize the potentially cytotoxic effects of reactive oxidants. The defenses that directly decompose or scavenge O_2^-, H_2O_2 and OH radicals are known as primary antioxidant defenses. Secondary antioxidant defenses consist of repair mechanisms that act on biomolecules subjected to oxidative damage.

Enzymatic antioxidant defenses involve superoxide dismutase, catalase and glutathione peroxidase. Whereas non enzymatic antioxidants include α-tocopherol, β-carotene, ascorbate, glutathione, selenium, ubiquinol-10, bilirubin and plasma proteins.

Vitamin E

α-tocopherol (vitamin E) is important in protecting tissue from a variety of physiopathological insults which result in enhanced penetration of reactive oxygen species [13]. Vitamin-E deficient animals are more susceptible to tissue damage from (i) chemical and drug toxicity (e.g. CCl_4 and paracetamol), (ii) air pollutants (e.g. O_3, NO_2), (iii) sternous exercise (e.g. hypoxia) and (v) ultraviolet radiation.

Table 6. **Malondialdehyde, GSH and GSSG in liver of rats fed Cd with glutathione, α-tocopherol, and Se[a]**

Group No.	Treatment	Malondialdehyde (n moles/mg protein)	GSH (μg/g fresh liver)	GSSG (μg/g fresh liver)
A	Cd	0.9920 ± 0.23^b	1500 ± 5.45^b	140 ± 5.05^c
B	Cd + glutathione	0.0692 ± 0.05^c	3510 ± 7.45^c	290 ± 3.05^c
C	Cd + α-tocopherol	0.2210 ± 0.15^d	2890 ± 6.98^c	375 ± 3.76^c
D	Cd + Se	0.0913 ± 0.04^d	4050 ± 9.15^c	125 ± 2.05^c
E	Control	0.140 ± 0.02	1400 ± 4.68	56 ± 2.78

[a]Values are the mean of $\pm$ S.E. of five observations in each group.
[b]$p < 0.01$; [c]$p < 0.02$; [d]$p < 0.001$ (control vs experimental rats)
(from [64], reprinted with permission).

Vitamin E acts primarily as a lipophilic radical scavenging antioxidant and suppresses the chain initiation and/or chain propagation by donating it's phenolic hydrogen to the oxygen radicals [47]. For example when vitamin E reacts with lipid peroxyl radical, lipid hydroperoxide is formed together with vitamin E radical. One may argue that if this hydroperoxide is decomposed by iron to give alkoxyl radical which is more reactive than peroxyl radical. More important is that vitamin E reduces the amount of hydroperoxide formation by breaking chain propagation. Biochemical indices for malondialdelyde determined in the liver of cadmium fed rats showed significant protective effect of vitamin E [63].

Selenium

Dietary selenium can protect against the toxicity of several heavy metals such as mercury and cadmium and certain other xenobiotics viz. paraquat, howerver, the mechanism of the protective effect is not known. The discovery that selenium is a compound of the enzyme glutathione peroxidase, protection against oxidative stress either by catalysing the destruction of hydrogen peroxide or by catalysing the decomposition of lipid hydroperoxides can be envisaged. In the later role the fatty acyl hydroperoxide must be liberated by phospholipase A_2 action from the hydrophobic region of the biological membrane, before its reaction can by catalyzed by glutathione peroxidase [21]. Thus both these nutrients play separate but interrelated roles in the

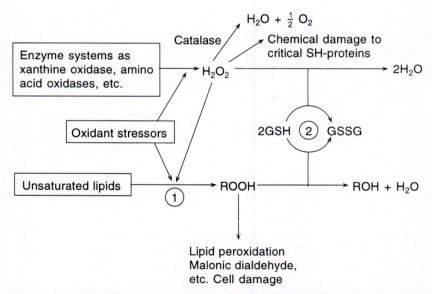

Fig. 1. Physiological role of selenium and its relationship to the antioxidant function of vitamin E. Modified from : Hoekstra [25]. ①—Vitamin E. terminated chain reaction of lipid peroxidation; ②—Se, as a component of GSH-peroxidase, catalyses reaction.

cellular defence mechanisms against oxidative damage. According to some authors Se-Hg and Se-Cd interaction is brought about be endogenous glutathione which reduces selenite to a selenide compound [31]. Rana and Boora [58] while studying the antioxidative mechanism offered by selenium against liver injury caused by cadmium and mercury suggested that one of the avenues through which selenium can antagonize with cadmium or mercury involves glutathione and glutathione peroxidase.

Table 7. Malondialdehyde, GSH and glutathione peroxidase in the liver of rats fed on cadmium and mercury with selenium

Group No.	Treatment	Malondialdehyde (n moles/mg protein)	GSH (µg/g fresh liver)	GSH peroxidase (n moles NADPH used/mg protein/min)
A	Cadmium	0.3900 ± 4.08***	1700 ± 2.93***	59.32 ± 2.90**
B	Cadmium + sodium selenite	0.3390 ± 4.00**	3800 ± 3.07***	26.40 ± 1.69***
C	Mercury	0.3280 ± 3.01**	1400 ± 2.69^{N.S.}	20.57 ± 0.97***
D	Mercury + sodium selenite	0.2825 ± 3.62*	1600 ± 1.94***	17.18 ± 0.83***
E	Control	0.1420 ± 2.64	1400 ± 2.68	43.40 ± 1.81

Values are mean ± S.E. of five observations in each group. *$p < 0.02$; **$p < 0.01$ ***$p < 0.001$ (control vs experimental rats). N.S.—Not significant. (From [59], reprinted with permission).

Selenium could protect liver against CCl_4 toxicity as it prevented lipid peroxidation [23]. It was helpful in maintaining intracellular levels of glutathione and the activity of glutathione peroxidase.

Skaare and Nafstad [74] evaluated the influence of vitamin E and selenium on the acute hepatotoxicity of dimethylnitrosamine (DMN) in rats. However, the mechanism by which selenium affect DMN toxicity could not be clarified.

It has been reported that selenium may play an important role in reducing the toxicity, mutagenicity and carcinogenicity of a variety of toxic substances including cadmium, lead, mercury, benzene, CCl_4 and PCBs, the gaseous irritant ozone and α-irradiation.

Glutathione (GSH)

Glutathione (γ-glutamyl cysteinyl glycine) a tripeptide found in abundance in most cells, is known to have key functions in protective processes. The reduced form (GSH) becomes readily oxidized (GSSG) on interacting with free radicals. GSSG is then reduced by the appropriate enzyme and becomes available again for further scavenging of free radicals [36, 49].

Glutathione participates in detoxication reactions of electrophilic substances, such as carcinogen-peroxide metabolites and certain drugs by conjugation between nucleophilic thiol of glutathione and an electrophilic site on another molecule. Hydrogen peroxide and lipid peroxides are also detoxified by reduced glutathione. Both types of reactions can occur chemically and enzymatically. In mammals GSH conjugates are often further metabolized by hydrolysis and N-acetylation, either in gut or in the kidney, to give N-acetylcysteinyl conjugates known as mercapturic acids which are excreted in the urine [10].

The importance of GSH conjugation in the detoxication of a xenobiotic depends on the extent to which the xenobiotic is metabolized to electrophiles. The generation of a soft, but not weak electrophile should lead to high levels of GSH conjugation. Several suggestive correlations between increased GSH content and enhanced resistance to cell injury have been drawn. GSH itself is a late preventive agent against CCl_4 hepatotoxicity [18, 20]. An inereased lipid peroxidation has been reported after chronic ethanol feeding and it has been suggested that this could be partly related to the depletion of liver glutathione.

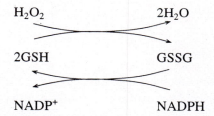

Detoxication of hydrogen peroxide by the glutathione redox cycle.

The enhancement of hepatotoxicity by GSH depletion has been noted during the metabolism of several compounds. GSH is rapidly depleted by bromobenzene [79], paraquat [24]. Exogenous glutathione protects intestinal epithelial cells from oxidative injury caused by t-butyl hydroperoxide or menadione [4]. The ability of cadmium and other heavy metals to interact with SH groups is widely appreciated and has been reviewed [14]. A sulfydryl carrier may be involved in cadmium uptake by hepatocytes. Furthermore, protection can be afforded at an extracellular level even after intracellular exposure to toxic concentrations of cadmium [75]. Rana and Verma [63] hypothesized that GSH fuctions as a cadmium chlelator. Naganuma et al [46] suggested that methylmercury is transported into the kidney as a complex with GSH, and then incorporated into the renal cells after degradation of the GSH moiety by γ-glutamyl transpeptidase and dipeptidase, although the methyl mercury bound to extracellular GSH can be reversibly transferred to plasma proteins in the blood-stream. It is concluded that the mode of antioxidant action of GSH in the heterogenous bilayer/aqueous system is due to reaction with the initiating aqueous peroxyl radicals

$$GSH + ROO^*(aq) \rightarrow GS^* + ROOH^*$$

GSH and vitamin E function separately in the prevention of peroxidation of liver microsomes.

Metabolic Zonation with Special Reference to GSH

There is mounting evidence that many metabolic processes are heterogenously distributed within the liver acinus [80]. The metabolism of xenobiotics also appears to be zonally distributed. The activation of numerous xenobiotics to potentially toxic metabolites predominates in the perivenous region of the acinus owing to higher activities of the microsomal mixed function oxidase enzymes as compared with the periportal region. There are some reports that the content of GSH is lower in the perivenous region of the acinus. Kera et al [34] suggested that cells from the perivenous region accumulate GSH more slowly, and to a lower final content, then do cells from the periportal region.

They suggest that there are constitutive differences between the cell types with respect to glutathione metabolism. Under certain conditions the rate of production of reactive intermediates exceeds the capacity of perivenous hepatocytes for glutathione mediated detoxication. The resulting imbalance may contribute to the greater vulnerability of the hepatic perivenous region to chemical damage.

Ascorbic Acid

In comparison to glutathione, the action of ascorbate in preventing damage from oxygen derived free radicals in biological systems in less well understood. However, interactions between α-tocopherol and ascorbate and glutathione and ascorbate are well known. α-tocopherol reacts with OH or lipid peroxyl radicals (LOO) to from a long lived α-tocopheroxyl radical which can be reduced back to α-tocopherol by ascorbate which in turn is transformed into ascorbyl radical. By this mechanism, a high concentration of α-tocopherol is maintained at the expense of ascorbate [48].

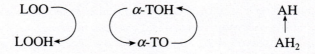

Where α-TOH is α-tocopherol, α-To is α-tocopheroxyl radical, LOOH is lipid-hydroperoxide, LOO is lipid peroxyl radical, AH_2 is ascorbate and AH is ascorbyl radical.

Similarly, glutathione and ascorbic acid can function in the destruction of reactive oxygen compounds. Glutathione functions in the reduction of hydrogen peroxide and other peroxides in reactions catalyzed by the glutathione peroxidase. Ascorbic acid can also iteract with hydrogen peroxide and other forms of reactive oxygen. Reaction of hydrogen peroxide with ascorbic acid is catalysed by an enzyme ascorbic acid peroxidase. Although ascorbate peroxidase has been known to occur in plant tissue, possibly animal tissue also contain ascorbate acid peroxidase activity.

Thus glutathione (and other thiols) can replace ascorbic acid in several

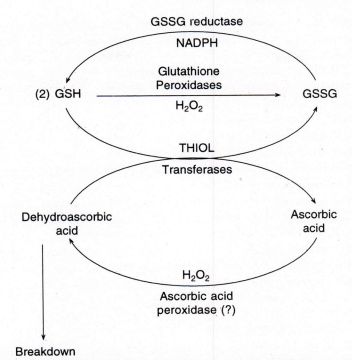

Fig. 2. Destruction of peroxides and related active oxygen forms by ascorbic acid and glutathione (GSH). Glutaredoxin and protein disulfide isomerase catalyze GSH-dependent reduction of dehydroascorbate. GSSG-glutathione disulfide.

hydroxylation reactions [16]. Administration of ascorbic acid can increase the availability of glutathione for various functions by sparing the glutathione requirement for the reduction of dehydroascorbic acid. Similarly the increased availability of glutathione in glutathione monoester treated ascorbic acid deficient guinea pigs may increase efficiency of recovery of dehydro ascorbic acid and thus the availability of ascorbic acid.

Ascorbic acid is an electron donor and reacts with superoxides and hydroxyl ions. The concentration of this water soluble vitamin has been reported to be low in certain pathological conditions like cancer, diabetes and alcoholic liver disease [73].

B Vitamins and Vitamin-Like Compounds

Several vitamins including vitamin C, E and β-carotene are known anti-oxidants that may protect against human disease and aging. However, a vitamin may function as a pro-oxidant depending on the availability of metal ions [26].

Hu et al [30] investigated the antioxidant and/or pro-oxidant activities of some B-vitamins (B-vit) and vitamin like compounds (VLC) including the thymine hydrochloride, nicotinic acid, pyridoxal, pyridoxins, calcium pantothenate, choline chloride, carnitine and myo-inositol. They have reported that microsomal lipid peroxidation induced by $FeCl_3$/ascorbate was inhibited in a concentration dependent manner by pentothenate and pyridoxal. In contrast, thiamin, pyridoxine and carnitine enhanced lipid peroxidation dose-dependently with pyridoxine being most effective.

Combined Effects of Antioxidants

Studies indicate that a combination of individual antioxidants could significantly reduce the oxidative damage to animal tissues [40].

A combination of vitamin E, selenium and β-carotene gave a high protective effect of heme proteins against oxidative damage. However, it is not clear whether the improvement of protective effect is due to the synergism among the antioxidants or the additive effect from the individual antioxidants. However, tocopherol and ascorbate are synergistic antioxidants in many *in vitro* models of lipid peroxidation. Further more GSH-dependent α-tocopherol regeneration remains an attractive hypothesis. Still more definitive answers are needed ragarding the possible metabolic participation of GSH in α-tocopherol redox cycles.

Gender Related Differences

There may be species specific, tissue specific and gender specific differences in the expression and characteristic of antioxidant enzymes. Three distinct classes of glutathione-S-transferases (GST EC 2.5.1.18) isozymes (α, μ and π) have long been recognized by several workers. Significant qualitative and quantitative gender specific differences in α, μ and π class of GST isozymes have been reported in mouse liver (Singhal et al, 1992). Variations in GST isozymes expression may determine tissue susceptibility to carcinogens and xenobiotics.

Species specific differences in the liver of fresh water fish *Channa punctatus* and *Clarias batrachus* were studied by Rana and Singh [64]. They concluded that the fish having higher activity can withstand oxidative stress more effectively.

Oxidative Injury and DNA

There is abundant evidence suggesting that DNA damage by endogenous free radicals does occur and accumulate *in vivo*. It has been estimated that genome of a human cell receives around 10^4 oxidative hits/day on an average and this process is likely to be critical for both cancer and ageing [82].

Under physiological conditions, neither O_2 nor H_2O_2 appear to produce modifications in DNA unless metal ions are present in the system. Thus much of the toxicity of O_2 and H_2O_2 is thought to result from their metal ion catalyzed conversion into the highly reactive $\cdot OH$. In normal cells a primary defence against oxidative damage is provided by antioxidants such as glutathione as well as DNA repair enzymes that participate in the excision repair process. However, these defence mechanisms can be subverted by xenobiotics that induce the production of excessive or untimely free radicals and result in damage to macromolecules, including DNA.

Two explanations of the DNA damage have been advanced. Mello-Filho et al [43] proposed that damage is due to OH radical formation. They envisaged that H_2O_2 which crosses biological membranes easily, can penetrate the nucleus and react with the iron and/or copper ions to form ·OH. Because of the high reactivity of ·OH and its resultant unability to diffuse significant distances within the cell (Halliwell and Gutteridge, 1990a), this mechanism is only feasible if the ·OH is generated from H_2O_2 by reaction with metal ions bound upon or very close to the DNA. A second possibility is that metal ions are released within the cell as a result of oxidative stress and then bind to DNA. Thus just as oxidative stress causes rises in intracellular free Ca^{++} [51], it may cause rises in intracellular free iron and/or copper ions by interfering with normal intracellular sequestration mechanisms. Some of these released ions may then bind to DNA and make it a target for oxidative damage.

Furthermore, the second explanation on the effect of oxidative stress on DNA damage is that stress triggers a series of metabolic events within the cell that leads to activation of nuclease enzymes that cleave the DNA backbone. Much has been written [17] that oxidative stress causes rises in intracellular free Ca^{++} which fragment DNA by activating Ca^{++} dependent endonucleases in a mechanism resembling apoptosis.

Both these mechanisms are not exclusive i.e. they both could take place. Menadione and other quinones appear to produce breaks in DNA strands in hepatocytes by Ca^{++} dependent activation of an endonuclease.

Oxidative stress imposed by a variety of chemicals and by a variety of mechanisms has been convincingly shown to be mutagenic to bacteria as well as mammalian cells [29]. Mutations induced by oxidative stress may lead to cancer. Low level of damage may be efficiently repaired with a minimal risk of error [7]. High levels of oxidative stress may lead to cell death.

For nuclear DNA, however the mammalian cells has three more levels of defence. First nuclear DNA is compartmentalized away from mitochondria and peroxisomes, where most oxidants are probably generated. Second, most nonreplicating nuclear DNA is surrounded by histones and polyamines that may protect against oxidants. Finally most types of DNA damage can be repaired by efficient enzyme systems. The net result of this multilevel defense is that nuclear DNA is very well protected but not completely protected from oxidants.

Conclusion

Oxidative stress, that is now known as a disturbance in the pro-oxidant-antioxidant balance in favour of the former, can induce damage to almost all bio-molecules. The use of model compounds to generate oxidative stress and a study on anti-oxidant defense capacity of selected compounds in the liver as discussed in foregoing pages help us to draw certain conclusions.

Processes disturbed by oxidative stress include calcium movements, modification of enzyme activities, formation of mixed disulphides with glutathione, damage to DNA and formation of excited species. In addition to the enzymatic defense mechanism, the role of nonenzymatic anti-oxidants (vit. E, ascorbate, vit. A. glutathione, selenium) cannot be ignored. A study on the combined effects of antioxidants seems attractive. Further, information on GST isozymes might be helpful in the elucidation of protective mechanisms. Species differences, gender differences, metabolic zonation of GSH and GSH dependent enzymes thus discussed suggest that liver possesses differential ability to detoxify various xenobiotics including carcinogens. The work is in progress in many laboratories and hepatocytes serve as a best model to study oxidative stress.

Acknowledgments

The work was supported by funds received from Council of Scientific and Industrial Research, University Grants Commission and Indian Council of Agriculture Research, New Delhi.

References

1. Albro, P.W., Corbett, J.T. and Schroeder, J.L. 1986. Generation of hydrogen peroxide by incidental metal ion catalyzed autooxidation of glutathione. *J. Inorg. Biochem.*, 27, 191–203.
2. Alleman, M.A., Koster, J.F., Wilson, J.H.P., Edixhoven Bosdijk, A., Slee, R.G., Kross, M.J. and Eijk, H.G.V. 1985. The involvement of iron and lipidperoxidation in the pathogenesis of HCB induced prophyria. *Biochem. Pharmacol.*, 34, 161–166.
3. Ames, B.M. 1993. Dietary carcinogens and anticarcinogens, oxygen radicals and degenerative diseases. *Science.*, 221, 1256–1264.
4. Andreoli, S.P., Mallett, C.P. and Berystein, J.M. 1986. Role of glutathione in protecting endothelial cells against hydrogen peroxide oxidant injury *J. Lab. Clin Med.*, 108, 190–198.
5. Bellomo, G., Jewell, S.A., Thor, H. et al, 1982. Regulation of calcium compartmentation in the hepatocyte studies with isolated hepatocytes and t-butyl-hydroperoxide. *Proc. Nat. Acad. Sci.* USA., 799, 6842–6846.
6. Bellomo, G., Thor, H. and Orrenius, S. 1984. Increase in cytosolic Ca^{2+} concentration during t-butyl hydroperoxide metabolism by isolated hepatocytes involves NADPH oxidation and mobilization of intracellular Ca^{2+} stores. *FEBS Lett.*, 168, 38–42.
7. Breimer, L.H. 1991. Repair of DNA damage induced by reactive oxygen species. *Free Radical Res. Commun.*, 14, 159.
8. Calvert, D.N. and Brody, T.M. 1960. Role of sympathetic nervous system in carbontetrachloride hepatotoxicity. *Am. J. Physiol.*, 198, 669–676.

9. Calvert, D.N. and Brody, T.M. 1961. The effects of thyroid function upon carbontetrachloride hepatotoxicity. *J. Pharmacol. Exptl. Therap.*, 134, 310.

10. Chasseaud, L.F. 1976. Conjugation with glutathione and mercapturic acid excretion. In "Glutathione Metabolism and Function." (I.M. Arias and W.B. Jakoby eds). Raven Press New York pp 77–114.

11. Chen, L.H., Hu, N. and Huang, T.L. 1992. Effects of acute alcohol intoxication on liver antioxidant defense systems in rats. *Biochemical Archives.*, 8, 95–100.

12. Chevion, M. 1991. Protection against free radical induced and transition metal mediated damage. The use of "pull" and "push" mechanisms. *Free Radic. Res. Commun.*, 13, 691–699.

13. Chow, K.C. 1991. Vitamin E and oxidative stress. *Free Rad. Biol. Med.*, 11, 215–232.

14. Christie, N.T. and Costa, M. 1984. *In vitro* assessment of toxicity of metal compounds. *Biol. Trace Elem.* Res., 6, 1399–1405.

15. Dillard, C.J. and Tappel, A.L. 1984. Lipid peroxidation and copper toxicity in rats. *Drug Chem Toxicol.*, 7, 477–487.

16. Englard, S. and Seifter, S. 1986. The biochemical functions of ascorbic acid. *Ann. Rev. Nutr.*, 6, 365–406.

17. Farber, J.L. 1990. The role of calcium in lethal cell injury. *Chem. Res. Toxicol.*, 3, 503.

18. Ferreyra, E.C. de., Bernacchi, A.S. and Castro, J.A. 1986. Increased glutathione (GSH) content in livers of control and CCl_4 poisoned rats treated with the anticalmodulin drug trifluoperayine (TFP). *Res Commun. Chem. Path. Pharmacol.*, 53, 399–402.

19. Fukino, H., Hirai, M., Hsuch, Y.M and Yamane, Y. 1984. Effect of zinc pretreatment on mercuric chloride induced lipid peroxidation in rat kidney. *Toxicol. Appl Pharmacol.*, 73, 395–401.

20. Gorla, N., Ferreyra, E.C. de., Villarruel, M.C., Fems, O.M. de. and Castro, J.A. 1983. Studies on the mechanism of glutathione prevention of carbontetrachloride induced liver injury. *Brit. J. Exptl. Pathol.*, 64, 388–395.

21. Grossman, A. and Wendel, A. 1983. Non-reactivity of the selenoenzyme glutathione peroxidase with enzymatically hydroperoxidized phospholipids. *Eur. J. Biochem.*, 135, 549–552.

22. Gustaffson, J.A., Eneroth, P., Hokfelt, T., Mode, A. and Morstedt, G. 1982. Studies on the hypothalomo-pituitary-liver axis: A novel concept in regulation of steroid and drug metabolism. In "The Endocrines and The Liver", Langer, Chiandussi, Chopra and Martini (eds). Academic Press, London & N.Y. pp. 9–34.

23. Hafeman, D.G. and Hoekstra, W.G. 1977. Protection against carbontetrachloride induced lipid peroxidation in rat by dietary vitamin E, selenium and methionine as measured by ethane evolution. *J. Nutr.*, 107, 656–665.

24. Hagen, T.M., Brown, L.A. and Jones, D.P. 1986. Protection against paraquat-induced injury by exogenous GSH in pulmonary alveolar type II cells. *Biochem. Pharmacol.*, 35, 4537–4542.

25. Hoekstra, W.G. 1975a. Biochemical function of selenium and its relation to vitamin E, *Fed. Proc.*, 34, 2083–2089.

26. Halliwell, B. and Gutteridge, J.M.C. 1989. In "Free radicals in biology and medicine," 2nd ed., Clarendon, Oxford.

27. Halliwell, B. 1981. In "Age Pigments", (R.S. Sohal ed.), pp 1–62, Elsevier/North Holland, New York and Amsterdam.

28. Halliwell, B. and Gutteridge, J.M.C. 1990. Role of free radicals and catalytic metal ions in human disease. *Methods Enzymol.*, 186, 1.

29. Halliwell, B. and Aruoma, O.I. 1991. DNA damage by oxygen-derived species. Its mechanism and measurement in mammalian systems. *FEBS Lett.*, 281, 99.

30. Hu, M.L., Chen, Y.K. and Lin, Y.F. 1995. The antioxidant and pro-oxidant activity of some B vitamins and vitamin like compounds. *Chem. Biol. Interaction.*, 97, 63–73.

31. Iwata, H., Masukawa, T., Kitto, H. and Hayashi, M. 1981. Involvement of tissue sulphydryls in the formation of a complex of methyl mercury with selenium. *Biochem. Pharmacol.*, 30, 3159–3163.

32. Jewell, S.A., Bellomo, G., Thor, H. et. al. 1982. Bleb formation in hepatocytes during metabolism is caused by disturbances in thiol and calcium homeostasis. *Science.*, 217, 1257–1259.

33. Jones, D.P., Thor, H., Smith, M.T. et al 1983. Inhibition of ATP dependent microsomal sequestration during oxidative stress and prevention by glutathione *J. Biol. Chem.* 258, 6390–6393.

34. Kera, Y., Penttila, K.E. and Lindros, K.O. 1988. Glutathione replenishment capacity is lower in isolated perivenous than in periportal hepatocytes. *Biochem. J.*, 254, 411–417.

35. Khan, M.F., Srivastava, S.K., Singhal, S.S., Chaubey, M., Awasthi, S., Petersen, D.R., Ansari, G.A.S. and Awasthi, Y.C. 1995. Iron induced lipid peroxidation in rat liver is accompanied by preferential induction of glutathione S-transferase 8-8 isozyme. *Toxicol. Applied Pharmacol.*, 131, 67–72.

36. Kosower, N.S. and Kosower, E.M. 1978. The glutathione status of cells. *Int. Rev. Cytol.*, 54, 109–160.

37. Kumar, S. and Rana, S.V.S. 1988a. Influence of testosterone and pregesterone on fatty liver of rats treated with few halogenalkanes. *Ind. J. Exp. Biol.*, 26, 811–813.

38. Kumar, S. and Rana, S.V.S. 1988b. Influence of sex hormones on serum transaminases during experimental liver injury in rats. *Curr. Sci.*, 20, 1259–1261.

39. Lehningr, A.L., Vercesi, A., Bababunmi, E. 1978. Regulation of Ca^{++} release from mitochondria by the oxidation-reduction state of pyridine nucleotides. *Proc. Nat. Acad. Sci.*, USA. 75, 1690–1694.

40. Leibovitz, B., Hu, M.L. and Tappel, A.L. 1990. Dietary supplements of Vitamin E, *b*-carotene, coenzyme Q 10 and selenium protect tissues against lipid peroxidation in rat tissue slices, *J. Nutr.*, 120, 97–104.

41. Levin, W., Wood, A.W., Lu, A.Y.H., Ryan, D., West, S., Conney, A.H., Thakker, D.R., Yagi, H. and Jerina, D.M. 1977. Role of purified cytochrome P-448 and epoxide hydrase in the activation and detoxication of benzo (o) pyrene. In Jerina, "Drug metabolism concepts, ACS symposium series No. 44", Jerina D.M. (ed), pp. 99–125.

42. Maki, A, Berezesky, I.K., Farejnoli, J. Holbrook, N.J. and Trump, B.F. (1992). Role of $(Ca^{2+})i$ in induction of c-fos, c-jun, and c-myc m-RNA in rat PTE after oxidative stress *FASEB, J.*, 6, 919–924.

43. Mello-Filho, A.C., Hoffman, R.E. and Meneghimi, R. 1984. Cell killing and DNA damage by hydrogen peroxide are mediated by intracellular iron. *Biochem. J.*, 218, 273.

44. Nebert, D.W. and Negishi, M. 1982. Multiple forms of cytochrome P.450 and the importance of moleculr biology and evolution. *Biochem. Pharmacol.*, 31, 2311–2317.

45. Meister, A. 1983. Selective modification of glutathione metabolism. *Science*, 220, 472–477.

46. Minotti, G. and Aust, S.D. 1987. The role of iron in the initiation of lipid peroxidation. *Chem. Phys. Lipid.*, 44, 191–208.

47. Naganuma, A., Vrano, N.O., Tanaka, T. and Imura, N. 1988. Possible role of hepatic glutathione in transport of methylmercury into mouse kidney. *Biochem. Pharmacol.*, 37, 291–296.

48. Niki, E. 1991. Antioxidant compounds. In "Oxidative damage and repair, chemical biological and medical aspects", K.J.A. Davies ed. Elmsford, N.Y. Pergamon Press. pp. 57–64.

49. Niki, E., Saito, T., Kawakami, A. and Kamiya, Y. 1984. Inhibition of oxidation of methyl linoleate in solution by vitamin E and vitamin C. *J. Biol. Chem.*, 259, 4177–4182.

50. Orrenius, S. and Moldeus, P. 1984. The multiple roles of glutathione in drug metabolism. *Trends in Pharmacol Sci.*, 5, 432–435.

51. Orrenius, S. and Nicotera, P. 1987. On the role of calcium in chemical toxicity. *Arch. Toxicol.*, *Suppl.* 11, 11–19.

52. Orrenius, S., Meconkey, D.J., Bellomo, G. and Nicotera, P. 1989. Role of Ca^{++} in toxic cell killing. *Trends Pharmacol Sci.*, 10, 281.

53. Pathiratne, A., Puyear, R.L. and Brammer, J.D. 1986. A comparative study of the effects of benzene, toluene and xylenes on their *in vitro* metabolism and drug metabolizing enzymes in rat liver. *Toxicol. Appl. Pharmacol.*, 82, 272–280.

54. Pavoine, C., Brechler, V., Roche, B., Lotersztajn S. and Pecker, F. 1989. Calcium et hepatotoxicite. *Gastroenterol Clin Biol.*, 13, 720–724.

55. Powell, S.R. and Tortolani, A.J. 1992. Recent advances in the role of reactive oxygen intermediates in ischemic injury. Evidence demonstrating presence of reactive oxygen intermediates. II. Role of metals in site specific formation of radicals. *J. Surg. Res.*, 53, 417–429.

56. Rana, S.V.S. and Kumar, A. 1984. Significance of lipid peroxidation in liver injury after heavy metal poisoning in rats. *Curr. Sci.*, 53, 933–934.

57. Rana, S.V.S. and Kumar, S. 1987a. Effect of sex hormones on lipid peroxidation in the mecrotic liver of rat. *Gegenbaurs morphol. Jahrb. Leipzig.*, 133, 657–663.

58. Rana, S.V.S. and Rastogi, S. 1991. Effect of parathyroidectomy on calcium and phosphoipase A_2 in the liver of carbontetrachloride treated rats. *Physiol. Chem. Phys. and Med. NMR.*, 23, 173–176.

59. Rana S.V.S and Boora, P.R. 1992. Antiperoxidative mechanisms offered by selenium against liver injury caused by cadmium and murcury. *Bull. Env. Cont. and Toxicol.*, 48, 120–124.

60. Rana, S.V.S. and Rastogi, S. 1993. Antioxidative enzyme in the liver of rat treated with carbontetrachloride after perathyroidectomy. *Physiol. Chem. Phys. and med. NMR.*, 25, 41–47.

61. Rana, S.V.S. and Kumar, S. 1994. Lipid-peroxidation in liver, kidney and brain of rats after combined exposure to xylene, toluene and methyl alcohol. *Ind. J. Exp. Biol.*, 32, 919–921.

62. Rana, S.V.S. and Kumar, S. 1995. Antioxidative enzymes in the liver of rats after exposure of tolune, toluene and methyl alcohol separately and in combination. *Physiol. Chem. Phys and Med. NMR.*, 27, 25–29.

63. Rana, S.V.S., Singh, R. and Verma, S. 1995. Mercury induced lipid peroxidation in liver, kidney, brain and gills of a fresh water fish *Channa punctatus.* *Jap. J. Ichthyol.* 42, 255–259.

64. Rana, S.V.S. and Verma, S. 1996. Protective effets of GSH, vitamin E and selenium on lipid peroxidation in cadmium-fed rats. *Biol. Trace. Elem. Res.*, 51, 161–168.

65. Rana, S.V.S. and Singh, R. 1996. Species differences on glutathione dependent enzymes in liver and kidney of two fresh water fish and their implications in cadmium toxicity. *Ichthyological. Res.*, 43, 223–229.

66. Rasmussen, H. 1981. Calcium and c-AMP as synarchic messengers. John Wiley and Sons. N.Y. pp. 370.

67. Recknagel, R.O., Stalder, J. and Litteria, M. 1958. Biochemical changes accompanying development of fatty liver. *Federation Proc.*, 17, 129.

68. Recknagel, R.O. 1983. A new direction in the study of carbontetrachloride hepatotoxicity. *Life Sciences.*, 33, 401–408.

69. Reynolds, E.S. and Moslem, M.T. 1980. Free radical damage in liver. In "Free Radicals in Biology," Pryor, W.A. ed. Academic Press, San Diego, pp. 499.

70. Shafiq-ur-Rehman 1984. Lead induced regional lipid peroxidation in brain. *Toxicol. Lett.*, 21, 233–337.

71. Singhal, S.S., Saxena, M., Awasthi, S., Ahmad, H., Sharma, R. and Awasthi, Y.C. 1992. Gender related differences in the expression and characteristics of glutathione-s-transferases of human colon. *Biochem., Biophys. Acta.*, 1171, 19–26.

72. Sunderman, F.W. Jr., Marzouk, A., Hopfer, S.M., Zaharia, O. and Reid, M.C 1985. Increased lipid peroxidation in tissues of nickel chloride treated rats. *Ann. Clin. Lab. Sci.*, 15, 229–236.

73. Sunderman, F.W. Jr. 1986. Metals and lipid peroxidation. *Acta Pharmacol Toxicol.*, 59 (Suppl 7) 248–255.

74. Sinclair, A.J., Barnett, A.H. and Lunic, J. 1991. Free-radicals and auto-oxidant systems in health and disease. *J. Appl. Med.*, 17, 409.

75. Skaare, J.V. and Nafstad, I, 1978. Interaction of vitamin E and selenium with the hepatotoxic agent dimethylnitrosamine. *Acta Pharmacol. Toxicol.*, 43, 119–128.

76. Stacey, N.H. 1986. The amelioration of cadmium induced injury in isolated hepatocyte by reduced gluthione. Toxicology., 42, 85–93.

77. Stacey, N.H., Cantilena, L.R. Jr. and Klaassen, C.D. 1980. Cadmium toxicity and lipid peroxidation in isolated rat hepatocytes. *Toxicol. Appl. Pharmacol.*, 53, 470–480.

78. Stohs, S.J., Hassan, M.Q. and Murray, W.J. 1984. Effect of BHA, d-tocopherol and retinol acetate on TCDD mediated changes in lipid peroxidation. glutathione peroxidase activity and survival. *Xenobiotica.*, 14, 533–537.

79. Tappel, A.L. 1978. Glutathione peroxidase and hydroperoxides. Methods in Enzymol. L II, Part C, 506–513.

80. Thor, H., Smith, M.T., Hartyell, P. et al 1982. The metabolism of menadione (2-methyl 1-1, 4 naphthoquinone) by isolated hepatocytes. *J. Biol. Chem.* 257, 12419–12425.

81. Thurman, R.G., Kowffman, F.C. and Jungermann, K. (eds). 1986. Regulation of hepatic metabolism: Intra and intercellular compartmentation. Plenum Press, New York, pp. 321–382.

82. Trump. B.F. and Berezesky, I.K. 1992. The role of cytosolic calcium (Ca^{2+}) in cell injury, necrosis and apoptosis. *Curr. opin. Cell. Bol.*, 4, 227–232.

83. Wang, Y.J., Ho, Y.S., Lo M.J. and Lin, J.K. 1995. Oxidative modification of DNA bases in rat liver and lung during chemical carcinogenesis and aging. *Chem. Biol. Interaction.*, 94, 135–145.

84. Yamamoto, N., Maki, A., Swann, J.D., Berezesky, I.K. and Trump, B.F. 1993. Induction of immediate early and stress genes in rat proximal tubular epithelium following injury. The significance of cytosolic ionized calcium. *Ren. Fail.*, 15. 163–171.

Liver and Environmental Xenobiotics
S.V.S. Rana and K. Taketa (Eds)
Copyright © 1997, Narosa Publishing House, New Delhi, India

11. Experimental Hepatocarcinogenesis and Its Prevention

Kiwamu Okita, Isao Sakaida and Yuko Matsuzaki

First Department of Internal Medicine, Yamaguchi University School of Medicine,
Ube, Yamaguchi-Pref., 755, Japan

Introduction

In Japan, hepatocellular carcinoma (HCC) is mainly caused by viruses such as HBV and HCV. Twenty cases per 100,000 population suffer from HCC.

A close association between HCC and food contaminated with aflatoxin B_1 has been noted in Far East Asia. These are called as aflatoxin-type HCC. Therefore environmental hepatocarcinogens pose a serious threat to human health.

Experimental hepatocarcinogenesis using small animals as model has allowed the monitoring of sequential changes in the liver during hepatocarcinogenesis. Therefore, a study on hepatocarcinogenesis in rats fed on 2-acetylaminofluorene (AAF) or a choline defficient L-amino acid-defined (CDAA) diet was followed.

This chapter would focus on natural history of neoplastic development during hepatocarcinogenesis and its prevention by chemicals.

Hepatocarcinogens and Their Metabolism

Table 1 shows that there are a number of chemicals that can induce liver cancer in animals. Most hepatocarcinogenesis do not appear to be by carcinogens per se, but by metabolically converted highly reactive derivatives, so-called ultimate carcinogens [1]. All such reactive compounds have been found to be positively charged "electrophilic reactants" or free radicals that can react with many nucleophilic groups found in the macromolecules (DNA, RNA, protein) and small molecular weight compounds in many different organelles of the target cells [2].

We have used AAF or CDAA diet as the hepatocarcinogen. Metabolism of each carcinogen will be shown briefly.

(1) 2–Acetylaminofluorene

Metabolism of AAF consists of alternative pathways one leading to activation and the other to inactivation (Fig. 1). Activated carcinogen, N-hydroxy-

Table 1.   Representative hepatocarcinogens in experimental animals [2]*

A. Natural Occurring
    Aflatoxins
    Sterigmatocystin
    Pyrrholizidine alkaloids
    Cycasin and its aglycon
    Safrole
    Griseofulvin
    Luteoskyrin
    Tannic acids
    Thiourea

B. Nitr
    Dimethylnitrosoamine
    Diethylinitrosamine
    N-Nitropsomorpholine
    N-Nitrosopiperidine
    N-nitrosodihydrohydrourouracil

C. Aromatic Amines
    p-Dimethylaminoazobenzene
    o-Aminoazotoluene
    2-Acetylaminofluorene
    m-Toluenediamine
    2-Anthramine

D. Chlorinated Hydrocarbones
    Carbon tetrachloride
    Chloroform

E. Miscellaneous
    Ethionine
    Aramite
    Thioacetamide
    Acetamide
    Hycanthone
    Urethan
    7, 12-Dimethylbebzanthracene
    3-Hydroxyxanthine
    Dieldrin
    Polychlorophenols
    Choline-defficint L-amino acid-defined
    diet

*Partially modified by authors.

2AAF induces double strand breaks in DNA with repair shortly after. Initiation is induced in hepatocytes by an activated from of carcinogen, presumably via interaction with DNA. These initiated hepatocytes have capacity to grow and are resistant to necrotic agents [2]. This resistance may be due to a loss of cytochrome p-450 activity in the initiated cells [3]. The clonal expansion of the initiated hepatocytes leads to the formation of nodules which are called hyperplastic nodules.

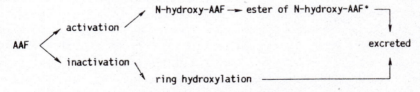

*Ester form of N-hydroxy-AAF interacts with various cell constituents.

Fig. 1.   Metabolism of AAF.

(2) Choline-Deficient L-Amino Acid-Defined (CDAA) Diet

The nuclear lipid peroxidation induced by the CDAA diet is followed shortly by some change in liver DNA that makes the DNA smaller than control DNA on alkaline sucrose gradient centrifugation [4]. The DNA change, like the nuclear lipid peroxidation, is prevented by extra Ca^{2+} and by the administration of free radical scavengers, i.e. tertnitrosobutane and N-p-methoxyphenylacetyl-dehydroalanine [5].

Neoplastic Development

Since the original discovery of an experimental model of liver carcinogenesis with o-aminoazotoluene (4-amino-2', 3-dimethylazobenzene) by Sasaki and Yoshida [6], focal proliferative areas of liver cells termed "hyperplastic nodules" (Fig. 2) have received major attention as ultimate precursors of cancer [7, 8, 9]. In addition to histological characterisitcs, phenotypic expression seen in hyperplastic nodules is different from normal hepatocytes. Presence of following markers in the nodules such as α-fetoprotein [10], epoxide hydrolase [11, 12] and HAM 7 [13] which could not be detected immunohistochemically in the normal liver provide experimental evidence. Moreover, Sato and co-workers discovered placenta form of glutathione-S tranferase (GST-p) (see Fig. 13) to be very specific marker for hyperplastic nodules [14].

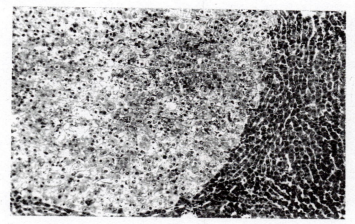

Fig. 2. **Hyperplastic liver nodule seen in the early stage of hepatocarcinogenesis. Hyperplastic nodule is composed of proliferating larger hepatocytes with a ground glass like cytoplasm and a large nucleoli. Note hyperplastic nudule is distinctly different from cirrhotic nodule. (H-E stain, × 240).**

Interestingly, an apparently similar type of hyperplastic lesion has been suggested as a precursor of liver cancer in human cirrhosis [15, 16, 17] (Fig. 3).

There are at least two types of hyperplastic nodules; an early reversible nodules and a later irreversible nodules. When we observed morphological changes in the liver of rats fed intermittently AAF-containing diet by the method of Epstein et al (Fig. 4) [18] by the 13th week, many large-sized hyperplastic nodules could not be seen on the surface of the liver (Fig. 5). However, shift to the basal diet after the 13th week reduced remarkably the

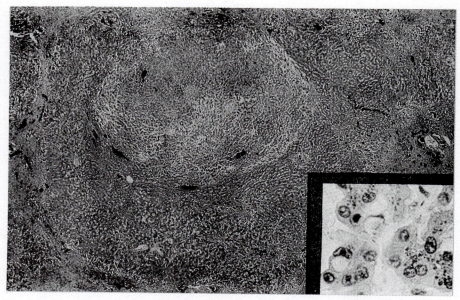

Fig. 3. Adenomatous hyperplasia seen in the patient of liver cirrhosis. Proliferating small hepatocytes with large nuclei form a nodule. Adenomatous hyperplasis has been focused as one of ultimate precursor lesion, because well-differentiated HCC are often included in this lesion. (H-E stain, × 120).

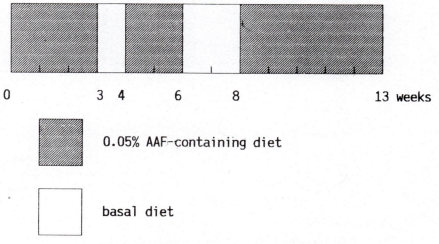

Fig. 4. Feeding protocol of 0.05 AAF-containing diet [18].

number of hyperplastic nodules. By the 25th week liver cancer could be detected (Fig. 6). Mechanism of its reversibility has been unclear. There is an observation that apoptosis in the regressing livers is at least as frequent in such hyperplastic nodules as it is in surrounding tissues [19]. That is, apoptosis could act to reduce the cellular balance in foci.

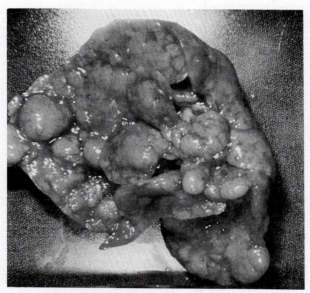

Fig. 5. Gross appearance of the liver of a rat killed at 13th week of hepatocarcinogenesis. Many large to small nodules are seen on the liver surface.

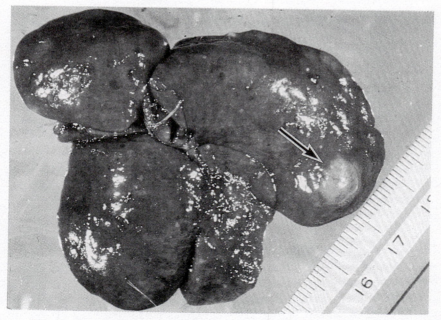

Fig. 6. Gross appearance of the liver of a rat killed at 25th week of hepatocarcinogenesis. A white nodule indicated by arrow is seen on the liver surface. Histological study revealed moderately differentiated HCC. Note large hyperplastic nodules observed in the early stage of carcinogenesis have almost disappeared.

Histology of a late hyperplastic nodule seen between the 13th and the 25th week during hepatocarcinogenesis shows accumulation of fat in the hepatocytes, thin trabecular arrangements of small hepatocytes and increased N/C ratio with dense chromatin (Fig. 7).

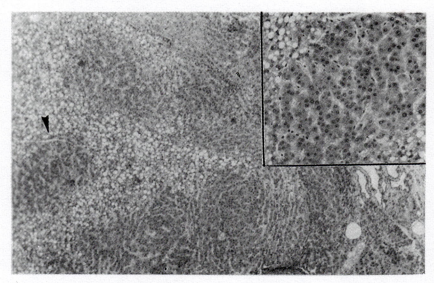

Fig. 7. Hyperplastic liver nodule seen in the late stage of hepatocarcinogenesis Nodule is composed of small hepatocytes. Note increase of N/C ratio, thin trabecular arrangement and remarkable fatty deposit of the hepatocytes. Those features are similar to atypical adenomatous hyperplasia which has been recognized to be a boaderline lesion between HCC and precancerous lesion in men (H-E stain, ×120 and ×240).

Hepatocarcinogenesis with CDAA diet is quite different from that with AAF or other aromatic amines. In the rats fed AAF liver cirrhosis was never observed and HCC appeared in the non-cirrhotic liver. On the other hand, in the rats fed CDAA diet at first fatty liver appeared and subsequently hyperplastic nodules and HCC appeared in the cirrhotic liver (Figs. 8 and 9).

The natural history of neoplastic development during hepatocarcinogenesis is shown in Fig. 10.

Inhibition of Hepatocarcinogenesis with Chemicals

According to Williams, there are two fundamental types of prophylaxis; one is causation prophylaxis, in which the causative agent is reduced or eliminated, often through behavioural changes and other is interventive prophylaxis, in which and agent is administered to deter the effects of carcinogen exposure [20]. An interventive agent interrupts either the first step of carcinogenesis i.e. conversion of normal hepatocytes to neoplastic cells or the second step i.e. conversion of neoplastic population to cancer.

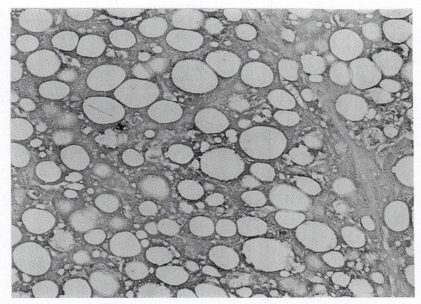

Fig. 8. Fatty deposition seen in the hepatocytes of rat ingested CDAA for one month. Large fatty droplets are seen in all hepatocytes (H-E stain, ×240).

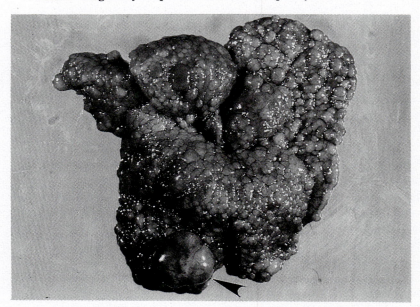

Fig. 9. Gross appearance of the rat liver ingested CDAA diet for one year. Cancer nodule (arrow) is observed on the surface of cirrhotic liver.

Inhibitors of chemical hepatocarcinogenesis in rodents are summarized in Table 2. Among them, 3-methylcholanthrene [21]. β-naphtoflavone [22]

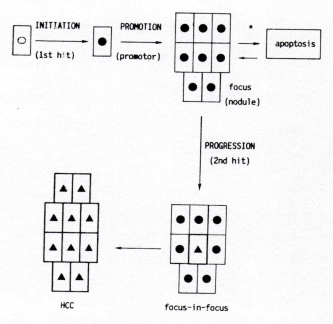

*Removal of promoting agent leads majority of cells to death. Therefore, nonodules show normal appearance of hepatocytes during remodeling process, whereas those escaped from cell death may have a proliferative activity.

Fig. 10.   Natural history of neoplastic development during hepatocarcinogenesis.

and phenobarbital [23] are inducers of detoxification of carcinogens, whereas selenium [24], p-methoxybenzeneselenol [25], benzylselenocyante [26] and acetaminophene [27] are known to be inhibitors of activation of carcinogens. Antioxidants are classified as agents that block carcinogen effects [28, 29, 30].

It seems that suppressive agents for neoplastic development are important for us because they might be applied to chemoprevention of the HCC in humans. Retinoids, derivatives of vitamin A, have been found to inhibit cancer development in a veriety of tissues including liver [31, 32, 33, 34]. Particularly, Muto et al [32] and our group [33] have revealed independently that E5166 (3,7,11,15-tetramethyl-2,4,6,10,14-hexadecapentaenoic acid), a new synthetic vitamin A derivative, inhibited induction of liver tumors and hyperplastic nodules in rats fed 3′-Me-DAB and AAF.

Recently, we could find 2 agents which blocked induction of hyperplastic nodules and also HCC in the rats. Briefly, their pharmacological actions will be discussed.

Sho-saiko-to (Xiao-chai-hu-tang)

Sho-saiko-to is traditional Chinese medicine which contains spray-dried aqueous extracts of seven kings of herbs, as follows; Bepleurum fulcatum

Table 2. **Representative inhibitors of chemical hepatocarcinogens in experimental animals**

Inhibitor	Carcinogen	Reference
A. Inducers of detoxification		
3-Methylcholanthrene	3'-Me-DAB	[21]
β-Naphthoflavone	AFB_1	[22]
Phenobarbital	AFB_1	[23]
B. Inhibitors of activation		
Selenium	3'-Me'-DAB	[24]
p-Methoxybenzeneselenol	Azoxymethane	[25]
Benzylselenocyanate	Azoxymethane	[26]
Acetaminophene	AAF	[27]
C. Antioxidants		
Butylated hydroxyanisole	AFB_1	[28]
Butylated hydroxytoluene	AAF	[29]
Vitamin E	DEN	[30]
D. Retinoids		
13-cis-Retinoic acid	3'-Me'-DAB	[31]
E5166	3'-Me'-DAB	[32]
	Solt & Farber Model	[33]
Retinyl acetate	3'-Me'-DAB	[34]
E. Others		
Sho-sakio-to	AAF	[39]
	n-Nitrosomorpholine	[42]
HOE 077	CDAA	[45]

3'-Me'-DAB: 3'-methyl-4-dimethylaminoazobenzene, AFB_1: aflatoxin B_1 DEN: diethylnitrosamine.

L., Pinellia ternata Ten. et Breit., Scutellaria baiclensis Georg., Zizyphus vulgaris Lamk., Panax ginseng Meyer, Glycyrrhiza glabra L., and Zingiber officinale Rosc. It has been reported that Sho-saiko-to can protect livers from injury [35], accelerate the hepatic regeneration after partial hepatectomy [36] and modify host immune response so as to combat against cancers [37]

These pieces of evidence have led Sho-saiko-to to be used in treating chronic liver diseases in Japan. Interestingly, a controlled study conducted to evaluate the potential of Sho-saiko-to for preventing HCC in patients with liver cirrhosis has found that treatment with Sho-saiko-to prevented or delayed the induction of HCC [38]. However, mechanism of cancer prevention with Sho-saiko to is still unknown. Therefore, the chemopreventive effect of this compound on hepatocarcinogenesis was investigated using rats fed AAF [39, 40, 41].

1. Sho-saiko-to and Prevention of Chemical Carcinogenesis in Rat
As shown in Fig. 11, ninety male Wistar rats were distributed in three

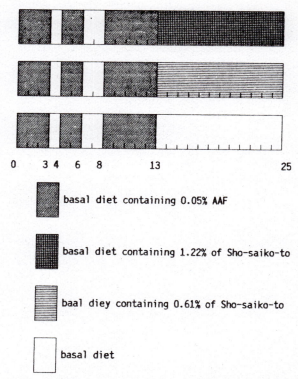

0   3 4   6   8   13   25

■ basal diet containing 0.05% AAF

▨ basal diet containing 1.22% of Sho-saiko-to

▤ baal diey containing 0.61% of Sho-saiko-to

☐ basal diet

**Fig. 11.   Experimental design for administration of Sho-saiko-to
to rats fed a diet containing AAF.**

groups. All animals were fed a basal diet containing 0.05% AAF, with
intermittent intervals of a basal diet alone, as previously described by Epstein
et al [18]. Starting from 14th week, the control animals were fed a basal
diet alone for additional 12 weeks, whereas animals in gorup A were fed
a basal diet containing 1.22% Sho-saiko-to (kindly gifted by Tsumura Co.,
Tokyo, Japan), and animals in group B received a basal diet containing
0.61% Sho-saiko-to. Animals from all the three groups were sacrificed at
the end of the 25th week.

Comparative histology of the liver reveled that the degree of inhibition
of development of liver fibrosis, hyperplastic nodule and HCC depended
on the dose of Sho-saiko-to (Table 3) [39]. Tatsuta et al also got similar
results in n-nitrosomorpholine-treated rats [42].

2. Pharmacologic Action of Sho-saiko-to for Chemoprevention

As mentioned above, Sho-saiko-to is composed of spray-dried aqueous
extracts of seven kinds of herbs and the main components are classified into
two families: saponins, such as saikosaponin, ginsenoside and glycyrrhizine,
and flavonoids, such as baicalein, baicalin and wogonin. Therefore, we
studied the proliferation of human HCC-derived cultured cell line, HuH-7,

Table 3. **Effects of HOE on inhibitions of liver fibrosis and GST-p positive Foci**

Treatments	Hydroxyproline (μg/g wet wt) (Rat #)	No. of Foci/cm^2 (Rat #)
CDAA	938 ± 136 (20)	13.2 ± 8.3 (30)
CDAA/HOE 077[1]		9.8 ± 5.3 (30)
CDAA/HOE077[2]		9.6 ± 6.4 (30)
CDAA/HOE 077[3]	642 ± 75[a] (20)	9.8 ± 4.7 (30)[a]

[1]CDAA diet with HOE 077 concentrations of 50 ppm.
[2]CDAA diet with HOE 077 concentrations of 100 ppm.
[3]CDAA diet with HOE 077 concentrations of 200 ppm.
[a]CDAA/HOE 077 (3) vs CDAA, $P \leq 0.01$.

using each of six purified components of Sho-saiko-to, namely baicalein, baicalin, saikosaponin-a, saikosaponin-c, ginsenoside Rb1, ginsenoside Rg1 and glycyrrhizine [40]. Different concentrations of the above six chemicals were added to the culture media, and changes of the growth curve were assayed by counting the number of cells every 24 hrs using a Coulter counter. Among the six chemicals tested, baicalein, baicalin and saikosaponin-a showed a dose dependent inhibitory effect on the growth curves of HuH-7 cells (Fig. 12). Cell kinetics revealed that baicalein and baicalin elongated the total cell cycle time without changing the relative rates among G_1, S and G_2M phase, whereas saikosaponin-a was regarded as cell-killing rather than an inhibitory agent. Recently, we found that baicalein could induce apoptosis in some human HCC derived cells, particularly in the cells in which mutation of p53 was not observed. These results indicate that Sho-saiko-to might act directly on the proliferation of cells and inhibited their growth.

Interestingly, no effect of baicalein on primary cultured rat hapatocytes was observed,

Recently, Yano et al found Sho-saiko-to itself inhibited the growth of human HCC-derived cultured cell line (Kim-1) [43]. Therefore, there is no doubt that Sho-saiko-to has a potent growth inhibitory effect on cancer cells. If Sho-saiko-to can mutate those cells that grow as hyperplastic nodules, action of Sho-saiko-to for chemoprerntion can be understood. However, we have not yet developed a suitable methods to study this effect of Sho-saiko-to on cancer cels and normal hepatocytes.

However, our results together with those of other investigations, might provide some scientific bases for better understanding the mechanism of chemoprevention of hepatocarcinogenesis with Sho-saiko-to, both in humans and animals.

Prolyl 4-Hydroxylase Inhibitor

A new prolyl 4-hydroxylase inhibitor, 2.4-pyridine dicarboxylic acid bis(2-methoxyethyl amide) (HOE 077) has been designed as a pro-drug for treatment

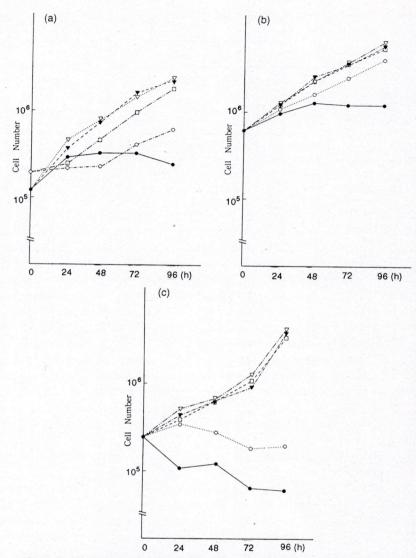

Fig. 12. Growth curves of HuH-7 cells treated with (a) 1 (□), 10 (○) or 50 (●) μg/ml baicalein, (b) 2 (□), 20 (○) or 100 (●) μg/ml baicalin and (c) 15 (□), 30 (○) or 50 (●) μg/ml saikosaponin-a. As the control study, HuH-7 cells were cultured with (∇) or without (▲) addition of (a) 0.5 and (b) and (c) 0.25 μml DMSO [40].

of liver fibrosis. It could significantly prevent the liver fibrosis induced by CCl_4 in rats [44] CDAA diet leads to the development of liver cirrhosis in 100% of male rats after 16 weeks and subsequently causes liver cancer [5]. Therefore, we examined whether HOE077 could prevent liver fivrosis and induction of enzyme altered foci in the liver wich correspond to putative premalignant lesions. Enzyme altered foci were detected to be GST-p positive foci (Fig. 13) which have been used as a marker of preneoplastic lesions.

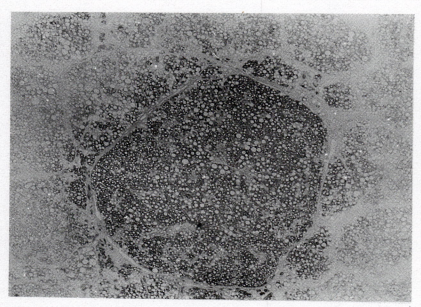

Fig. 13. GST-p positive focus. Hyperplastic liver nodules are always positive for GST-p. The GST-p positive focus was stained immunohistochemically using monoclonal antibody against GST-p. (ABC method, × 120).

Briefly, eight experimental groups consisting of 20-30 rats each for assessing the effect of HOE (Courtesy: Hechst, Germany) on hydroxyproline content and hepatocarcinogenesis. Four groups of 20 rats received a CDAA diet with HOE 077 concentrations of 200, 100, 50 or 0 ppm. For groups of 20 rats received a cholin-supplemented L-amino acid-defined (CSAA) diet at the same concentration of HOE 077. After feeding for 16 weeks, all rats were killed. Hydroxyproline content and frequency of GST-p positive foci were investigated using rat livers which received diets (CSAA). Results are shown in Table 4. In the group fed CDAA diet alone for 16 weeks, many GST-p positive lesions were observed in the liver. On the other hand, HOE 077 reduced, in a dose dependent manner, the number and size, as well as the percent area, of GST-p positive lesions. The inhibition of the formation of GST-p positive lesions by this antifibrous agent finds agreement with hydroxyproline content of the liver. Our results thus suggest that the inhibition of fibrosis may limit the development of liver neoplasms in a CDAA diet model [45].

Conclusion

Chemically induced hepatocarcinogenesis can be treated as a good model for understabding human hepatocarcinogenes is. Moreover, the experimental models introduced here might be useful in studies with the inhibition of HCC.

References

1. Miller, J.A. (1970). Carcinogenesis by chemicals: an overview. GHA Clowes Memrial Lecture. Cancer Res **30:** 559–576.
2. Farber, E. (1976). The pathogenesis of experimental hepatocellular carcinoma. In "Hepatocellular Carcinoma", ed. by K. Okuda & R.L., Peters, A Wiley Medical Publication, New York, pp. 3–22.
3. Okita, K., Noda, K., Fukumoto, Y., Takemoto T. (1976). Cytochrome p-450 in hyperplastic liver nodules during hepatocarcinogenesis with N-2-Fluorenylacetamide in rats. Gann (Jap J Cancer Res) **67:** 899–902.
4. Rushmore, T.H., Farber, E., Ghoshal, A.K., Parodi, S., Pala, Mlk Taningher, M. (1996). A cholin-devoid diet, carcinogenic in the rat, induces DNA damage and repair. Carcinogenesis **7:** 1677–1680.
5. Ghoshal, A.K. and Farber, E. (1993). Cholin deficiency, lipotrope deficiency and the development of liver disease inducing liver cancer: a new perspective. Lab Invest **68:** 255–260.
6. Sasaki, T. and Yoshida, T. (1935). Experimentelle Erzeugung des Lebercarcinoms durch Futterung mit o-amidoazotoluol. Virchows Arch Pathol Anat Physiol **295:**175 –200.
7. Farber, E. (1956). Similarities in the sequence of early histological changes induction the liver of the rat by ethionine, 2-acetylaminofluorene and 3-methy1-4-dimethylaminoazobenezene, Cancer Res **16:** 142–148.
8. Farber, E. (1973). Hyperplastic liver nodules. Methods Cancer Res **7:** 345–373,
9. Farber, E. (1973) Carcinogenesis-cellular evolution as a unifying thread: Presidential address. Cancer Res **33:** 2537–2550.
10. Okita, K., Gruenstein, M., Klaiber, M., Farber, E. (1974). Localization of α-fetoprotein by immunofluorescence in hyperplastic nodules during hepatocarcinogenesis induced by 2-acetylaminofluorene. Cancer Res **34:** 2758–2763.
11. Okita, K., Kligman, L.H., Farber, E. (1975). A new common marker for premalignant and malignant hepatocyte induced in the rat by chemical carcinogenesis. JNCI **54:** 199–202.
12. Ogino, M., Okita, K., Tsubota, W., Numa, Y., Kodama, T., Takemoto, T. (1982). Some biochemical properties of the preneoplastic antigen in rat liver hyperpalstic nudules. Gann (Jap J Cancer Res) **73:** 349–353.
13. Okita, K., Esaki, T., Kurokawa, F., Takemoto, T., Fujicura, Y., Fukumoto, T. (1988). An antigen specific to hyperplastic nodules defined with monoclonal antibody: a new marker for preneoplastic cells in rat chemical carcinogenesis. Tumor Bio **9:** 170–177.
14. Sato, K., Kitahara, A., Soma, Y., Inaba, Y., Hatayama, I., Sato, K., (1985). Purification, induction and distribution of placental glutathione transferase: A new marker enzyme for preneoplastic cells in the rat chemical hepatocarcinogenesis. Proc Natl Acad Sci USA **82:** 3964–3968.
15. Watanabe, S., Okita, K., Harada, T., Kodama, T., Numa, Y., Takemoto, T., Takahashi, M. (1983). Morphologic studies of the liver cell dysplasia. Cancer **51:** 2197–2205.

16. Arakawa, M., Kage, M., Sugihara, S., Nakashima, T., Suenaga, M., Okuda, K. (1986): Emergence of malignant lesions within an adenomatous hyperplastic nodule in a cirrhotic liver: observation in five cases. Gastroenterology **91:** 198–208.

17. Takayama, T., Makuuchi, M., Hirohashi, S., Sakamoto, M., Okazaki, N., Takayasu, K., Kosuge, T., Motoo, Y., Yamazaki, S., Hasegawa, H. (1990). Malignant transformation of adenomatous hyperplasia to hepatocellular carcinoma. Lancet **336:** 1150–1153.

18. Epstein, S.M., Ito, N., Markow, L., Farber, E. (1967). Cellular analysis of liver carcinogenesis: The induction of large hyperplastic nodules in the liver with 2-fluorenylacetamide or ethionine and some aspects of their morphology and glycogen metabolism., Cancer Res **27:** 1702–1711.

19. Bursch, W., Lauer, B., Timmermann-Trosiener, I., Barthel, G., Schuppler, J., Schulte-Hermann, R. (1984). Controlled cell death (apoptosis) of normal and putative preneoplastic cells in rat liver following withdrawal of tumor promoters. Carcinogenesis **5:** 453–458.

20. Williams, G.M. (1994). Interventive prophylaxis of liver cancer. Eur J Cancer Prev **3:** 89–99.

21. Richardson, H.L., Stier, A.R., Borsos-Nachatnebel, C. (1952). Liver tumor inhibition and adrenal histologic responses in rats to which 3-methyl-1,4-methylaminoazobenzene and 3-methylcholanthrene were simultaneously administered. Cancer Res **12:** 356–361.

22. Gurtoo,. H.L., Koser, P.L., Bansal, S.K. (1995). Inhibition of aflatoxin B_1-hepatocarcinogenesis in rats by β-naphthtoflavon. Carcinogenesis **6:** 675–678.

23. McLean, A.E.M. and Marshall, A. (1971). Reduced carcinogenic effects of aflatoxin in rats given phenobarbitone. Br J Exp Pathol **52:** 322–329.

24. Clayton, C.C. and Baumann, C.A. (1949). Diet and azotumors: effect of dietry period when the diet is not fed. Cancer Res **9:** 675–582.

25. Tanaka, T. and Reddy, B.S., El-Bayoumy, K. (1985). Inhibition effect of dietry p-methoxybenzeneselenol of hepatocarcinogenesis induced by azoxymethane in rats. Jap J Cancer Res (Gann) **76:** 462–467.

26. Sugie, S., Reddy, B.S., El-Bayoumy, K., Tanaka, T. (1989). Inhibition by dietry benzylselenocyanate of hepatocarcinogenesis induced by azoxymethane in Fischer 344 rats. Jap J Cancer Res (Gann) **80:** 952–957,

27. Yamamoto, R.S., Williams, G.M., Richardson, H.L., Weisburger, E.K., Weisburger, J.H. (1973). Effect of P-hydroxyacetanilide on liver cancer induction by N-hydroxy-N-2-fluorenylacetamide. Cancer Res **33:** 454–457.

28. Williams, G.M. (1986). Epigenetic promoting effects of butylated hydroxyanisole. Fd Chem Toxicol **24:** 1163–1166.

29. Ulland, B.J., Weisburger, J.H., Yamamoto, R.S., Weisburger, E.K. (1973). Antioxidants and carcinogenesis: butylated hydroxytoluene, but not diphenyl-p-phenylenediamine, inhibits cancer induction by N-2-fluorenylacetamide in rats, Fd Cosmet Toxicol **11:** 199–207.

30. Ura, H., Denda, A., Yokose, Y., Tsutsumi, M., Konishi, Y. (1987). Effect of vitamine E on the induction and evolution of enzyme-altered foci in the liver of rats treated with diethylinitrosamine. Carcinogenesis **8:** 1595–1600.

31. Daoud, A., Griffin, A.C. (1980). Effect of retiomic acid, butylated hydroxytoluene, selenium and sorbic acid on azodye hepatocarcinogenesis. Cancer Lett **9:** 299–304.

32. Muto, Y. and Moriwaki, A. (1984). Antitumor activity of vitamin A and its derivatives. JNCI **73:** 1389–1393.

33. Murata, M., Okita, K., Oka, S., Tanaka, S., Yamamoto, K., Kinukawa. K., Noda, K., Takemoto, T. (1985). Study on the mechanism of inhibition of chemical hepatocarcinogenesis by polyprenoic acid. Acta Hepatol Jpn. **47: 26:** 605–612.

34. Mack, D.O., Reed, V.L., Smith, L.D. (1990): Retinyl acetate inhibition of 3-methyl-4-dimethyl-aminoazobenzene induced hepatic neoplasia. Int J Biochem **22:** 359–365.

35. Abe, H., Sakaguchi, M., Yamada, M., Arichi, S., Odashima, S. (1980). Pharmacological action of saikosaponins isolated from *Bupleunem falcatum* L. (1) Effects if saikosaponins on liver function. Planta Med **40:** 366–372.

36. Usami, S., Duan, Y-S., NIshimatsu, S., Shiraiwa, H., Ohyanagi, H. (1990). Experimental investigation of the effect on hepatectomy with the Pringle method. Kanpo-Igaku **4:** 121–127.

37. Mizoguchi, Y. and Shibata, Y. (1986). The effect of Sho-saiko-to on tumor immunology. Kanpo-Igaku **3:** 58–64.

38. Yamamoto, S., Oka, H., Kanno, T., Mizoguchi, Y., Kobayashi, K., (1989). Controlled prospective trial to evaluate Sho-saiko-to for the prevention of hepatocellular carcinoma in patients with cirrhosis of the liver. Jpn J Cancer Chemother **16:** 1519–1524.

39. Okita, K., Kurokawa, F., Yamazaki, T., Furukawa, T., Li, Q., Murakami, T., Takahashi, M. (1994). The use of Sho-saiko-to (TJ-9) for chemoprevention of chemical hepatocarcinogenesis in rats and discussion of its possible pharmacologic action. J Clin Biotech **1:** 39–44.

40. Okita, K., Li, Q., Murakami, T., Takahashi, M. (1993). Anti-growth effects with components of Sho-saiko-to (TJ-9) on cultured human hepatoma cells. Eur J Cancer Prev **2:** 169–176.

41. Li, Q., Murakami, T., Kimura, Y., Takahashi, M. Okita, K. (1995). Saikosaponin A-induced cell death of a human hepatoma cell line (HuH-7): The significance of the 'sub-G_1 peak' in a DNA histogram. Pathology Int **45:** 207–214.

42. Tatsuta, M., Ishii, H., Baba, M., Nakaizumi, A., Uehara, H. (1991). Inhibition by Xiao-chai-hu-tang (TJ-9) of development of hepatic foci induced by N-nitrosomorpholine in Sprague-Dawley rats. Jap J Cancer Res (Gann) **82:** 987–992.

43. Yano, H., Mizoguchi, A., Fukuda, K., Haramaki, M., Ogasawara, S., Momosaki, S., Kojiro, M. (1994). The herbal medicine Sho-saiko-to inhibits proliferation of cancer cell lines by inducing apoptosis and arrest at the G_0/G_1 phase. Cancer Res **54:** 448–454.

44. Bickel, M., Baader, E., Brocks, D.G., Engelbart, K., Gunzer, V., Schmids, H.L., Vogel, G.H. (1991). Beneficial effects of inhibitors of prolyl 4-hydroxylase in CCl_4-induced fibrosis of the liver in rats. J. Hepatol 13 (Suppl. 3): 26–24.

45. Sakaida, I., Kubota, M., Kayano, K., Takenaka, K., Mori, K., Okita, K. (1994). Prevention of fibrosis reduces enzyme-altered lesions in the rat liver. Carcinogenesis **15:** 2201–2206.

Liver and Environmental Xenobiotics
S.V.S. Rana and K. Taketa (Eds)
Copyright © 1997, Narosa Publishing House, New Delhi, India

12. Oncogene Expression in Liver Injury

**Yutaka Sasaki, Norio Hayashi, Masayoshi Horimoto,
Toshifumi Ito, Hideyuki Fusamoto and Takenobu Kamada**

First Department of Medicine, Osaka University School of Medicine,
Suita, Osaka 565, Japan

Introduction

The past decade has seen important advances in our comprehension of the molecular basis of cellular proliferation and transformation. Especially, the discovery and characterization of oncogenes provided one of the most promising avenues in the research on tissue regeneration and carcinogenesis.

Oncogenes are traditionally defined as dominant genes that are capable of inducing or maintaining cellular transformation. They are often related to known normal cellular genes, termed proto-oncogenes, with critical functions in cell growth and/or differentiation. These proto-oncogenes may turn out to be oncogenes, if their expression becomes out of regulation.

This chapter will focus on how proto-oncogenes and oncogenes participate in cell growth and cellular transformation in the liver.

Proto-Oncogene Expression During Liver Regeneration

Two types of liver regeneration models have been established so far. Liver regeneration after partial hepatectomy (PH) exhibits a primary regeneration, while liver regeneration induced by chemical perturbation provides a compensatory model. The former model has been most widely studied, and the proliferative response develops not adjacent to the wound margin but in quite separate portions of the liver. Chemical perturbation as a model for liver regeneration has not been a common choice for physiologists; inability to induce a reproducible amount of death from one animal to another and sublethal effects on the remnant cells provide two good reasons for avoiding this type of experiment. However, it is worth to investigate the response of the liver treated with the hepatotoxins such as carbon tetrachloride (CCl_4), since cell injury followed by regenerative process takes place side by side so that the possibility may exist for the influence of a local wound hormone or growth factor.

The degree of synchrony of the growth response is remarkable for an *in vivo* phenomenon after partial hepatectomy (PH) [1]. It can be, therefore, expected that some cellular genes may become active in the regenerative liver, if expression of these genes is directly or indirectly associated with non-neoplastic cell proliferation. While early studies indicate that the whole amount of mRNAs of normal and regenerative livers are nearly identical, obvious quantitative differences have been revealed in the abundance of some specific mRNAs between normal and regenerating liver. Among the thousands of mRNAs present in liver polysomes, two types of cellular genes were specially spotlighted; onco-developmental genes such as α-fetoprotein (AFP), and cellular oncogenes (i.e., proto-oncogenes).

The proportion of AFP mRNA in liver polysomal RNA increases approximately 2 fold prior to the wave of DNA synthesis, whereas that of albumin mRNA exhibits little change during liver regeneration [2]. These findings indicate that de-differentiation state may participate in the regenerative process of the liver.

With regard to proto-oncogene expression during liver regeneration, there is no common pattern for the expression of cellular oncogenes; some proto-oncogenes exhibit dramatic change in expression, while other proto-oncogenes show no change or are undetectable. Previous data evaluated by Northern blot analysis describe that c-myc, c-Ha-ras proto-oncogenes sequentially increase their transcription during regenerative growth induced by PH or treatment with chemical hepato-toxin(s) [3, 4, 5]. The timing of the change in proto-oncogene expression roughly parallels the major wave of DNA synthesis during liver regeneration; c-myc and c-Ha-ras proto-oncogenes begin to increase their transcripts at around 1–3 hrs and 18 hrs after PH, respectively, prior to the major wave of DNA synthesis which is taking place at 24 hrs after PH (Fig. 1) [5]. In the regenerative process induced by CCl_4, the peak of DNA synthesis occurs around 1 day later than in regeneration induced by PH. The c-myc and c-Ha-ras transcripts also increase in parallel with DNA synthesis; c-myc and c-Ha-ras begin to increase their transcripts at around 12 hrs and 24–48 hrs after the treatment, respectively [6, 7]. In addition, c-fos proto-oncogene and c-jun proto-oncogene expression precede the c-myc and c-Ha-ras gene expression [8]. The c-fos gene expression peaks at 30 min following PH or 1hr after CCl_4 administration, and declines rapidly thereafter towards the baseline level. In contrast, enhancement of c-jun gene expression lasts longer; the expression increases within 30 min after PH, and this increase is sustained through 4 hrs, returning to the baseline level at 12 hrs after PH.

On the other hand, the c-met gene encoding hepatocyte growth factor receptor (HGFR) increases in expression during rat liver regeneration [9].

Transcripts of other proto-oncogenes such as c-mos, c-myb, c-abl and c-src, however, either show no change or are undetectable during liver regeneration regardless of the etiology [3].

An *in situ* hybridization technique can provide an important qualitative information regarding the proto-oncogene expression at the tissue as well as the cell level during regenerative process.

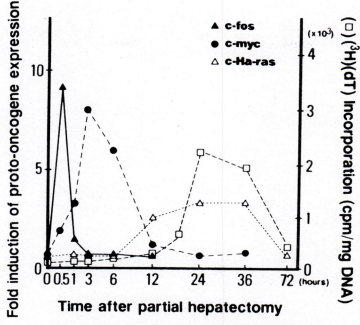

Fig. 1. Proto-oncogene expression during rat liver regeneration after two-third partial hepatectomy.

In a normal rat liver, only a few hepatocytes are expressing the above proto-oncogene mRNAs including c-fos, c-jun, c-myc, c-Ha-ras and c-met mRNA [6, 7]. These expressing cells are sparsely distributed, and no preferential localization can be detected within the hepatic lobule. After PH, number of the expressing cells is increased, and these expressing cells are distributed homogeneously in the hepatic lobules. In contrast, expression of these proto-oncogenes after CCl_4 administration is enhanced in a heterogeneous fashion (Figs. 2 and 3); expression of these proto-oncogenes is predominantly enhanced in the pericentral zone and around the areas where necrosis or fatty change can be observed after CCl_4 treatment. Zonal heterogeneity in the level of c-myc and c-Ha-ras mRNAs parallel that in the level of the respective proteins.

The c-met mRNAs are also highly expressed with a peak at 24 hrs after the treatment on the cells around damaged areas. In contrast, the c-met protein is detected in cytoplasm of the hepatocytes at 72 hrs after the administration. Since the c-met protein is localized in the cell membrane, cytoplasmic localization of the c-met protein indicates enhancement of protein synthesis [9]. Taking these findings together, it can be speculated that the c-met mRNAs expression followed by the c-met protein expression may compensate for degradation of the c-met protein occurred after auto-phosphorylation in the early stage of rat liver regeneration.

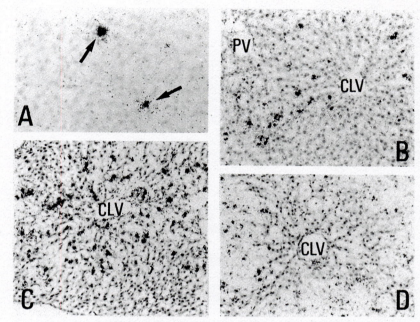

Fig. 2. Tissue distribution of the cells expressing c-myc mRNAs in the rat liver after CCl₄ administration. A few hepatocytes expressing c-myc mRNAs are sparsely distributed in normal rat liver (A, arrows). Zonal heterogeneity of the hepatocytes expressing c-myc mRNAs first becomes evident at 6 hrs after CCl₄ administration (B). At 12 hrs after the treatment, expression of the c-myc gene become maximal with the development of zonal heterogeneity (C), and is decreased at 18 hrs after the administration (D), PV, portal vein; CLV, centrilobular vein.

Furthermore, non-parenchymal cells of the liver also participate in expression of proto-oncogenes [6]. Although implication of these proto-oncogene expression in non-parenchymal cells is poorly defined, there has been a piece of evidence suggesting that non-parenchymal cells may be involved in the regulation of normal and abnormal liver growth [10]. It has been clearly demonstrated that a striking feature of early stage of hepato-carcinogenesis induced by some chemical carcinogens is the proliferation of small non-parenchymal cells, called oval cells [11], and that these oval cells can be also induced by prolonged severe liver damage. Oval cells are distinct morphologically from hepatocytes and staine for γ-GTP [12]. These findings lead us to speculate that expression of c-myc and c-Ha-ras gene may be relevant to the differentiation of oval cells, which are considered to be stem cells, that mature into that hepatocytes during liver regenration.

Although the cell population is not clearly identified, the c-jun gene expression is also observed in non-parenchymal cells after PH [8].

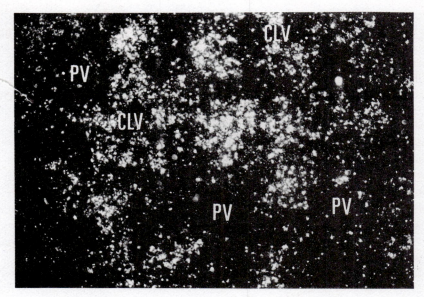

Fig. 3. Tissue distribution of the cells expressing c-Ha-ras mRNAs in the rat liver at 24 hr after CCl$_4$ administration. White grains, corresponding to the hybridization signals, are located throughout the hepatic lobule in a heterogeneous fashion. PV, portal vein; CLV, centrilobular vein.

Regulation of Proto-Oncogene Expression

The mechanism whereby these proto-oncogenes are expressed during liver regeneration are not fully understood. One of the earliest nuclear response of quiescent cells exposed to growth factors is a rapid and transient increase in c-fos and c-jun expression. c-fos mRNA is Swiss 3T3 cells, which is virtually absent from quiescent cells, can be detected as early as 5 min following the addition of growth factor, peaks at 30 min and declines rapidly thereafter towards the baseline levels [13]. The transcriptional regulation of c-fos gene is complicated. Using *in vitro* assay, a number of *cis* acting DNA sequences have been identified which stimulate c-fos gene expression in a signal-specific manner [13, 14]. Protein kinase C (PKC), Ca^{2+} mobilization, cyclic AMP accumulation act synergistically to regulate c-fos gene expression. However, it is important to recognize the existence of additional pathway involved in c-fos gene induction. In this context, the effect of EGF is particularly interesting. This growth factor does not activate PKC, nor mobilize Ca^{2+} nor increase cyclic AMP level, yet it can induce c-fos gene expression. Growth factor signals are mostly transmitted through SH$_2$ domain-containing molecules [15]. Grb2, which can bind to EGF receptor through SH$_2$ domain, can transmit EGF signal to activate Ras/raf/MEKK/ MAP kinase pathway [16]. Interestingly, MAP kinase activity is enhanced with a peak at 1 hr after partial hepatectomy [17], just prior to c-fos gene expression. EGF can also induce c-jun expression and subsequent cell proliferation in fibroblast [18], and TGFα, which acts through the EGF receptor, induces c-jun expression leading to cell division in adult rat hepatocytes [19]. These findings indicate that Ras/raf/MEKK/MAP kinase pathway, which can be activated by EGF as well as TGFα, may induce c-jun gene expression as is the case with c-fos expression. Thus, growth factor signal(s) can modulate c-fos and c-jun gene expression through MAP kinase activation during liver regeneration.

Little is known about the regulation of expression of growth factor receptors. Recent study on transcriptional regulation of c-met gene describes that the promoter fragment of this gene contains the cis-acting elements responsible for PKC induction [20]. It has been found that partial hepatectomy or CCl₄-induced hepatocellular necrosis, cause a dramatic rise in the level of circulation HGF [21]. Furthermore, c-met/HGF receptor can associate with PLCγ, resulting in activation of PKC through the PI turnover during liver regeneration [9]. Indeed, there has been a report regarding PKC activation during rat liver regeneration [22]. Taking all findings together, it is likely that HGF itself may modulate c-met gene expression through PKC activation during liver regeneration.

Physiological Implication of Proto-Oncogene Expression

What is the physiological implication of proto-oncogene expression during liver regeneration? May these two events be linked and be important for control of DNA synthesis, or simply take place at the same time and have no functional association whatsoever?

It is worthy to note that most oncogenes encode proteins whose location and action strongly suggest a role in signal transduction pathway involved in cell growth as well as transformation. According to the cellular location and functional roles, components of the signal transduction pathways are classified into growth factor receptors, cytoplasmic second messengers, and membrane-associated or cytoplasmic proteins. Principally, proto-oncogenes fall into two major categories, encoding : (1) transcriptional factors, (2) membrane-associated or cytoplasmic proteins which function in signal transduction pathway (Table 1).

For the first category, the physiological roles of three proto-oncogenes including c-fos, c-jun and c-myc have been extensively examined. The fos/jun family of leucine zipper-containing transcriptional factors are including c-fos, c-jun, jun B, jun D, fra-1, fra-2 and fos b [23, 24]. The multiple heterodimeric FOS/JUN complexes are revealed to activate the transcription of delayed early genes; the transcriptional factor AP-1, coded by c-jun gene in combination with c-fos protein exert a direct effect on AP-1 responsive genes that are important in the transduction of cell proliferation. For example, replication-dependent histone gene has been demonstrated to bear an AP-1 binding site, and it is suggested that c-jun protein (AP-1) may play an important role in the expression of this gene essential to G0 to G1

Table 1. Functional classification of proto-oncogenes

Category	Oncogene	Homologous cellular gene
1. Transcription factors	c-myc, N-myc, L-myc, mos, jun, myb, ski	
2. Components of signal transduction pathway		
(a) Transmembrace growth factor receptors	c-erbB, c-met, c-fms	EGF receptor HGF recepor
(b) Membrane-asociated tyrosine kinases	c-abl, c-src family, c-fes, c-fps	
(c) Membrane-associated guanine nucleotide binging proteins	c-Ha-ras, c-ki-ras, N-ras	
(d) Cytoplasmic serine-threonine kinases	c-raf-1/c-mil, c-raf-2 c-mos	

transition. Furthermore the functional significance of c-jun protein can be also demonstrated in the activation of the genes critical to extra cellular aspects of regeneration such as matrix remodeling. During matrix remodeling after PH, collagen content briefly decreases. Transin, which acts as a procollagenase activator and bears a AP-1 responsive element, increases its expression with c-jun activation, resulting in catalyzing the breakdown of laminin and type IV collagen [25]. Thus, c-jun protein in combination with c-fos protein may play an important role in initiating the extracellular matrix remodeling necessary for the accommodation of cell proliferation in the liver.

Interestingly, in the later phase of liver regeneration, the c-jun protein (AP-1) in combination with LRF-1 (liver regeneration factor 1), which is also one of the leucine zipper containing proteins [26], can strongly activates cyclic AMP-responsive elements (CREs). Many liver specific genes such as PEPCK and TAT contains CRE sites in their promoters. In this regard, c-jun can induce the liver-specific phenotype as well in the later stage of liver regeneration.

The myc family contains three members, c-myc, N-myc and L-myc. These genes encode related but distinct nuclear proteins that can contribute to tumorigenic conversion both *in vitro* and *in vivo*. Although the actual role of myc family genes has not been determined, the nuclear localization of myc family and the affinity for DNA *in vitro* suggest that they may function as specific DNA binding proteins *in vivo*, possible as modulators of gene expression. This hypothesis is supported by the evidence that myc family proteins share two regions of homology with DNA-binding transcriptional regulatory proteins [27]. The first region, termed the leucine zipper domain, is shared with a group of proteins that include the fos and the jun proto-oncogenes. Mutational analysis indicated that the leucine zipper region is important for the activity of c-myc protein, possibly functioning in multimer formation. The myc proteins also contains a basic amino acid-rich region, termed the helix-loop-helix (HLH) domains. This region is also detected in a number of cell determination genes, including myogemic determination genes myoD1 and myogenin.

A role for c-myc protein in normal cellular growth has been proposed based on the rapid induction of c-myc gene expression that accompanies the *in vitro* exposure of quiescent cells to mitogenic stimuli. The importance of c-myc expression for cellular proliferation is further indicated by the observations that c-myc antisense oligonucleotides inhibit the proliferation of the promyelocytic HL-60 cell line and motogen-stimulated peripheral T cells [28]. Furthermore, the introduction of high levels of exogenous c-myc into cell lines results in the induction of growth factor-independent DNA synthesis [29]. These *in vitro* studies described above indicate that c-myc proteins may play a crucial role in cell proliferation. However, specific binding sites for c-myc protein has not been so far identified except a positive enhance region upstream of its own promoter. In order to reveal the exact nature of c-myc protein in hepatocyte growth, specific binding sites for c-myc protein in the upstream of the genes involved in hepatocytes cell growth.

In this way, proto-oncogenes whose products are considered to bind DNA may play their physiological roles during liver regeneration.

Some proto-oncogenes encode the growth factor receptors with tyrosine kinase activity. As mentioned above, upon the binding of growth factor to the respective receptor, the receptor is auto-phosphorylated (activated) by the endogenous tyrosine kinase, followed by the activation of intracellular signaling pathways. Transduction of the growth factor stimulus from the receptor to the cytoplasmic second messengers is absolutely dependent on a functional kinase domain in the receptor. Thus, the physiological significance of the proto-oncogenes encoding growth factor receptors depend on not the amount of protein but the auto-phosphorylation of receptors. The c-met oncogene encodes a transmembrane tyrosine kinase identified as the receptor for hepatocyte growth factor (HGF) [30]. Although expression of c-met protein is increased about 2 fold over the baseline level, c-met protein is auto-phosphorylated 30 fold over the initial level during rat liver regeneration after CCl_4 administration. Consequently, signal transduction pathways are activated through auto-phosphorylated HGF receptor/c-met protein during the rat liver regeneration [9]. The Src homology 2 (SH2) domains are conserved sequences found among a series of signal transducing molecules [15]. Proteins with SH2 domains bind specifically phosphotyrosine-containing sequences in growth factor receptors. In this context, PLCγ, PtdIns 3-kinase are highly associated with tyrosyl-phosphorylated c-met protein during rat liver regeneration, and these association change in parallel with the state of tyrosyl phosphorylation of c-met protein (Fig. 4) [9]. PLCγ, breaks down phosphoinositides to activate PKC. Whereas the cellular functions of PtdIns 3-kinase remain to be elucidated, it has been considered that the PtdIns 3-kinase may play an important role in cell growth in responses to mitogen. Thus, association of c-met proein with PLCγ, or PtdIns 3-kinase may provide one of the possible explanations of HGF action on hepatocyte growth. Interestingly, association of c-met protein with PLCγ, is followed by association with PtdIns 3-kinase during liver regeneration. These findings indicate that HGF simulation may be transmitted, dependent on the stage of liver regeneration, into different intracellular signal transduction pathways responsible for the programmed processes in liver regeneration.

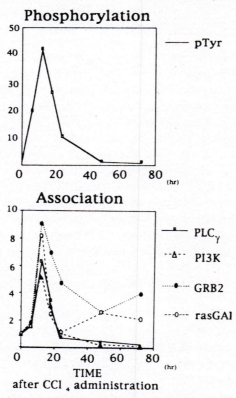

Fig. 4. Tyrosyl-phosphorylation of the c-met protein and its association with signal transducing molecules during rat liver regeneration after the CCl$_4$ administration. Upper panel describes tyrosyl-phosphorylation of the c-met protein after CCl$_4$ administration. Lower panel demonstrates association of c-met protein with SH2 domain-containing signal-transducing molecules including PLCγ, PI3K (PtdIns 3-kinase), Grb2 and ras GAP. Numbers along the vertical line indicate extent of induction fold over the initial level.

On the other hand, the ras family including c-Ha-ras, c-ki-ras, rho encodes a 21KDa membrane-associated protein (p21ras) that exhibits limited sequence homology to the Gs subunit of G protein [31]. The ras protein binds the guanidine nucleotides GDP and GTP, creating the inactive (GDP bound) and active (GTP bound) states. Following the binding of normal ras protein to GTP, a further protein, GTPase-activating protein (GAP), interacts with the ras/GTP complex, promoting GTP hydrolysis and returning ras to the inactive state. The GTP-bound ras protein was most likely to have a positive effect on cellular growth. In contrast, the trasforming ras oncogenes exist as mutant of the proto-oncogene. Mutant ras forms a complex with GAP but the interaction is incomplete, with no increase in hydrolytic activity, leading to allow ras to escape down-regulation. Consequently, mutant ras remains in the GTP-bound state, providing a constant stimulus to downstream of the signal transduction pathways [32]. The last few years have provided us with many insights into the role of ras protein in signal transduction pathway. The complete signaling pathway including upstream and downstream of ras protein, emerges now. Downstream elements have been discovered with raf-1 kinase [33] and erks [34], and immediate upstream partners have been identified as SOS, a nucleotide exchanger [35]. In addition, GRB2 can link growth factor receptor and SOS as an adapter protein [16]. Stimulation of cells by binding of growth factors to their respective receptors leads to the auto-phosphorylation of the receptors, which can interact with GRB2-SOS complex. This in turn leads to activation of ras protein. Activation of p21 ras (GTP-bound state) results in activation of raf-1, which in turn can activate MAPKK (MEK-1). MEK-1 can activate erk1 and erk2 (MAP kinases). As mentioned before, these latter kinases are considered to be involved in the activation of a variety of transcriptional factors including c-jun, c-myc and other serine/threonine kinases. These findings indicate that physiological significance of ras protein depends not on protein expression itself but on active state of this protein. Although there is no way available to determine active state of ras protein *in vivo*, the raf-1 activity may reflect ras activation *in vivo*.

The raf family including c-raf-1 and A-raf-1 encode closely related cytoplasmic proteins with serine/thereonine kinase activity [33]. The raf-1 kinase activity is enhanced at 0.5 hr after PH [21], followed by enhancement of the raf-1 gene expression [36], indicating that ras protein is activated during liver regeneration.

On the other hand, heterogeneous expression of the proto-oncogenes during liver regeneration after CCl_4 administration may provide a clue to comprehend the physiological implications of proto-oncogenes. Previous works have revealed that the contribution of each acinar zone to liver regeneration depends on the zonal distribution of the damage. Whereas the periportal zone is responsible for the 70 to 80% of the DNA synthesis after PH [37], selective pericentral injury due to bromobenzene or CCl_4 is accompanied by the predominant contribution of the pericentral and midlobular zones to DNA synthesis [38–40]. Distribution of the cells expressing the above proto-oncogene is essentially similar to that of the cells expressing PCNA, which indicates DNA synthesis. In addition, expression of proto-oncogene mRNAs precedes that of PCNA during liver regeneration. Based on the functions of the proto-oncogenes and the observations on how these genes are expressed, proto-oncogenes may play roles in a programmed sequence of interacellular events involved in hepatocyte growth during liver regeneration.

Oncogene Expression Induced by Chemical Carcinogens

The liver is a frequent site for the development of chemically induced carcinogenesis [41]. This is primarily owing to the capacity of the liver to activate many kinds of exogenous chemicals metabolically to reactive electrophilic species that can covalently interact with cellular DNA and other macromolecules.

Recent studies on the molecular basis for cancer development have revealed potential targets in the cell genome for the reactive forms of chemical carcinogens. Primary among such potential targets are proto-oncogenes. In experimental animal models of hepatocarcinogenesis, exposure to carcinogens induces focal areas of preneoplastic cells which exhibit a variety of morphological, biochemical and proliferative alterations that distinguish them from normal hepatocytes. These focal areas have been considered to represent an early stage of the multistep process of carcinogenesis and are detected histochemically by γ-GTP (γ-glutamyltranspeptidase) [12]. Wheareas γ-GTP positive preneoplastic cells, isolated from the livers 6 months after the treatment with low dose of diethylnitrosamine (DEN), showed no difference from normal hepatocyte in expression of c-myc and c-Ha-ras gene, slight increase in c-myc expression can be detected in γ-GTP-positive cells after 11 months [42]. In contrast, treatment with higher dose of DEN demonstrated increased level of c-Ha-ras gene in γ-GTP-positive focal cells in the rat liver [42]. Recent study may provide a possible explanation for the discrepancy mentioned above. Cells isolated from altered foci of animals treated with low dose (non-necrotizing) of DEN reveal no chromosomal abnormalities, while those from animals treated with high dose (necrotizing) of DEN exhibit significant chromosomal breaks. These observations are implicating that the focal areas observed after the administration of high dose of DEN may already be advanced further in multistage of hepatocarcinogenesis, presumably into the stage of progression, whereas those observed following low dose of DEN may be in the stage of initiation.

In rats and mice, primary liver tumors are also induced by 3-methyl-4-dimethyl-aminoazobenzene [43], aflatoxin B1 [44], or a diet deficient in choline and containing 0.1% ethionine [45], and they vary considerably in their expression of the c-Ha-ras and the c-myc proto-oncogenes. These findings are implicating that continuously increased expression of c-myc or c-Ha-ras gene may not be necessary for the growth to the maintenance of hepatic neoplasms, and also suggest that increased expression of these genes in neoplasms may result from one or more secondary alterations during hepato-carcinogenesis.

The activation of proto-oncogenes may occur in cells by a number of theoretically as well as experimentally proven mechanisms. In general, transcriptional activation of proto-oncogene may take place as a result of: (1) mutations not within exons of the proto-oncogenes, (2) hypomethylation of DNA, (3) gene amplifications and (4) chromosomal translocation.

With regard to mutations in liver tumors, evidence have revealed that different mutations in c-Ha-ras gene arise in liver DNA from rats and B6C3F1 mice, which exhibit a 30% spontaneous hepatoma incidence, soon after the treatment with the structurally distinct carcinogens [46]. Such distinct patterns of c-Ha-ras gene mutations demonstrate that the direct activation of c-Ha-ras induced by carcinogen is an early event of hepato-carcinogenesis. In fact, ras family genes acquire transformation-inducing properties by single point mutations within their coding sequence. In this context, mutations impairing the intrinsic GTP hydrolysis, like valine 12, can enhance the potency to induce ras transformation [32]. However, the presence of mutations in liver adenoma [47] may indicate that such mutations are necessary but not themselves are sufficient to induce the malignant transformation. Furthermore, given that liver carcinogenesis is a multistep process, other proto-oncogenes may be involved in the conversion of hepatocytes to neoplastic cells. The finding that two or more proto-oncogenes may act in concert to transform normal hepatocytes seem to be compatible with the multistep hypothesis of carcinogenesis.

A number of studies have shown that proto-oncogene overexpression may play a role in transformation. For instance, the transforming efficiency of mutated-activated ras oncogenes is known to be influenced by their level of expression.

On the other hand, DNA hypomethylation of a particular gene often precedes its expression, leading to the proposal that specific gene hypomethylation may play an important role in carcinogenesis through altered gene regulation. For example, hypomethylation of oncogenes during hepatocarcinogenesis has been observed in the c-Ha-ras and the c-Ki-ras genes in B6C3F1 mouse liver tumor, where loss of stringent control of gene expressions is detected. In contrast, the methylation state of c-myc gene is unaltered, although this gene appears to be amplified in the liver tumors [48].

These results indicate that a component of mechanism, whereby these two oncogene are activated, involves loss of stringent control of expression through hypomethylation of c-Ha-ras gene and via amplification of c-myc gene.

In addition, Phenobarbital-induced B6C3F1 mouse liver tumors exhibit hypomethylation of c-raf oncogene, facilitating the elevated gene expression [49]. Since c-raf gene may act in the signal transduction pathway involved in cell growth as described before, it is likely that elevated c-raf may induce activation of signal pathways, resulting in the progression of carcinogenesis.

In this way, it is possible to place the importance of proto-oncogenes as critical targets for carcinogenesis on the context of the stages of neoplastic development.

Conclusion

Proto-oncogenes are expressed in a programmed manner during liver regeneration. Interestingly, these proto-oncogenes encode proteins, whose location and biological action strongly suggest that they have a role in the signal transduction pathway. Cell proliferation of the liver requires the intracellular signal pathways which mediate the transfer of the growth signals, and in this context the induction of proto-oncogenes may play a crucial role in mitogenesis of the liver. On the other hand, induced alterations in the structure and/or in the regulation of proto-oncogenes may induce aberrant signal transduction, eventually resulting in continuous growth stimuli which are considered to exist in malignant cells.

In this way, proto-oncogenes have recently been focused in terms of their relevance to signal transduction pathways involved in cell growth as well as transformation of the liver. However, signal transduction pathways are composed of a number of elements. Roles of proto-oncogenes have been so far studied individually, and proximal and/or distal elements remain unrecognized.

In order to establish the physiological role of proto-oncogenes in hepatic cell growth and transformation, a study on the contribution of proto-oncogenes in signal transduction is warranted.

References

1. Bucher NLR, Malt RA. (1971). Modifying influences. In Bucher NLR, Malt RA, eds. Regeneration of liver and kidney. Boston, Little Brown and Co., 143–159.
2. Petropoulos C, Andrew G Tamaoki T et al. (1983). α-fetoprotein and albumin mRNA levels in liver regeneration and carcinogenesis. J Biol Chem 258: 4901–4906.
3. Gayety M, CJ, Shank PR et al. (1983). Expression of a cellular oncogene during liver regeneration. Science 219: 510–512.
4. Fausto N, Shank PR. (1983). Oncogene expression in liver regeneration and hepatocarcinogenesis. Hepatology 3: 1016–1023.
5. Yashima T, Hayashi N, Kasahara A, Furusawa S, Sasaki Y et al. (1988). Inhibition of liver regeneration through decreased proto-oncogene expression by ethanol.

In: Kuriyama K, Tadada A and Ishii H (eds). Biomedical and Social Aspects of Alcohol and Alcoholism. Amsterdam, NY, Oxford: Excerpta Medica. pp. 737–740.

6. Sasaki Y, Hayashi N, Morita Y, et al. (1989). Cellular analysis of c-Ha-ras gene expression in rat liver after CCl_4 administration. Hepatology 10: 494–500.

7. Sasaki Y, Hayashi N, Kamada T. (1990). Heterogeneous activation of protein kinase C during rat liver regeneration. In Yasutomi Nishizuka et al., eds. The Biology and Medicine of Signal Transduction. New York, Ravin Press. pp 345–351.

8. Alcorn JA, Feitelberg SP and Brenner DA. (1990). Transient induction of c-jun during hepatic regeneration. Hepatology 11: 909–915.

9. Horimoto M, Hayashi N, Sasaki Y, et al. (1995). Expression and phosphorylation of rat c-met/hepatocyte growth factor receptor during rat liver regeneration. J of Hepatology 23: 174–183.

10. Sell S and Leffert HL. (1982). An evaluation of cellular lineage in the pathogenesis of experimental hepatocellular carcinoma. Hepatology 2: 77–86.

11. Farber E. (1956). Similarities in the sequence of early histological changes induced in the liver of the rat by ethionine, 2-acetylaminofluorene, and 3-methyl-4 dimethyl-aminoazobenzene. Cancer Res 16: 142–155.

12. Grisham JW. (1980). Cell types in long term propagable cultures of rat liver. In Borek C, Williams GM, eds. Differentiation and carcinogenesis in liver cell culture. New York: New York Academy of Science, 128–137.

13. Curran T. (1988). The fos oncogene. In Reddy EP, Skalka AM, Curran T, eds. The oncogene handbook. Amsterdam: Elsevier. pp. 307–325.

14. Prywes R, Fisch TM, Roeder RG. (1988). Transcriptional regulation of c-fos. Cold Spring Harbor Symp Quant Biol 53: 739–748.

15. Pawson T and Gish GD. (1992). SH2 and SH3 domains: From structure to function. Cell 71: 359–362.

16. Lowenstein EJ, Daly RJ, Batzer AG et al. (1992). The SH2 and SH3 domain-containing protein GRB2 links receptor tyrosine kinases to ras signaling. Cell 70: 431–442.

17. Horimoto M, et al. (in preparation).

18. Quantin B and Breathnach R. (1988). Epidermal growth factor stimulates transcription of the c-jun proto-oncogene in rat fibroblast. Nature 334: 535–537.

19. Brenner DA, Koch KS and Leffert HL. (1989). Transforming growth factor-α stimulates proto-oncogene c-jun expression and a mitogenic program in primary cultures of adult rat hepatocytes. DNA cell Biol 8: 279–285.

20. Bocaccio C, Gaudino G, Gambarotta G et al. (1994). Hepatocyte growth factor (HGF) receptor expression is inducible and is part of the delayed-early response to HGF. J Biol chem 269: 12846_12851.

21. Lindoroos PM, Zarnegar R and Michalopoulos GK. (1991). Hepatocyte growth factor rapidly increases in plasma before DNA synthesis and liver regeneration stimulated by partial hepatectomy and carbon tetrachloride administration. Hepatology 13: 743–750.

22. Sasaki Y, Hayashi N, Ito T et al. (1989). Heterogeneous activation of protein kinase C during rat liver regeneration induced by carbon tetrachloride administration. FEBS Lett 254: 59–65.

23. Kerppola TK and Curran T. (1991). Transcriptional factor interactions: basics on zippers. Curr. Opin. Struct 1: 71–79

24. Ransone LJ and Verma IM. (1989). Association of nuclear oncoproteins fos and jun. Curr Opin Cell Biol 1: 536–540.

25. Murphy G, Nagase H, Brinckkerhoff CE. (1988). Relationship of procollagenase activator, stromelysin and matrix metalloproteinase 3. Collagen Rel Res 8: 389–391.

26. Hsu J, Bravo R and Taub R. (1992). Interactions amomg LRF-1, Jun B, c-Jun, and c-Fos define a regulatory program in the G1 phase of liver regeneration. J Biol Chem 12: 4654–4665.

27. Landschultz W, Johnson P and McKnight S. (1988). A hypothetical structure common to a new class of DNA binding proteins. Science, 240: 1759–1764.

28. Heikkila R, Schwab, G, Wickstrom E et al. (1987). c-myc antisense oligodeoxynucleotide inhibits entry into S phase but not progress from G0 to G1. Nature 328: 445–449.

29. Iguchi-Ariga S, Itani T, Kiji Y et al. (1987)). Possible function of the c-myc product: promotion of cellular DNA replication, EMBO J 6: 2365–2371.

30. Bottaro DP, Rubin JS, Faletoo DL et al. (1991), Identification of the hepatocyte growth factor receptor as the *c-met* proto-oncogene product. Science 251: 802–804.

31. Wiesmuller L and Wittinghofer F. (1994). Signal transduction pathways involving Ras. Cellular Signaling 6: 247–267.

32. Kitayama H, Matsuzaki T, Ikawa Y et al. (1990). Genetic analysis of the Kirsten-ras-revertant 1 gene: Potentiation of its tumor suppresser activity by specific point mutations. Proc Natl Acad Sci (USA) 87: 4284–4288.

33. Rapp UR. (1991). Role of Raf-1 serine/threonine protein kinase in growth factor signal transduction. Oncogene 6: 495–500.

34. Anderson NG, Maller JL, Tonks NK. et al. (1990). Requirement for integration of signals from two distinct phosphorylation pathways for activation of MAP kinase. Nature 343: 651–653.

35. Egan SE, Giddings BW, Brooks MW et al. (1993). Association of sos, ras exchange protein, with Grb2 is implicated in tyrosine kinase signal transduction and transformation. Nature 363: 45–51.

36. Silverman JA, Zurlo J, Watson MA et al (1989). Expression of c-raf-1 and A-raf-1 during regeneration of rat liver following surgical partial hepatectomy. Mol Carcinogen 2: 63–67.

37. Robes HM, Juczek JV, Wirschug R. (1973). Kinetics of hepatocellular proliferation after partial hepatectomy as a function of structural and biochemical heterogeneity of the rat liver. In Lesch R, Reutfler W, eds. Liver regeneration after experimental injury III workshop. New York: Stratton International Medical Book Corp., 35–52.

38. Nostrant TT, Miller DL, Appelman HD, et al. (1978). Acinar distribution of liver cell regeneration after selective zonal injury in the rat. Gastroenterology. 75: 181–186.

39. Leevy CM, Hollister RM, Schmnid R et al. (1959). Liver regeneration in experimental carbon tetrachloride intoxication. Proc Soc Exp Bio Med. 102: 672–675.

40. Recknagel RO, Glende EA. (1973). Carbon tetrachloride hepatotoxicity: an example of lethal cleavage. Crit Rev Toxical. 2: 263–270.

41. Miller EC. (1978). Some current perspectives on chemical carcinogenesis in humans and experimental animals. Cancer Res 38: 1479–1496.

42. Beer DG, Schwarz M, Sawada N et al. (1986). Expression of c-Ha-ras and c-myc proto-oncogenes in isolated γ-glutamyl transpeptidase-positive rat hepatocytes and in hepatocellular carcinomas induced by diethylnitrosamine. Cancer Res 46: 2435–2441.

43. Makino R, Hayashi K, Sato S et al. (1984). Expression of the c-Ha-ras and c-myc genes in rat liver tumors. Biochem Biophys Res Commun 119: 1096–1102.

44. Tashiro F, Morimura K, Hayashi R et al. (1996). Expression of the c-Ha-ras and c-myc genes in aflatoxin B1-induced hepatocellular carcinomas. Biochem Biophys Res Commun 138: 858–864.

45. Yaswen P, Goyette M, Shank PR et al. (1985). Expression of c-Ki-ras, c-Ha-ras and c-myc in specific cell types during hepatocarcinogenesis. Mol Cell Biol 5: 780–786.

46. Wiseman RW, Stowers SJ, Miller EC et al. (1987). Activating mutations of the c-Ha-ras proto-oncogene in chemically induced hepatomas of the male B6C3F1 mouse. Proc Natl Acad Sci (USA) 83: 5285–5289.

47. Reynolds SH, Stowers SJ, Maronpot RR et al. (1986). Detefction and identification of activated oncogenes in spontaneously occurring benign and malignant hepatocellular tumors of the B6C3F1 mouse. Proc Natl Acad Sci (USA) 83: 33–37.

48. Vorce RL and Goodman JI. (1991). Hypomethylation of ras oncogenes in chemically induced and spontaneous B6C3F1 mouse liver tumors. J Toxicology and Environmental Health 34: 367–384.

49. Ray JS, Margaret L, Harbison R et al. (1994). Alterations in the methylation status and expression of the raf oncogene in Phenobarbital-induced and spontaneous B6C3F1 mouse liver tumors. Molecular Carcinogen 9: 155–166.

Liver and Environmental Xenobiotics
S.V.S. Rana and K. Taketa (Eds)
Copyright © 1997, Narosa Publishing House, New Delhi, India

13. Undifferentiated Gene Expression as the Entity of Liver Injuries

Kazuhisa Taketa

Department of Public Health, Okayama University Medical School, Okayama, Japan

Introduction

In a series of studies analyzing enzyme activities of carbohydrate and related metabolism in injured livers as well as serum levels of α-fetoprotein (AFP) and its sugar chain in acute liver injury, undifferentiated phenotypes were noted as a common feature of hepatic injuries of different etiologies [1–8].

Some of these changes in phenotypes, particularly those showing positive responses, such as the increased levels of fetal-type liver enzymes or AFP, were once considered as reflecting the regenerating process or phase following hepatocyte necrosis rather than hepatic injury *per se*. Since the chronological sequence of the events leading to hepatocyte death and regeneration has been elucidated recently at the molecular level, it becomes now clear that the undifferentiated gene expressions are directly caused by the liver injury or as an immediate consequence of the action of hepatotoxins.

The undifferentiated phenotypical expressions caused by liver injuries are reviewed in this article in the light of currently available evidence at the molecular level, which appears in different chapters of this volume.

Enzyme Profiles of Injured Livers

Relative enzyme activities of carbohydrate metabolism in livers of rats treated with different xenobiotics and under other conditions are given in Fig. 1. Different xenobiotics cause different types of liver injuries. Carbon tetrachloride induces extensive hepatocyte necrosis with marked elevation of serum levels of liver enzymes, such as alanine aminotransferase (ALT) or aspartate aminotransferase (AST). DL-ethionine causes marked fatty deposition of hepatocytes without serum enzyme elevation, and α-naphthylisothiocyanate induces liver injury characterized by cholestasis. The enzyme activities in Fig. 1 are given in the increasing order of parenchymal liver cell damage as reflected by serum ALT elevation. Increased activities of fetal-type liver enzymes, low-Km hexokinases (HK)-I, -II and -III, pyruvate kinase (PK)-M$_2$ and glucose 6-phosphate dehydrogenase (G6PD), were observed roughly in this order and decreased activities of

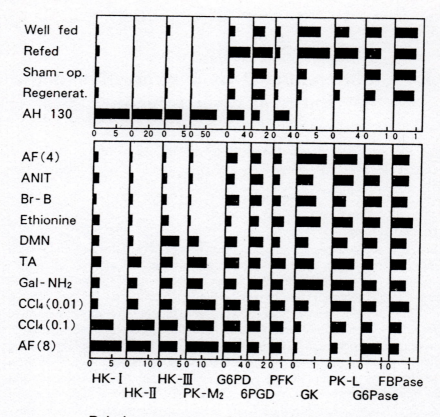

Relative enzyme activities in control liver units

Fig. 1. Activities of key carbohydrate-metabolizing enzymes in livers of rats treated with different xenobiotics and under other conditions. Sham-op—sham operated; Regenerate— regeneration afeter partial hepatectomy; AH 130— a rat hepatoma cell line; *AF* [4, 8]—allyl formate (4, 8 μl/100 g body weight), respectively; Br-B. bromobenzene; DMN—dimethyl-nitrosamine; TA— thioacetamide; Gal-NH₂—D-galactosamine; CCl₄ (0.01, 0.1)—carbon tetrachloride (0.01, 0.1 ml/100 g body weight), respectively; 6PGD—6-phosphogluconate dehydrogenase; PFK— phosphofructokinase-1 and G6Pase—glucose 6-phosphatase. Reproduced from Fig. 4 in [9] with permission.

adult-type liver enzymes, glucokinase (GK), PK-L and fructose 1,6-bisphosphatase (FBPase), in the opposite order. When the patterns of enzyme deviation are compared with those of regenerating liver and hepatoma, AH 130, it may be readily recognized that the enzyme profiles resulting from liver injuries resemble those of hepatoma as an extreme example of malignant profile since AH 130 is the most dedifferentiated hepatoma cell line. Deviation of liver phosphorylase isozymes toward those of fetal liver and AH130 is also seen in carbon tetrachloride treatment of rats [10] as is schematically shown in Fig. 2.

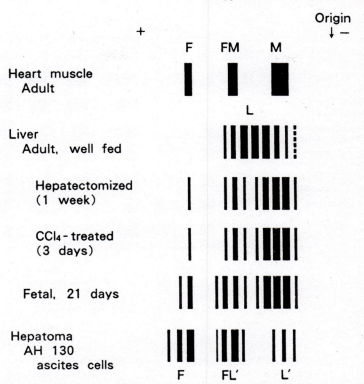

Fig. 2. **Phosphorylase isozyme patterns of rat liver and other tissues. F— fetal type; M—muscle type; L—adult liver type; and L′—fetal liver type. Reproduced from Fig. 10 in [9] with permission.**

Similar undifferentiated profiles of carbohydrate-metabolizing enzymes have been found in acute hepatitis of viral etiology [11] and in liver injuries of metabolic disorders as shown in Fig. 3 and Table 1, respectively. The increased activites of low-Km HK, PK-M$_2$ and G6PD and decreased activities of high-Km HK or GK, PK-L, G6Pase and FBPase may be compared to those of hepatocellular carcinoma or fetal liver. It is now readily understood that the undifferentiated profiles of injured livers are caused not only by decreased activities of differentiated adult-type liver enzymes but also by increaed activities of undifferentiated fetal-type liver enzymes.

Re-Expression of α-Fetoprotein by Liver Injury

Another typical example of the undifferentiated gene expression in liver injury is the re-expression of AFP, which is a specific marker of hepatocellular carcinoma, by acute liver injuries caused by viral hepatitis [13], xenobiotics [7] and congenital metabolic disorders, such as tyrosinosis (see Table 1) or ataxia-telangiectasia [14].

In experimental hepatic injury induced by carbon-tetrachloride treatment of rats, the extent of AFP rise was much greater than that attained after

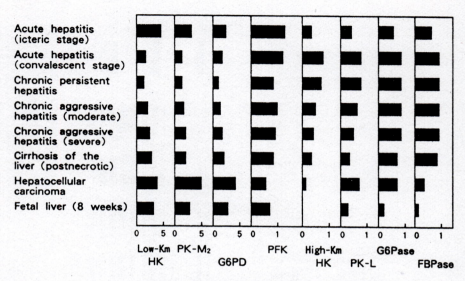

Relative enzyme activities in control liver units

Fig. 3. Activities of key carbohydrate-metabolizing enzymes in livers of patients with acute hepatitis, chronic hepatitis, cirrhosis, hepatocellular carcinoma and a fetus. Symbols and enzyme activities, see the legend to Fig. 1. Reproduced from Fig. 3 in [9] with permission.

Table 1. Carbohydrate-metabolizing enzyme activites and AFP concentrations of liver tissues in tyrosinosis (unpublished observations by Taketa, Shimamura, Bélanger and Grenier)

	Enzyme activities (U/g protein)									AFP
	HK-I	HK-II	HK-III	GK	G6PD	G6Pase	FBPase	PK-M2	PK-L	(ng/ml*)
Control adult	0.7	0	2.2	10.6	20.3	45.5	109	182	471	/
liver ($\bar{x} \pm$ SE)	±0.2	0	±0.4	±0.9	±1.0	±3.0	±13	±20	±46	
J.R. (11 M)	9.9	0	4.3	0	15.6	47.7	113	401	189	60
D.M. (12 Y)	8.7	0.3	3.2	0	35.2	21.7	137	526	341	400
C.T. (1.5 M)	7.6	0.5	6.9	0	52.4	5.7	49	1081	115	560
M.T. (11 M)	7.0	0	2.7	0	27.6	14.5	122	100	367	80
M.-J.C. (18 M)	6.6	1.0	1.1	0	57.3	14.0	61	1008	281	74
N.B. (13 M)	14.9	0	5.5	0	76.9	10.5	44	2030	0	200
D.D. (13 M)	15.9	1.3	3.4	2.6	93.1	6.1	14	1531	74	2000
N.P. (11 M)	19.5	0	3.7	0	56.5	6.8	49	956	64	1800
S.M. (6 Y)	9.8	0	6.5	0	13.5	5.9	74	1358	146	5000

*Liver cell sap. Enzyme activities were determined on frozen livers by our methods [6]. HK isozymes were separated by the method of Ueda [12].

partial hepatectomy (Fig. 4.), even though the time courses of AFP elevation are similar with respect to the onset of AFP rise, which was observed in 2 days, and also with respect to the peak of AFP rise, which was observed in 4 days after the treatments. The extents of DNA synthesis in carbon tetrachloride liver injury and partial hepatectomy were similar, although DNA synthesis started 1 day earlier in partial hepatectomy than in carbon tetrachloride treatment [15]. The peak of serum GPT elevation was observed in 24 to 48 hrs, when there was already a significant increase in serum AFP level, indicating that the trigger of increased AFP synthesis in carbon tetrachloride treatment is not the decreased viable hepatocyte mass as for partial hepatectomy but the intracellular process that is directly involved in the liver injury. This would be readily understood from the protooncogene activation (expression of c-myc mRNAs) related to regeneration starting in 6 to 12 hrs after carbon tetrachloride treatment (see the chapter under oncogene expression in liver injury of this volume by Sasaki et al.). Hepatocyte growth factor (HGF) mRNA also increases as early as 5 hours after carbon terrachloride treatment of rats [16, 17]. Similar results are obtained on the c-met/HGF [18]. In extension of these observations, it may be readily

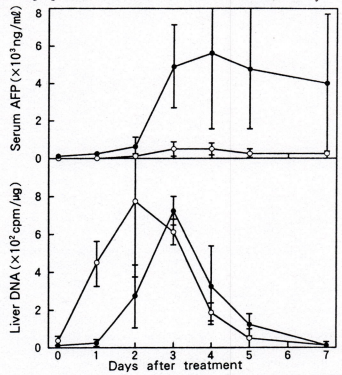

Fig. 4. Serum levels of AFP and liver DNA synthesis in rats following carbon tetrachloride treatment or partial hepatectomy. ●—CCl₄ and ○—partial hepatectomy. Vertical lines represent standard deviation. Modified from Charts 1 and 2 in [15] with permission.

understood that hepatocyte regeneration is not triggered by hepatocyte necrosis, but by hepatic injury or metabolic alteration induced by the hepatotoxin before liver cell death and that this applys also to increased AFP synthesis and even to hepatocyte necrosis. Injured hepatocytes which are initiated to synthesize increased amounts of AFP may sustain and enter into a regenerative phase or die as a result of severer functional damage as illustrated in Fig. 5. In fact, there is no increase in serum AFP level after

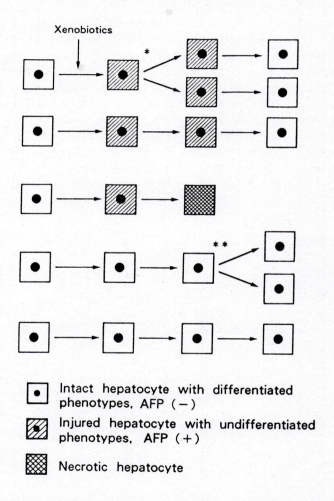

Fig. 5. Schematic illustration of chronological changes of injured hepatocytes in relation to AFP production, cell division and cell death (the common trigger theory of Taketa). *—dedifferentiated or the step-down regeneration, corresponding to restitutive (Sell) or reparative (Taketa) proliferation [23, 24]. **—differentiated regeneration, such as that following partial hepatectomy. Ratio of injured hepatocytes to necrotic hepatocytes may differ depending on the kind and severity of the injury. Reproduced from Fig. 1 in [22] with permission.

partial hepatectomy in human [19]. Thus, the increased serum level of AFP in acute liver damage reflects the extent or severity of hepatic injury and not the extent of hepatocyte regeneration as generally believed [20]. Collazos et al [21] have a view supporting this common trigger theory proposed by Taketa [22].

Undifferentiated Types of AFP Sugar Chain

The above contention that the undifferentiated expression of injured hepatocytes is not a reflection of hepatocyte regeneration but liver injury *per se* was consolidated by the finding that the fetal-type sugar chain of AFP was demonstrated from the beginning of liver injury. In other words, AFP which has sugar chains reacting with lentil lectin, namely AFP-L3, and that reacting with erythroagglutinating phytohemagglutinin, namely AFP-P4, both of which are specific markers of hepatocellular carcinoma [25], were already increased when peptide portion of AFP started to rise in acute hepatitis at the time of AST and ALT elevations far before hepatocyte regeneration. A representative case of fulminant hepatitis is shown in Table 2. The increased proportions of AFP-L3 and AFP-P4 were observed irrespective of the types of acute liver injury, type A, B, C and E hepatitises and drug-induced hepatic injuries [26, 27]. Since AFP-L3 and AFP-P4 are the most specific markers of hepatocellular carcinoma, the increased proportions of AFP-L3 and AFP-P4 in acute liver injuries again support the contention that injured hepatocytes are undifferentiated with respect not only to the peptide portion of AFP but also to the sugar chain moiety of AFP.

Table 2. **Time courses of liver function tests, elevation of total AFP and percentages of AFP-L3 and AFP-P4 in a case of type A fulminant hepatitis (acute form)***

Days after onset	T-Bilirubin (mg/dl) [1.0]	GOT (IU/I) [27]	GPT (IU/I) [33]	AFP (ng/ml) [10]	AFP-3 (%) [15]	AFP-P4 (%) [12]
5	3.64	10260	5530	2	/	/
8	7.47	970	2140	27	54.7	12.3
10	8.65	212	610	224	59.6	13.4
16	14.59	49	148	1046	55.6	10.5

*The grade 2 coma was observed on days 7–8. [ ] , cutoff levels.

Integrated Mechanisms

Recent studies on transcription factors in man and rat have shown that hepatic nuclear factor 1 (HNF1) and other liver-enriched transcription factors, such as HNF3, HNF4, CCAAT/enhancer binding protein (C/EBP), D site of albumin promoter binding protein (DBP) [28–33], or enhancer AT motif binding factor 1 (ATBF1) [34], account for the differentiated state of hepatocytes. Thus, the undifferentiated phenotypes in liver injuries and in hepatocellular carcinoma could result from an impaired production and/or binding of these regulators [35]. Translational mechanisms also appear to play a role as in the induction of G6PD by carbon terachloride [36]. This kind of dysregulation probably occurs in a more concerted manner in injured hepatocytes than in hepatocellular carcinoma in view of the fact that the phenotypic alteration in liver injury is more or less uniform in contrast with the heterogeneity of individual phenotypes in malignancy [23, 25]. This will be an attractive research area in future in xenobiotic-induced liver injuries. Cytokines may also play a direct role in altering phenotypes in inflammatory as well as neoplastic changes. Altered sugar chains of glycoproteins induced by interleukins in inflammatory diseases are documented [37–40]. Increased serum levels of interleukin-8 in hepatocellular carcinomas have been demonstrated by Okada et al [41].

The fundamental difference in undifferentiated phenotype between liver injury and malignant transformation lies in the fact that the undifferentiated phenotypes in acute liver injury are reversible and relatively concordant with the extent or severity of injury, while the undifferentiated phenotypes in hepatocellular carcinomas are heterogeneous and irreversible as might be seen in the stable phenotypes of cultured cell line HuH-7 [42].

Acknowledgement

The author wishes to thank Miss Yuki Kuchiba for preparing manuscript.

References

1. Taketa, K. (1973). *Electrophoretic multiplicity of phosphofructokinase in rat liver and other tissues and effect of carbon tetrachloride intoxication,* Acta Med Okayama, Vol. 27, pp. 205–209.
2. Watanabe, A. and Taketa, K. (1973). *Actinomycin D-insensitive induction of rat liver glucose-6-phosphate dehydrogenase by carbon tetrachloride injury,* J. Biochem, Tokyo, Vol. 73, pp. 771–779.
3. Taketa, K., Watanabe, A. and Kosaka, K. (1973). *Biochemical mechanisms of increased AFP production by injured livers,* Tumor Res, Vol. 8 pp. 108–113.
4. Ueda, M., Taketa, K. and Kosaka, K. (1975). *Hexokinase isozyme pattern in CCl_4-injured rat liver,* Clin Chim Acta, Vol. 60, pp. 77–84.
5. Taketa, K., Watanabe, A. and Kosaka, K. (1975). *Different mechanisms of increased a-fetoprotein production in rats following CCl_4 intoxication and partial hepatectomy,* Ann N.Y.Acad Sci, Vol. 259, pp. 80–84.
6. Taketa, K., Tanaka, A., Watanabe, A., Takesue, A., Aoe, H. and Koşaka, K. (1976). *Undifferentiated patterns of key carbohydrate metabolizing enzymes in injured livers, I. Acute carbon tetrachloride intoxication of rat,* Enzyme, Vol. 21, pp. 158–173.
7. Watanabe, A., Taketa, K., Kosaka, K. and Miyazaki, M. (1976). *Mechanisms of increased alpha-fetoprotein production by hepatic injury and its pathophysiological significance,* Onco-Developmental Gene Expression, W. H. Fishman and S. Sell, eds., Academic Press, New York, pp. 209–217.

8. Taketa, K., Watanabe, A. and Kosaka, K. (1976). *Undifferentiated gene expression in liver injuries*, Onco-Developmental Gene Expression, W.H. Fishman and S. Sell, eds., Academic Press, New York, pp. 219–226.

9. Taketa, K., Shimamura, J., Mori, O., Watanabe, A., Ueda, M., Kobayashi, M. and Nagashima, H. (1979). Onco-fetal proteins in liver injuries and preneoplastic livers—*Alteration of carbohydrate-metabolizing key isozymes*, Oncofetal Protein, Particularly on Hepatoma, H. Hirai and Y. Tsukada, eds., Nankoudou Publisher, Tokyo, pp. 308–322 (Japanese).

10. Kobayashi, M. (1978). *Studies of liver phosphorylase in hepatic injuries II. Alteration in isozyme pattern*, Acta Med Okayama, Vol. 32, pp. 319–330.

11. Taketa, K., Shimamura, J., Takesue, A., Tanaka, A. and Kosaka, K. (1976). *Undifferentiated patterns of key carbohydrate-metabolizing enzymes in injured livers, II. Human viral hepatitis and cirrhosis of the liver*, Enzyme, Vol. 21, pp. 200–210.

12. Ueda, M. (1975). Hexokinase isozyme in human liver: altered isozyme distribution among liver diseases, Acta Hepatol Jpn, Vol. 16, pp. 503–510 (Japanese).

13. Nishi, S. and Hirai, H. (1973). *Radioimmunoassay of a-fetoprotein in hepatoma, other liver diseases, and pregnancy*, Gann Monogr Cancer Res, Vol. 14, pp. 79–87.

14. Ishiguro, T., Taketa, K. and Gatti, R.A. (1986). *Tissue of origin of elevated alpha-fetoprotein in ataxia-telangiectasia*, Disease Markers, Vol. 4, pp. 293–297.

15. Watanabe, A., Miyazaki, M. and Taketa, K. (1976). Differential mechanisms of increased a_1-fetoprotein production in rats following carbon tetrachloride injury and partial hepatectomy, Cancer Res, Vol. 36, pp. 2171–2175.

16. Kinoshita, T., Tashiro, K. and Nakamura, T. (1989). *Marked increase of HGF mRNA in non-parenchymal liver cells of rats treated with hepatotoxins*, Biochem and Biophys Res Communs, Vol. 165, pp. 1229–1234.

17. Okajima, A., Miyazawa, K. and Kitamura, N. (1990). *Primary structure of rat hepatocyte growth factor and induction of its mRNA during liver regeneration following hepatic injury*, Eur J. Biochem, Vol. 193, pp. 375–381.

18. Ito, T., Hayashi, N., Horimoto, M., Sasaki, Y., Tanaka, Y., Kaneko A., Fusamoto, H. and Kamada, T. (1993). *Expression of the c-met/hepatocyte growth factor receptor gene during rat liver regeneration induced by carbon tetrachloride*, Biochem Biophys Res Communs, Vol. 190, pp. 870–874.

19. Alpert, E. and Feller E.R. (1978). *a-Fetoprotein (AFP) in benign liver disease: evidence that normal liver regeneration does not induce AFP synthesis*, Gastroenterology, Vol. 74, pp. 856–858.

20. Karvountizis, G.G. and Redeker, A.G. (1974). *Relation of alpha-fetoprotein in acute hepatitis to severity and prognosis*, Ann Intern Med, Vol. 80, pp. 156–160.

21. Collazos, J., Genolla, J. and Ruibal, A. (1992). *Preliminary study of alpha-fetoprotein in nonmalignant liver diseases. A clinicobiochemical evaluation*, Int J Biol Markers, Vol. 7, pp. 97–102.

22. Taketa, K. and Sekiya, C. (1993). *Liver injury marker (9), Tumor marker*, Practical Gastroenterology, A. Okub, eds., Bunkou-dou Publisher, Tokyo, pp. 144–147 (Japanese).

23. Taketa, K., Shimamura, J., Ueda, M., Shimada, Y. and Kosaka, K. (1988). *Profiles of carbohydrate-metabolizing enzymes in human hepatocellular carcinomas and preneoplastic livers*, Cancer Research, Vol. 48, pp. 467–474.

24. Taketa, K. (1990). *a-Fetoprotein: reevaluation in hepatology*, Hepatology, Vol. 12, pp. 1420–1432.

25. Taketa, K., Sekiya, C., Namiki, M., Akamatsu, K., Ohta, Y. and Endo, Y. (1990). *Lectin-reactive profiles of alpha-fetoprotein characterizing hepatocellular carcinoma and related conditions*, Gastroenterology, Vol. 99, pp. 508–518.
26. Taketa, K., Ikeda, S., Sekiya, C. and Shimamura, J. (1994). *a-fetoprotein*, Kan-Tan-Sui, Vol. 29, pp. 621–627 (Japanese).
27. Du, M.Q., Hutchinson, W.L., Johnson, P.J. and Williams, R. (1991). *Differential alpha-fetoprotein lectin binding in hepatocellular carcinoma, Diagnostic utility at low serum levels*, Cancer, Vol. 67, pp. 476–480.
28. Szpirer, C., Riviere, M., Cortese, R., Nakamura, T., Islam, M.Q., Levan, G. and Szpirer, J. (1992). *Chromosomal localization in man and rat of the genes encoding the liver-enriched transcription factors C/EBP, DBP, and HNF1/LFB-1 (CEBP, DBP, and transcription factor 1, TCF1, respectively) and of the hepatocyte growth factor/scatter factor gene (HGF)*, Genomics, Vol. 13, pp. 293–300.
29. Tronche, F. and Yaniv, M. (1992). *HNF1, a homeoprotein member of the hepatic transcription regulatory network*, Bioessays, Vol. 14, pp. 579–587.
30. Cuif, M.H., Porteu, A., Kahn, A. and Vaulont, S. (1993). *Exploration of a liver-specific, glucose/insulin-responsive promoter in transgenic mice*, J Biol Chem, Vol. 268, pp. 13769–13772.
31. Wu, K.J., Wilson, D.R., Shih, C. and Darlington, G.J. (1994). *The transcription factor HNF1 acts with C/EBP alpha to synergistically activate the human albumin promoter through a novel domain*, J Biol Chem, Vol. 269, pp. 1177–1182.
32. Nagy, P., Bisgaard, H.C. and Thorgeirsson, S.S. (1994). *Expression of hepatic tracscription factors during liver development and oval cell differentiation*, J Cell Biol, Vol. 126, pp. 223–233.
33. Stumpf, H., Senkel, S., Rabes, H.M. and Ryffel, G.U. (1995). *The DNA binding activity of the liver transcription factors LFB1 (HNF1) and HNF4 varies coordinately in rat hepatocellular carcinoma*, Carcinogenesis, Vol. 16, pp. 143–145.
34. Yasuda, H., Mizuno, A., Tamaoki, T. and Morinaga, T. (1994). *ATBF1, a multiple-homeodomain zinc finger protein, selectively down-regulates AT-rich elements of the human alpha-fetoprotein gene*, Mol Cell Biol, Vol. 14, pp. 1395–1401.
35. Panduro, A., Shalaby, F. and Shafritz, D.A. (1987). *Liver-specific gene expression in various pathophysiologic states*, Hepatology, Vol. 7, pp. 10S–18S.
36. Watanabe, A. and Taketa, K. (1972). *Actinomycin D-insensitive induction of rat liver glucose-6-phosphate dehydrogenase by carbon tetrachloride injury*, J Biochem, Vol. 73, pp. 771–779.
37. Bręborowicz, J. and Mackiewicz, A. (1989). *Affinity electrophoresis for diagnosis of cancer and inflammatory conditions*, Electrophoresis, Vol. 10, pp. 568–573.
38. Hansen, J.E.S., Bøg-Hansen, T.C., Pedersen, B. and Neland, K. (1989). *Microheterogeneity of orosomucoid in pathological conditions*, Electrophoresis, Vol. 10, pp. 574–578.
39. Mackiewicz, A., Rose, J.S., Schooltink, H., Laciak, M., Gorny, A. and Heinrich, P.C. (1992). *Soluble human interleukin-6-receptor modulates interleukin-6-dependent N-glycosylation of a_1-protease inhibitor secreted by HepG2 cells*, Febs Lett, Vol. 306, pp. 257–261.
40. Hanasaki, K., Varki, A., Stamenkovic, I. and Bevilacqua, M.P. (1994). Cytokine-induced β-galactoside $\alpha 2,6$-sialyltransferase in human endothelial cells mediates $\alpha 2,6$-sialylation of adhesion molecules and CD22 ligands, J Biol Chem, Vol. 269, pp. 10637–10643.

41. Okada, K., Shimizu, Y., Tsukishiro, T., Minemura, M., Nishimori, H., Higuchi, K. and Watanabe, A. (1994). *Serum interleukin-8 levels in patients with hepatocellular carcinoma*, Int Hepatol Commun, Vol. 2, pp. 178–182.
42. Nakabayashi, H., Taketa, K., Miyano, K., Yamane, T. and Sato, J. (1982). *Growth of human hepatoma cell lines with differentiated functions in chemically defined medium*, Cancer Res, Vol. 42, pp. 3858–3863.

Liver and Environmental Xenobiotics
S.V.S. Rana and K. Taketa (Eds)

14. Standard Liver Function Tests and Their Limitations: Selectivity and sensitivity of individual serum bile acid levels in hepatic dysfunction

Samy A. Azer[1], Geoffrey W. McCaughan[2], Neill H. Stacey[3]

[1]The Department of Medicine, [2]A.W. Morrow Gastroenterology and Liver Center
Liver Transplant Unit, [3]National Institute of Occupation Health and Safety
Royal Prince Alfred Hospital Sydney, NSW, Australia

Introduction

Numerous laboratory tests have been employed for the early detection, differential diagnosis and assessment of prognosis of hepatobiliary dysfunction. Based on the physiologic principles and the pathophysiological abnormalities that can affect liver functions during various disorders, these tests can be classified into three main groups. The first group includes biochemical tests which measure the ability of the hepatocytes for organic anion transport and representatives of this group may include: total and individual serum bile acid (SBA) concentrations [19, 98, 152], total serum bilirubin [49, 71] and dye tests such as sulfobromophthalein [160] and indocyanine green clearance [33, 73, 104]. The second group of tests reflects the metabolic capacity of the liver as measured by aminopyrine clearance (aminopyrine breath test) [18, 103, 149] galactose elimination [103, 125] and lidocaine disposition [19, 118]. The third group includes tests concerned with the capacity of the liver to synthesize certain serum proteins such as albumin [154] and clotting factors.

It is important to note that till now most of these tests have no accepted clinical significance. What is really used in routine practice is a battery of serum markers for hepatocellular necrosis or bile stasis rather than testes for liver function *per se*. These tests have become widely known as the "standard liver function tests" and include: aspartate aminotransferase (AST) and alanine aminotransferase (ALT) (both of which reflect hepatocellular necrosis); alkaline phosphatese (AP) and γ-glutamyltranspeptidase (γ-GT) (may relate to bile stasis and enzyme induction, respectively); total serum bilirubin (may reflect hepatocellular damage as well as bile stasis); prothrombin time and serum albumin (both may reflect chronicity of

Standard Liver Tests

The Aminotransferases

The activities of AST (previously designated serum glutamic oxaloacetic transaminase or SGOT) and ALT (previously designated serum glutamic pyruvic transaminase or SGPT) in the serum have been the most frequently measured indicators of liver disease for more than 35 years [80]. These enzymes catalyze the transfer of the alpha amino group of aspartate and alanine, respectively, to the alpha keto group of ketoglutaric acid, resulting in the formation of oxaloacetic acid and pyruvic acid. Pyridoxal-5′-phosphate (phosphopyridoxal; P-5′-P) functions as a prosthetic group in the amino transfer reactions.

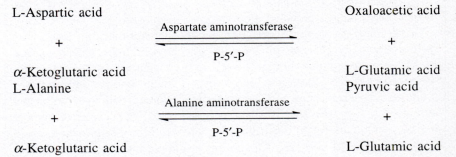

The P-5′-P bound to the apoenzyme accepts the amino group from the first substrate, aspartate or alanine, to form enzyme-bound pyridoxamine-5′-phosphate and the first reaction product, oxaloacetate or pyruvate, respectively. The coenzyme, then transfers its amino group to the second substrate, α-ketoglutarate to form the second product, glutamate. Pyridoxal-5′-phosphate is thus regenerated [108].

Spectrophotometric assay methods (linked to NAHD absorbance at 340 nm) are most commonly used for the measurement of these enzymes. It is important to note that these assay measure enzyme activity and not the true enzyme level. Because activity of an enzyme is a function of multiple factors including concentration of enzyme/substrate, temperature, serum solutes that interfere with or enhance absorption and control standards, inherent inaccuracies of enzyme activity need to be noted. Also, exact factors for normal ranges need to be set in each laboratory because of the variability of reagents and standards [136].

It must be borne in mind that the increases in serum enzyme activities often seen following liver damage do not indicate an increase in the liver's ability to synthesize that enzyme [159]. In addition, detection of substantial activities of AST or ALT in the serum are not necessarily a result of cell death. As well as being present in liver, AST is found in a wide variety of tissues including heart, skeletal muscles, kidney and brain, whereas ALT appears to be located primarily in the liver. This may explain the non-

Alkaline Phosphatase

Alkaline phosphatase actually comprises a group of enzymes that hydrolyse organic phosphate esters in an alkaline environment, generating an organic radical and inorganic phosphate [123]. Alkaline phosphatase (AP) has a dimeric structure in serum and exists in the same form when released form the liver plasma membrane by phospholipases or proteases [62, 63]. The enzyme is anchored to the plasma membrane by a glycosyl-phosphatidylinositol structure [95] and when solublized from the membrane with nonionic detergent Triton X-100 or with butanol treatment at higher pH, the hydrophobic phosphatidylinositol anchor remains covalently attached to the C-terminal amino acid residue of the enzyme [64]. Recently, it has been shown that the covalent attachment of the hydrophobic phosphatidylinositol membrane anchor cause the amphiphilic forms of the enzyme to behave anomalously on electrophoresis and affects certain catalytic and physical properties of the enzyme [83].

Several physiological factors have been reported to affect serum AP activity, including age, sex and gestation [126]. Pathologically, the activity of AP in the serum was first reported, more than sixty years ago, and found to be elevated in patients with hepatobiliary disorders [127]. Since then, it has been considered as the major indicator of cholestatic liver disease. However, besides the liver, AP is also present in many organs including intestine, placenta, kidney and leukocytes, but particularly in bone [50]. Thus, elevations of serum AP could be expected to be associated with a wide variety of pathogenic lesions besides those associated with the liver. In other words, diseases that do not directly involve the liver may show elevation of AP serum levels. These include myeloid metaplasia, intraabdominal infections and osteomyelitis [24]. This non-specificity of the activity of serum AP to discriminate hepatic from non hepatic disorders did not improve even with the measurement of serum liver isoenzyme [24]. Also, the present knowledge of amphiphilic and hydrophilic forms of AP [83] and their different physical properties and affinity to monoclonal antibodies did not bolster the clinical validity of this enzyme as a test for liver function.

The problem with serum AP activities as a test for assessment of hepatic functions limited not only by its low specificity but also its lack of sensitivity. In focal hepatic lesions and in cases with complete unilateral occlusion of the biliary tree, for example, the activities of AP in the serum were normal [59]. Interestingly, in some individuals the activity of serum AP has been reported to be elevated in the absence of liver disorders or any other disease possibly due to genetic causes [158].

γ-Glutamyltranspeptidase

γ-glutamyltranspeptidase (γ-GT) catalyzes the transfer of gamma glutamyl group from one pepatide to another or to an L-amino acid. Apart from the use of γ-GT in screening for alcoholic liver disease [72] and in the confirming the hepatic origin of an elevated AP, γ-GY may be useful in the diagnosis of hepatobiliary disorders in pregnancy [81]. However, γ-GT is found in many tissues other than the liver, such as kidney, seminal vesicles, spleen, heart and brain [55]. This may explain its low specificity as a marker for liver disorders [25]. Abnormally high values, for example, may occur in conditions such as pancreatic disease, renal disease, chronic obstructive pulmonary disease, diabetes mellitus and postmyocardial infarction [54]. Thus, a finding of elevated γ-GT has limited usefulness beeause the enzyme elevation is in not specific to hepatic disorders. Furthermore, the enzyme is inducible by alcohol and numerous drugs have been reported to induce this enzyme [82, 102, 120]. In conclusion, γ-GT is of high sensitivity but poor specificity for detection of liver diseases.

Total Serum Bilirubin

Bilirubin is derived mainly from the haem moiety of haemoglobin liberated when effete red cells are removed from the circulation by the reticuloendothelial system [100]. Other sources of unconjugated bilirubin include myoglobin and the cytochromes. Thus, haemolysis, haematological disorders and massive muscle injuries could significantly raise total serum bilirubin without associated hepatic injury indicating its low specificity in detecting hepatobiliary disorders. Unconjugated bilirubin is not water-soluble and is transported in blood bound to albumin. At least in humans, but not in the rat, the liver is the only organ that removes bilirubin from plasma [37].

Inside the hepatocytes, bilirubin is transported to the smooth endoplasmic reticulum where it undergoes conjugation, particularly with glucuronic acid, to form a diglucuronide, this process being catalysed by the enzyme bilirubin-diphosphate glucuronyl transferase. Conjugated bilirubin formed in the liver is water soluble and is efficiently excreted by the hepatobiliary system into the small intestine [100]. A small fraction of estrified bilirubin normally refluxes to plasma, where conjugates constitute approximately 4% of the total serum pigment in humans and 10% in the rat [142].

It may be of interest to note that partition of bilirubin into its conjugated and unconjugated fractions does not signigicantly improve the low specificity of bilirubin and only rarely serves any useful clinical purpose in the evaluation of liver disease [68]. In addition to its low specificity, hyperbilirubinemia is an insensitive index for early detection of parenchymal liver disease [76]. This is because the normal liver is capable of conjugating up to 1500 mg bilirubin/day while less than 500 mg of unconjugated bilirubin is normally produced each day from the breakdown of haem. Thus, in the early stages of liver disorders, no rise in serum bilirubin is expected to occur [76]. Another reason for the low sensitivity of serum bilirubin may be related to the smaller pool size of bilirubin compared to bile acids. Although both bilirubin and bile acids are excreted in bile, only the bole acids undergo enterohepatic recycling and storage in the gall bladder. Sine the load of bile acids or bilirubin excreted daily by the liver is a function of pool size and cycling frequency, bile acid flux is approximately 100-fold greater than the flux of bilirubin. Thus, a slight defect in excretion of either organic anion will be reflected in a larger increase in serum bile acids in bilirubin [142].

Pathrombin Time and Serum Albumin

The serum albumin concentration and prothrombin time may be regarded as indicators of the synthetic capacity of the liver [102]. Following chronic hepatic damage, the capacity to synthesize albumin, fibrinogen, prothrombin and other proteins is reduced. However , serum albumin concentrations is affected not only by hepatic synthesis but also by the nutritional and catabolic state of the patient and by loss from the diseased gastrointestinal or renal tract [154]. Leakage of plasma proteins into ascites and the extravascular compartment and dilution due to fluid retention are also important contributing factors. Furthermore, half lives of serum albumins are much longer than enzymes, and the rate of synthesis required to maintain plasma level is much lower [121]. This may partly explain the lack of effect on serum albumin concentration in acute hepatic injuries. It is worth noting that a normal serum albumin concentration in patients with chronic liver disease does not necessarily imply adequate hepatic function. It has shown recently that 15% of cirrhotic patients have albumin concentration within the normal range indicating low sensitivity of serum albumin even in chronic liver disorders [154]. Furthermore, a reversal of globulin/albumin ratio is not specific for liver disease and may occur in any inflammatory state or renal disease. Prothrombin time which may reflect the hepatic synthesis of clotting factor I, II, V, VII and X [102] is also not a specific indicator for hepatic injury or disease process. The test is altered by several factors such as: nutrition, drugs, hepatic synthesis and consumption of clotting factors in local or disseminated coagulopathies.

Limitations of Standard Liver Tests

As Screening Tools for Chemical-induced Hepatic Dysfunction in Humans

Liver injury induced by chemicals has been recognized as a toxicological problem for more than 100 years [162]. Examples for these chemicals which are known to induce hepatotoxicity may include: arsenic, inorganic salts, beryllium, carbon tetrachloride, methylene dianiline, dioxane, yellow phosphorus, tetrachloroethane, tetrachloroethylene and vinyl chloride. The marked vulnerability of the liver to chemical-induced damage is a function of several factors: (1) anatomical proximity of the liver to the blood supply from the digestive tract (2) the ability of the liver to biotransform foreign chemicals and (3) the role of the liver in excretion of xenobiotics and chemical metabolites into the bile [122, 140]. The liver response to such toxicants is determined by a variety of factors such as dose, duration and route of exposure, age, simultaneous exposure to other drugs or toxicants, the presence or lack of established liver disease and inherent sensitivity of the exposed individual to the noxious agents.

Thus, regular monitoring of these workers may be appropriate for the detection of early hepatic dysfunction induced by these chemicals. For many years, biological markers such as blood lead, urinary phenol levels in benzene exposure and liver tests have been used in monitoring workers exposed to toxicants. Although standard tests for liver function have also been reported to be a useful screening tool [130, 148], interpretation of these tests in hazard-exposed workers and in those with potential exposure to hepatotoxicants is difficult. Several reasons may account for these difficulties: (1) standard liver tests are not sensitive and specific indicators for detection of hepatic dysfunction, (2) the true positive predictive value of these tests in the assessment of the functional status of the liver is not generally known as the prevelance value of the liver disease in most populations is unknown, (3) the long-term prognosis of minor or transient elevation of standard liver tests is undefined and (4) concomitant exposure to other hepatotoxicants such as drug and alcohol may not allow early recognition hepatic dysfunction in response to other chemicals [69].

Lundberg and Hakansson [96], for example, examined the serum activities of the liver enzymes ALT, AST, ornithine carbamyl transferase and γ-GT in 47 paint industry workers and unexposed age matched control individuals. The workers were exposed to a mixture of industrial solvents, of which xylene was the main component in most cases. The median total exposure was about 50% of Swedish 1981 threshold limit values. No significant difference in the liver enzyme activities was shown either when the whole exposed and control groups were compared or when the five workers with outstanding solvent exposure of five times the threshold limit values or more were compared with their controls. The authors concluded that the liver remains largely unchanged by exposure to commonly occurring mixtures of predominantly non-chlorinated solvents. However, this study did not consider other parameters and screening tools for the assessment of the functional status of the livers of these workers before reaching this conclusion. Recently, it has been shown that the concentrations of SBA were consistently higher in apprentice spray-painters than their age matched control individuals within each year of follow up and the glycine-conjugated SBA showed a significant increase in the third year of follow up [16]. Comparison of high to low solvent exposure groups for these apprentices showed increased levels of SBA in the high exposure group [94]. None of the standard liver tests showed singnificant differences outside the normal range. The data indicate the limitation of these tests as a screening tool in these workers and the higher sensitivity of SBA in spray-painters exposed to solvent mixtures. However, the biological significance of these results remains to be fully evaluated by more comprehensive studies that consider a large number of subjects and a longer period of follow up. It may also be important to correlate the early change in individual SBA and bile acid ratios with any subsequent hepatic pathology provided that other causses of liver damage have been excluded.

Other studies have shown that alcohol consumption may potentiate perhloroethylene-induced hepatotoxicity in dry cleaners and that concomitant exposure to the two compounds may confound early detection of hepatic dysfunction induce by this industrial solvent [144].

Standard liver tests have also been criticised for lacking sensitivity and spe icity as screening tools in the workplace [146] and were inferior to individual SBA when workers exposed to chlorinated aliphatic hydrocarbons [41], styrene [42], organic solvents [51], toluene and xylene [52] were screened. These studies, taken together, suggest that standard liver tests are not an ideal screening tool in workers exposed to various hepatotoxicants and also demonstrate that SBA may provide an improved indicator of hepatic alterations both at earlier stage and at exposures to lower concentrations of hepatotoxicants.

In Predicting Early Hepatic Dysfunction in Experimental Animals

Standard liver tests have been used in the assessment of hepatic injury in experimental animals and in clinical settings for the last 35 years. However, it has been reported that these tests are of limited value in the assessment of early hepatic dysfunction induced by single or low exposure to chemicals. For example, it has been reported that treatment of rats with a single dose of chloroform at 34 or 180 mg/kg is associated with morphologic changes of the centrilobular hepatocytes. At these doses, plasma enzyme activities of AST and ALT were not elevated and did not show any changes associated with these early histological lesions. At a higher dose (477 mg/kg), chloroform was clearly hepatotoxic as evidenced from the histological lesions as well as elevation of the serum activities of transaminases [90]. The data suggest that transaminases do not reflected early hepatic lesions induced by smaller doses of chemicals and the rise in the serum activities of transaminases was only detected with marked hepatic damage induced by higher doses.

Cadmium has also been shown to induce alterations in the expression of hepatic gene products *in vivo* as evidenced by enhanced stress protein synthesis. These changes in liver protein synthesis occurred prior to overt hepatic injury, based on historical evidence and two biochemical assays to assess hepatic injury [53]. The failure of liver tests to detect early changes in hepatic function has also been demonstrated in rats treated with a single oral dose (150 mg/kg) of α-naphthylisothiocyanate [86]. These authors have demonstrated significant increases in hepatocellular tight junction permeability, serum bile acid concentrations and decreased bile acid excretion 16 hours after α-naphthylisothiocyanate administration. At 24 hr, bile flow decreased together with increases in serum 5′-nucleotidase and ALT activities as well as scattered small foci of hepatocellular necrosis accompanied by inflammatory cell responses observed under light microscopic examination. The findings suggest that the changes in SBA antedated the histological changes and other biochemical tests for assessment of the functional status of the liver by at least 8 hr.

In Predicting Severity of Injury Following Hepatotoxicant Exposure

Recent studies have shown that conventional liver tests are not always able to predict severity of hepatic damage induced by chemicals. For example, single exposure of B6C3F1 mice to 500 ppm styrene have been associated with a singnificant rise in the serum activities of sorbitol dehydrogenase and ALT within the first day of exposure [107]. The activities of these two enzyme, however, returned to control levels by the third day at which time severe necrosis was detected in the livers of all mice included in the study. The finding indicate that any decline in the serum activities of these enzyme is not a sign of hepatic lesion recovery and should no be used as an index in the assessment of hepatic lesion outcome. Such limitations have also been observed in rats treated with CCl_4, $MnSO_4$ or 2, 4-xylidine [56]. Serum bilirubin concentrations remained unaltered in each of the treated groups. Similarly the activity of AP was not altered with either $MnSO_4$-induced cholestasis or in xylidine hepatoxicity. Although the serum levels of glutamic dehydrogenase and ALT were elevated in the treated animals, these enzymes were not able to provide specific biochemical evidence for the extent and severity of hepatic dysfunction.

In Predicting Prognosis in Patients with End-stage Liver Disease

Emergence of liver transplantation as a successful therapeutic modality for the patient with end-stage liver disease has dramatically changed evaluation and treatment strategies [116, 141]. Continuous improvement in patient survival is due to several factors, including better selection of patients, improvement in operative techniques, the availability of selective immunosuppressive agents such as cyclosporin A and a greater understanding of postoperative management. Thus, a major goal in caring for these patients is to identify when they become optimal candidates for liver transplantation. Optimal timing of liver transplantation is defined as intervention with transplantation in the course of the disease when quality of life is sufficiently diminished and life threatening complications of portal hypertension are likely to occur. The patient at such a time has the best chance of achieving maximal survival success with minimal complications related to the original disease process [156]. Therefore, different prognostic markers [44, 115] and composite mathematical indices have been proposed and extracted from large patient populations using Cox models [39, 58, 129].

Serum bilirubin is the single most useful prognostic factor in primary biliary cirrhosis [70]. The importance of this factor was emphasised in a review of 55 patients [135]. Nevertheless, because of its wide variation in confidence limits as a prognostic factor, serum bilirbuin has been replaced by composite mathematical prognostic models based on established independently predictive clinicopathological variables. Examples of these prognostic models that have been validated for large population groups include: The Child-Turcotte classification [30], the Pugh modification [124] and the Mayo score [39, 85, 155]. The Child-Pugh classification is derived from clinical data, bilirubin, serum albumin and prothrombin time while the Mayo prognostic index for primary biliary cirrhosis is based on patient's age, total serum bilirubin, serum albumin concentrations, prothrombin time and severity of edema [39]. The use of these model is simple and of considerable clinical value and their validation has been reported from several centers [58, 62, 129, 153]. However, the Child-Pugh criteria have several limitations [31, 34]; for example, serum bilirubin can be elevated by increased haemolysis or obstruction of the biliary tract [34], the serum albumin concentration does not necessarily reflect a decrease in the rate of albumin synthesis [154] and hypoalbuminaemia in these patients represents the result of multiple factors other than hepatic synthetic ability or prognosis. Furthermore, the predictive value of the Child-Pugh and Mayo scores is most accurate shortly before the patient's death. Moreover, their applicability to individual patients may be less than ideal [32, 75].

In patients with fulminant hepatitis, the King's College group [117] presented criteria based combinations of patient age, pathogenesis, duration of jaundice before onset of encephalopathy, prothrombin time and serum bilirubin level. These criteria were recently examined [119], and it was reported that the predictive values of these guidelines were not as good as had been expected.

More recently regression models for fulminant hepatitis B and fulminant non-A, non-B hepatitis have been considered [145]. These two models were based on patient history and routine laboratory data (total bilirubin level , white blood count, ALT activity, prothrombin time and the ratio of total to direct bilirubin) on the day of development of hepatic encephalopathy. These models were found to be of high reliability in the assessment and early reference for liver transplantation. However, these models were not applicable to drug- or halothane-induced fulminant liver failure.

Several independent prognostic markers have been commended as useful prognostic tools, such as serum hyaluronate and the N-terminal propeptide of type III procollagen [13]. Neither has yet achieved widespread popularity and the latter marker has been disputed and was found to have no prognostic value [110]. Other prognostic tests such as galactose elimination capacity [125], indocyanine green clearance and antipyrine clearance are still under investigation.

Serum Bile Acids in Hepatic Dysfunction

Introduction

The validity of SBA as an indicator of hepatic function has been shown by several laboratories [35, 48, 92, 114]. SBA concentrations have also been shown to be of value in the prediction of outcome in severe cirrhosis [98] and, in principle, portal systemic shunting [28, 36]. Furthermore, total SBA have been shown to be a useful marker of hepatic dysfunction in experimental liver transplantation in rats [150] and in pigs [106] and in orthotopic liver transplantation in humans [11, 109] as well as in α-naphthylisothiocyanate-induced hepatic cholestasis in rats [152, 159]. Similar conclusions concerning the utility of total SBA may also be drawn for the majority of hepatobiliary disorders in the dog and cat [29, 63, 77, 105, 133] and in the horse [43]. However, total concentrations of bile acids in the serum do not permit the distinction between major categories of disease process [66] and were of limited value in the assessment of early hepatic dysfunction in rats and humans exposed to industrial solvents [14, 15, 41, 60, 152]. It is important to note that the recently developed techniques such as high-performance liquid chromatography [4, 47, 57, 151] and gas-liquid chromatography and mass spectrometry [78, 91, 134] have made relatively easy the separation and quantitation of free- and conjugated-bile acids and the determination of bile acid ratios. This has the potential to overcome the limitations of total SBA levels and provide an increase in diagnostic and prognostic significance. For example, in a rat model for cirrhosis, we have recently shown that the ratio of serum cholic acid to serum chenodeoxycholic acid changes in temporal relationship to progression in the histological lesions in livers of these rats. Furthermore, unconjugated bile acids, particularly, cholic acid showed significantly higher levels at all stages except with the occurence of cirrhosis at 30 wk, at which time there was a significantly lower level for unconjugated bile acids and cholic acid. Thus, the hepatic pathological changes in cirrhotic rats were reflected by the changes in the individual SBA together with the ratio of serum cholic acid to serum chenodeoxycholic acid. On the other hand, total SBA levels were raised at all stages and failed to reflect progression in the hepatic lesion [12]. This superiority of individual SBA and certain bile acid ratios over total SBA concentrations has also been recently shown in patients who underwent orthotopic liver transplantation [11]. The data from this study indicate that patients with biopsy-confirmed graft malfunction due to rejection or nonrejection causes had significantly elevated serum concentrations of glycocholate plus glycochenodeoxycholate and the taurocholate/taurochenodeoxycholate ratio compared with non-complicated grafts. Furthermore, in acute rejection episodes there was a significant rise in the concentrations of glycodeoxycholate plus deoxycholate and a significant fall in the cholate/chenodeoxycholate ratio compared with non-refection graft malfunction. Both of these changes antedated any other biochemical parameters by 24 hr indicating the usefulness of individual SBA determination in the early postoperative period.

Sensitivity and Specificity of SBA

For screening the diagnostic purposes, a discriminative limit for the SBA levels and each of the individual SBA and bile acid ratios need to be set at two standard deviations above the mean value found in healthy subjects. New tests should also be analyzed in terms of their specificity (the percentage of unaffected persons with a negative test), sensitivity (the percentage of affected persons with a positive test) and predictive values of positive and negative results [65]. Thus, the use of SBA as an index of liver function necessiates an accurate evaluation of total, individual and bile acid ratios in this respect. Although little data are available with regard to the sensitivity and specificity of individual SBA and bile acid ratios, several studies have shown SBA are quite sensitive and specific in several hepatic disorders [46, 51]. For example, total SBA concentrations have been reported to have a sensitivity and specificity of 78 and 93% respectively. The predictive value for a positive test (corrected for the actual prevalence of hepatobiliary diseases in general population) was only 10% but was still better than any of the other tests examined, while that of a negative test was 74% again superior to any other liver test studied [46]. However, these authors reported that total SBA were not of singnificant value with respect to assessment of hepatic disease severity. In another study, total SBA levels were determined in workers exposed to a mixture of organic solvents mostly toluene, xylene, acetone, n-butylacetate, n-butanol and ethylacetate. Total SBA was found to have sensitivity of 74% and specificity of 94%. None of the standard liver function tests such as ALT, AST, γ-GT or direct bilirubin was able to show similar sensitivity [51]. It should be noted that total SBA levels have higher sensitivity for the presence of liver disease, but rises in total SBA are not helpful in differentiating one type of liver disorder from another. It is expected that individual SBA will show a much higher sensitivity and specificity compared to total SBA and will be able to specify the type and severity of the hepatic disorder. For example, using a choline-deficient rat model for cirrhosis, we have recently shown that total SBA levels have sensitivity of 86% and specificity of 81% for the development of cirrhosis at 30 wk of feeding. Cholic acid levels and the ratio of cholic acid to chenodeoxycholic acid were of high specificity and sensitivity, with each giving values of 94% and 100%, respectively. Although other liver function tests were of comparable specificity, their sensitivity was 50% for ALT and AP and only 14% for bilirubin [12]. In another study we have shown that individual SBA (glycocholic acid+glycochenodeoxycholic acid levels and the ratio of taurocholate to taurochenodeoxycholate) were able to detect graft dysfunction with sensitivity and specificity of 100% for each. None of the standard liver tests (bilirubin, serum albumin, AP, AST, ALT or γ-GT) was able to match such values [11].

Serum Bile Acids in Chemical-induced Hepatic Dysfunction

Several chemicals have been reported to induce rises in SBA in experimental animals and in humans (Table 1). These studies have also shown that rises in total SBA concentrations were superior to standard liver tests for the early detection of hepatic dysfunction. For example, Wang and Stacey [152] reported that SBA were elevated in rats treated with trichloroethylene at 0.1 mmol/kg or α-naphthylisothiocyanate at 50 μmol/kg body weight. None of the other parameters of liver function (ALT, AP and sorbitol dehydrogenase) were increased at such doses. Also it has been shown that treatment of rats with 1,1,2,2-tetrachloroethylene at doses as low as 0.1 mmol/kg is able to cause rises in total SBA while none of the conventional liver tests (ALT, AST and AP) was affected at this dose [14].

Recently it has been shown that individual SBA were more sensitive indicators of hepatic dysfunction as compared with total SBA or conventional liver tests. For example, rats treated with cyclosporin A ip for four days at doses as low as 0.1 mg/kg/day showed a significant rise in serum cholic acid levels [7]. None of the standard liver tests or even total SBA was significantly changed at this dose. Similar conclusions could be drawn from studies with short-term exposure to ethinyl estradiol [9]. Similarly Bai et al [15] found that the levels of certain individual SBA, notably cholic acid, glycocholic acid and taurocholic acid, were sensitive indicators of liver dysfunction in rats treated with CCl_4. Sensitivity was greater compared with serum liver transaminases (AST and ALT), bilirubin or total SBA measurements. When a low dose of the hepatotoxicant CCl_4 (0.1 mmol/kg) was administered ip to rats, cholic acid and glycodeoxycholic acid in serum were significantly raised despite the absence of consistent pathological changes detectable by light or electron microscopy. Serum cholate levels are claimed to be more sensitive and discriminant than other routine liver function tests in detection of hepatobiliary diseases [23, 131, 132] and have been shown to be a valid index of the severity of the liver disease [101].

Serum cholic acid to serum chenodeoxycholic acid ratio has also been shown to be a sensitive indicator of heaptic injury in women treated with danazol [67] and in workers exposed to toluene and xylene [52]. This ratio has been shown to be a sensitive and specific indicator of progression of hepatic histological lesions in choline-deficient rat model for cirrhosis [12] and was able to differentiate acute graft rejection from graft dysfunction due to causes other than rejection following orthotopic liver transplantation [11].

Furthermore, SBA levels have been shown to be significantly raised in workers exposed to vinyl chloride [93], organic solvents [51], chlorinated aliphetic hydrocarbons [41], toluene and xylene [52] and styrene [42]. In these studies it has been shown that SBA and indocyanine green clearance provide a higher specificity and sensitivity for vinyl chloride hepatotoxicity [93] and higher concentrations of certain bile acids such as: taurocholic

Table 1. Use of serum bile acid concentrations in the assessment of chemical-induced hepatobiliary dysfunction in experimental animals and humans

Chemical Used	Dose (Route)	Species/ Sex	Duration	Raised SBA of exposure Total	Individual	Reference
Hornet Venom sac extract	5 mg/kg/day (ip)	Rat/M	2 wk	+++	ND	[112]
Cyclosporin A	0.1 mg/kg/day (ip)	Rat/M	4 days	—	CA	[6, 7]
MnSO$_4$	0.2 ml (iv)	Rat/F	Single dose	—	Conjugated Bile Acids	[56]
ANIT	5 mmol/kg (ip)	Rat/M	3 days	—	TCA	[152]
Aluminum	5 mg/kg (iv)	Rat/M	14 days	+++	ND	[84]
17α-Ethinylestradiol	5 mg/kg (sc)	Rat/M	5 days	+++	ND	[22]
Hexachloro-1, 3-Butadiene	0.2 mmol/kg (ip)	Rat/M	3 days	—	CA	[14]
1,1,2,2-Tetrachloro-ethylene	0.01 mmol/kg (ip)	Rat/M	3 days	++	CA, CDCA, GCA	[14]
Carbon tetrachloride	0.1 mmol/kg	Rat/M	3 days	—	CA, GDCA	[15]
Carbon tetrachloride	0.2 ml of 33% (v/v) (ip)	Rat/M	Twice/wk for 4 wk	+	GCA	[21]
	60 ml (ingested)	Human/F	Once	+++	ND	[26]
Trichloro ethylene	1 mmol/kg (ip)	Rat/M	Once	++	CA,TCA, DCA, TDCA, CDCA, TCDCA	[60]
Organic solvents	Occupational exposure	Humans/ Both	Over 2 years	++	ND	[51]
Chlorinated aliphatic hydrocarbons	Occupational exposure	Humans/M	8–17 years	++	TCA, CDCA, total CA	[41]
Vinyl chloride	Occupational exposure	Humans/ both	1 year more	ND	Conjugated CA, GCA	[93]
Toluene and Xylene	Occupational exposure	Humans/M	at least 2 years	ND	CDCA, CA/CDCA	[52]
Styrene	Occupational exposure	Humans/M	average 2.5 years	ND	CA and or CDCA	[42]
Danazol	600 mg/day	Humans/F	6 months	ND	CA, CA/ CDCA	[67]

ANIT: a-naphthylisothiocynate; CA: cholic acid; CDCA: chenodeoxycholic acid; DCA: deoxycholic GCA: glycocholic acid; GDCA: glycodeoxycholic acid; ND: not determined; TCA: taurocholic acid; TCDCA: taurochenodeoxycholic acid; TDCA: taurodeoxycholic acid

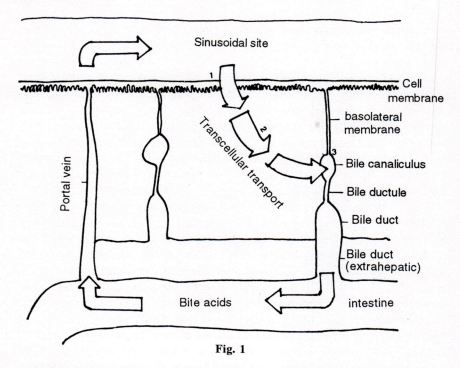

Sinusoidal site

Cell membrane

basolateral membrane

Bile canaliculus

Bile ductule

Bile duct

Bile duct (extrahepatic)

Portal vein

Transcellular transport

Bile acids

intestine

Fig. 1

tools for the early detection of hepatic dysfunction in workers exposed to industrial solvents. In addition, these conventional tests were unable to predict early hepatic dysfunction or indicate the extent of hepatic injury on chemical exposure. Although several prognostic indices are now available and are commonly used in the assessment of patients with end-stage liver disease, none has shown its ability to predict survival at an earlier stage and validity of these indices seems to be less than ideal with regard to their applicability to individual patients.

On the other hand, individual SBA assays using high performance liquid chromatography or gas-liquid chromatography mass and spectrometry have been shown to be of high sensitivity. Several recent studies indicate that, with an adequate assay, individual SBA and certain bile acid ratios are more sensitive and specific than conventional liver tests in detecting hepatic dysfunction, progress of pathological lesions and the nature of the hepatic disorders. This superiority of individual SBA has been shown in several hepatic disorders and in particular those induced by chemicals in the workplace. Future study may explain the molecular basis for the high sensitivity and specificity of individual SBA and certain bile acid ratios in hepatic disorders induced by chemicals.

serum bile acids. II In vitro and in vivo interference by trichloroethylene with bile acid transport in isolated rat hepatocytes. Toxicol Appl Pharmacol 1993; 121: 296–302.

18. Baker A, Kotake AN, Schoeller DA. Clinical utility of breath tests for the assessment of hepatic function. Semin Liver Dis 1983; 3: 318–329.

19. Balistreri WF, A-Kader HH, Setchell KDR, Gremse D, Ryckman FC, Schroeder TJ. New Methods for assessing liver function in infants and children. Ann Clin Lab Sci 1992; 22: 162–174.

20. Batta AK, Arora R, Salen G, Tint GS, Eskreis D, Katz S. Characterization of serum and urinary bile acids in patients with primary biliary cirrhoris by gas-liquid chromatography-mass spectormetry: effect of unsodeoxycholic acid treatment . J Lipid Res 1989; 30: 1953–1962.

21. Bolarin DM. Serum bile acid in the evaluation of colchicine treatment of carbon tetrachloride-induced liver injury. Exp Mol Pathol 1984; 41: 384–389.

22. Bossard R, Stieger B, O'Neill B, Fricker G, Meier PJ. Ethinylestradiol treatment induces multiple canalicular membrane transport alterations in rat liver. J Clin Invest 1993; 91: 2714–2720.

23. Bouchin IAD, Pennington CR. Serum bile acids in hepatobiliary disease. Gut 1978; 19: 492–496.

24. Brensilver HL, Kaplan MM. Significance of elevated liver alkaline phosphatase in serum. Gastroenterology 1975; 68: 1556–1562.

25. Burrows S, Feldman W, McBride F. Serum gamma–glutamyl transpeptidase. Elevation in screening of hospitalized patients. Am J Clin Pathol 1975; 64: 311–314.

26. Campbell CB, Collins DM, Tongeren AV. Serum bile acids and other liver fuction tests in hpato-cellular damage from carbon tetrachloride ingestion. NZ Med J 1980; 91: 381–384.

27. Campbell GR, Olding-Smee GW, Rowlands BS, Irvine GB. Determination of bile acids and their conjugates in serum by HPLC using immobilized 3 alpha-hydroxysteroid dehydrogenase for detection. Biomed Chromatogr 1989; 3: 75–80.

28. Center SA, Baldwin BH, de Lahunta A, Dietz AE, Tannant BC. Evaluation of serum bile acid concentrations for the diagnosis of portosystemic venous anomalies in the dog and cat. J Am Vet Med Assoc 1985; 186: 1090–1094.

29. Center SA, Baldwin BH, Erb HN, Tennant BC. Bile acid concentrations in the diagnosis of hepatobiliary disease in the cat. J Am Vet Met Assoc 1986; 189: 891–896.

30. Child III CG, Turcotte JG. Surgery and portal hypertension. In. Child III CG ed. The liver and portal hypertension, Philadelphia: Saunders WB, 1964: 1–85.

31. Christensen E, Schlichting P, Fauerholdt, L, Gluud C, Andersen PK, Juhl E, Poulsen H, Tygstrup N. Prognostic value of Child-Turcotte criteria in medically treated cirrhosis. Hepatology 1984; 4: 430–435.

32. Christensen E. Prognostication in primary biliary cirrhosis: relevance to the individual patients. Hepatology 1989; 10: 111–113.

33. Clements D, Elias E, McMaster P. Preliminary study of indocyanine green clearance in primary biliary cirrhosis. Scand J Gastroenterol 1991; 26: 119–123.

34. Conn HO. A peak at the Child-Turcotte classification. Hepatology 1981; 1: 673–676.

35. Cravetto C, Molino G, Biondi AM, Cavanna A, Avagnina P, Frediani S. Evalution of the diagnostic value of serum bile acids in the detection and functional assessment of liver diseases. Ann Clin Biochem 1985; 22: 596–605.

36. Cravetto C, Molino G, Hofmann AF, Belforte G, Bona B. Computer stimulation of portal venous shunting and other isolated hepatobiliary defects of the enterohepatic circulation of bile acids using a physiological pharmacokinetic model. Hepatology 1988; 8: 866–878.

37. De Schpper J, Van der Stock J. Increased urinary biliubin excretion after elevated free plasma haemoglobin levels. I. Variations in the calculated renal clearance of bilirubin in whole dogs. Arch Int Physiol Biochim 1972; 80: 279–291.

38. Dhami MSI, Drangova R, Farkas R, Balazs T, Feuer G. Decreased aminotransferase activity of serum and various tissues in the rat after cefazolin treatment. Clin Chem 1979; 25: 1263–1266.

39. Dickson ER, Grambsch PM, Fleming TR, Fisher LD, Langworthy A. Prognosis in primary biliary cirrhosis: model for decision making. Hepatology 1989; 10: 1–7.

40. Diehl AM, Potter J, Boitnott J, Van Duyn MA, Herlong HF, Mezey E. Relationship between pyridoxal-5′-phosphate deficiency and aminotransferase levels in alcoholic hepatitis. Gastroenterology 1984; 86: 632–636.

41. Driscoll TR, Hamdan HH, Wang G, Wright PFA, Stacey NH. Concentrations of individual serum of plasma bile acids in workers exposed to chlorinated aliphatic hydrocarbons. Br J Ind Med 1992; 49: 700–705.

42. Edling C, Tagesson C. Raised serum bile acid concentrations after occupational exposure to styrene: a possible sign of hepatoxicity. Br J Ind Med 1984; 41: 257–259.

43. Engelking LR, Paradis MR. Evaluation of hepatobiliary disorders in the horse. Vet Clin North Am Equine Pract 1987; 3: 563–583.

44. Eriksson S, Zetteervall O. The N-terminal propeptide of collagen type III in serum as a prognostic indicator in primary biliary cirrhosis. J Hepatol 1982; 2: 370–380.

45. Farthing MJG, Clark ML, Pendry A, Sloane J, Alexander P. Nature of the toxicity of cyclosporin A in the rat. Biochem Pharmacol 1981; 30: 3311–3316.

46. Ferraris R, Colombatti G, Fiorentini MT, Carosso R, Arossa W, De La Pierre M. Diagnostic value of serum bile acids and routine liver function tests in hepatobiliary disease. Sensitivity, specificity and predictive value. Dig Dis Sci 1983; 28: 129–136.

47. Ferreira HECS, Elliott WH. Pre-column derivatization of free bile acids for high-performance liquid chromatographic and gas chromatographic-mass spetrometric analysis. J Chromatogr 1991; 562: 697–712.

48. Festi D, Labate AMM, Roda A, Bazzoli F, Frabboni R, Rucci P, Taroni F, Aldini R, Roda E, Barbara L. Diagnostic effetiveness of serum bile acids in liver disease as evaluated by multivariete statistical methods. Hepatology 1983; 3: 707–713.

49. Fevery J, Blanckaert N. What can we learn from analyses of serum bilirubin? J Hepatol 1986; 2: 113–121.

50. Fishman WH. Prespectives on alkaline phosphatase isoenzymes. Am J Med 1974; 56: 617–622.

51. Franco G, Fonte R, Tempini G, Candura F. Serum bile acid concentrations as a liver function test in workers occupationally exposed to organic solvents. Int Arch Occup Environ Health 1986; 58: 157–164.

52. Franco G, Santagostino G, Lorenas M. Imbriani M. Conjugated serum bile acid concentrations in workers exposed to low doses of toluene and xylene. Br J Ind Med 1989; 46: 141–142.

53. Goering PL, Fisher B, Kish CL. Stress protein synthesis induced in rat liver by cadmium precedes hepatoxicity. Toxicol Appl Pharmacol 1993; 122: 139–148.

54. Goldberg DM, Martin JV. Role of γ-glutamyl transpeptidase activity in the diagnosis of hepatobiliary disease. Digestion 1975; 12: 232–236.

55. Goldberg DM. Structural, functional and clinical aspects of gamma-glutamyl transferase. CRC Crit Rev Clin Lab Sci 1980; 12: 1–58.

56. Gopinath C, Prentice DE, Street AE, Crook D. Serum bile acid concentration in some experimental liveer lesions of rat. Toxicology 1980; 15: 113–127.

57. Goto J, Kato Y, Saruta Y, Nambara T. Separation and determination of bile acids in human bile by high-performance liquid chromatography. J. Liq Chromatogr 1980; 3: 991–1003.

58. Goudie BM, Burt AD, Macfarlane GJ, Boyle P, Gillis CR, MacSween RNM, Watkinson G. Risk factors and prognosis in primary biliary cirrhosis. Am J Gastroenterol 1989; 84: 713–716.

59. Hadjis NS, Blenkharn JI, Hatzis G, Adam A, Beachem J, Blumgart LH. Patterns of serum alkaline phosphatase activity in unilateral hepatic duct obstruction: a clinical and experimental study. Surgery 1990; 107: 193–200.

60. Hamdan H, Stacey NH. Mechanism of trichloroethylene-induced elevation of individual serum bile acids. I. Correlation of trichloroethylene concentrations to bile acids in rats serum. Txicol Appl Pharmacol 1993; 121: 291–295.

61. Hamilton BA, McPhee JL, Howrylak K, Stinson RA. Alkaline phosphatase releasing activity in human tissues. Clin Chim Acta 1990; 186: 249–254.

62. Hartmann AH, Bircher J, Creutzfeldt W. Superiority of the Child-Pugh classification to quantitative liver function tests for assessing prognosis of liver cirrhosis. Scand J Gastroenterol 1989; 24: 269–276.

63. Hauge JG, Abdelkader SV. Serum bile acids as an indicator of liver disease in dogs. Acta Vet Scand 1984; 25: 495–503.

64. Hawrylak K, Stinson RA. The solubilization to tetrameric alkaline phosphatase from human liver and its conversion into various forms by phosphatidylinositol phospholipase C or proteolysis. J. Biol Chem 1988; 263: 14368–14373.

65. Haynes RB. How to read clinical journal: II. to learn about a diagnostic test. Can Med Assoc J 1981; 124: 703–751.

66. Heaton KW. Bile salts. In: Wright R, Millward-Sadler GH, Alberti KGMM, Karran S, eds. Liver and biliary disease. London: Bailliere Tindall, 1985: 277–299.

67. Heikkinen J, Ronnberg L., Kirkinen P, Sotaniemi E. Serum bile acid concentrations as an indicator of liver dysfunction induced during danazol therapy. Fetil Steril 1988; 50: 761–765.

68. Helzberg JH, Spiro HM. 'LFTS' Test more than the liver. JAMA 1986; 21: 3006–3007.

69. Hodgson MJ, Goodman-Klein BM, Van Thiel DH. Evaluating the liver in harzaradous waste workers. Occup Med 1990; 5: 67–78.

70. Hoffbauer FW. Primary biliary cirrhosis observations in the natural course of the disease in 25 women. Ann J Dig Dis 1960; 5: 348–383.

71. Hootegem PV, Fevery J, Blanckaert N. Serum bilirubin in hepatobiliary disease: comparison with other liver function tests and changes in the postobstructive periods. Hepatology 1985; 5: 112–117.

72. Ivanov E, Adjarov D, Etarska M, Standhushev T, Braum barov K, Kerimova M. Elevated liver gamma-glutamyl transferase in chronic alcoholic. Enzyme 1980; 25: 304–308.

73. Izawa K, Sasaki M, Tomioka T, Oka S, Segawa T, Yamaguchi T, Tsunoda T, Kanematsu T. Evaluation of the maximal excretion rate of indocyanin green as a prognostic indicator in patients undergoing biliary decompression for obstructive jaundice. J Gastroenterol Hepatol 1993; 8: 557–564.

74. Jaeschke H, Trummer E, Krell H. Increase in biliary permeability subsequent to intrahepatic cholestasis by estradiol valerate in rats. Gastroenterology 1987; 93: 533–538.

75. Jeffrey GP, Hoffman NE, Reed WD. Validation of prognostic models in primary biliary cirrosis. Aust NZ J Med 1990; 20: 107–110.

76. Johnson PJ. Role of the standard 'liver function test' in current clinical practice. Ann Clin Biochem 1989; 26: 463–471.

77. Johnson SE, Rogers WA, Bonagura JD, Caldwell JH. Determination of serum bile acids in fasting dogs with hepatobiliary disease. Am J Vet Res 1985; 46: 2048–2053.

78. Jonsson G, Hedenborg G, Wisen O, Norman A. Presence of bile acid metabolites in serum, urine and faeces in cirrhosis. Scand J Clin Lab Invest 1992; 52: 555–564.

79. Kaplan MM. Laboratory tests In: Schiff L, Schiff ER, eds. Disease of the liver. Philadelphia: Lippincott JB, 1987: 219–260.

80. Karmen A, Worblewski F, LeDue JS. Transaminase activity in human blood. J Clin Invest 1955; 34: 126–133.

81. Kater RMH, Mistilis SP. Obsteric cholestasis and pruritus of pregnancy. Med J Aust 1967; 54: 638–642.

82. Keeffe EB, Sunderland MC, Gabourel JD. Serum gamma-glutamyltranspeptidase acdivity in patients receiving chronic phenytoin therapy. Dig Dis Sci 1986; 31: 1056–1061.

83. Kihn L, Rutkowski D, Nakatsui T, Stinson RA. Properties of amphiphilic and hydrophilic forms of alkaline phosphatse from human liver. Enzyme 1991; 45: 155–164.

84. Klein GL, Heyman MB, Lee TC, Miller NL, Marathe G, Gourley WK, Alfrey AC. Aluminum-associated hepatobiliary dysfunction in rats: relationships to dosage and duration of exposure. Pediatr Res 1988; 23: 275–278

85. Klion FM, Fabry TL, Palmer M, Schaffner F. Prediction of survival of patients with primary biliary cirrhosis. Examination of the Mayo clinic model on a group of patients with known endpoint. Gastroenterology 1992; 102: 310–313.

86. Kossor DC, Meunier PC, Handler JA, Sozio RS, Godstein RS. Temporal relationship of changes in hepatobiliary function and morphology in rats following *a*-naphthylisothiocyanate (ANIT) administration. Toxicol Appl Pharmacol 1993; 119: 108–114.

87. Kukongviriyapan V, Kukongviriyapan U, Stacey NH. Interference with hepatocellular substrate uptake by 1,1,1-trichloroethane and tetrachloroethylene. Toxicol Appl Pharmacol 1990; 102: 80–90.

88. Kukongviriyapan V, Stacey NH. Inhibition of taurocholate transport by cyclosporin A in cultured rat hepatocytes. J Pharmacol Exp Ther 1988; 247: 685–689.

89. Laker MF. Liver function tests. Br Med J 1990; 301: 250–251.

90. Larson JL, Wolf DC, Butterworth BE. Acute hepatotoxic and nephrotoxic effects of chloroform in male F-344 rats and female B6C3F1 mice. Fundam Appl Toxicol 1993; 20: 302–315.

91. Lawson AM, Setchell KDR. Mass spectrometry of bile acids In: Setchell KDR, Kritchevsky D, Nair PP, eds. The bile acids, chemistry physiology and metabolism Vol 4: Methods and applications. New York. Plenum Press, 1988: 167–267.

92. Linnet K, Keback H, Bahnsen M. Diagnostic values of fasting and postprandial concentrations in serum of hydroxy bile acids and gamma-glutamyl transferase in hepatobiliary disease. Scand J Gastroenterol 1983; 18: 49–56.

93. Liss GM, Greenberg RA, Tamburro CH. Use of serum bile acid in the identification of vinyl chloride hepatotoxicity. Am J Med 1985; 78: 68–75.

94. Liu JJY. Individual serum bile acids in spray painters exposed to different levels of solvents. MOHS Treatise. The University of Sydney, Australia, 1994.

95. Low MG. Biochemistry of the glycosyl-phosphatidylinositol anchor in membranes. Biochem J 1987; 244: 1–13.

96. Lundberg I, Hakansson M. Normal serum activities of liver enzymes in Swedish paint industry workers with heavy exposure to organic solvents. Br. J Ind Med 1986; 42: 596–600.

97. Mannes GA, Stellaard F, Paumgartner G. Increased serum bile acid in cirrhosis with normal transaminases. Digestion 1982; 25: 217–221.

98. Mannes GA, Thieme C, Stellaard F, Wang T, Sauerbruch T, Paumgartner G. Prognostic significance of serum bile acids in cirrhosis. Hepatopolgy 1986; 6: 50–53.

99. Manolio TA, Burke GL, Savage PJ, Jacobs DR Jr, Sidney S, Wagenknecht LE, Allman RM, Tracy RP. Sex-and race-related differences in liver-associated serum chemistry test in young adults in the CARDIA study. Clin Chem 1992; 38: 1853–1859.

100. Marshall WJ. Clinical chemistry. Philadelphia: Lippincott JB, 1988: 75–89.

101. McCormick WC III, Bell CC Jr, Swell L, Vlahcevic ZR. Cholic acid synthesis as an index of the severity of liver disease in man. Gut 1973; 14: 895–902.

102. McKenna JP, Moskovitz M, Cox J. Abnormal liver function tests in asymptomatic patient. Am Fam Physician 1989; 39: 117–126.

103. Merkel C, Bolognesi M, Bellon S, Bianco S, Honisch B, Lampe H, Angeli P, Gatta A. Aminopyrine breath test in the prognostic evaluation of patients with cirrhosis. Gut 1992; 33: 836–842.

104. Merkel C, Gatta A, Zoli M, Bolognesi M, Angeli P, Iervese T, Marchesini G, Ruol A. Prognostic value of galactose elimination capacity, aminopyrine breath test, and ICG clearance in patients with cirrhosis. Comparison with the Pugh Score. Dig Dis Sci 1991; 36: 1197–1203.

105. Meyer DJ. Liver function tests in dogs with portosystemic shunts: measurement of serum bile acid concentration. J Am Vet Med Assoc 1986; 188: 168–169.

106. Mora NP, Cienfuegos JA, Codoceo R, Jara P, Tendillo FJ, Menchaca C, Berisa F, Navidad R, Castillo-Olivares JL. Monitoring of serum total bile acids as an early indicator of graft function in clinical and experimental liver transplantation. Transplant Proc 1987; 19: 3840–3841.

107. Morgan DL, Mahler JF, O'Connor RW, Price HC Jr, Adkins B Jr. Styrene inhalation toxicity studies in mice I. hepatotoxicity in B6C3F1 mice. Fundam Appl Toxicol 1993; 20: 325–335

108. Moss DW, Henderson AR, Kachmar JF. Enzymes In: Tietz NW, ed. Fundamentals of clinical chemistry. 3rd ed. Philadelphia: Saunder WB, 1987: 346–421.

109. Muraca M, Kohlhaw K, Vilei MT, Ringe B, Bunzendahl H. Gubernatis G, Wonigeit K. Serum bile acids and estrified bilirubin in early detection and differential diagnosis of hepatic dysfunction following orthotopic liver transplantation. J Hepatol 1993; 17: 141–145.

110. Mutimer DJ, Bassendine MF, Kelly P, James OF. Is measurment of type III procollagen amin peptide usefull in primary biliary cirrhosis. J Hepatol 1989; 9: 184–189.

111. Nanji AA. Decreased activity of commonly measured serum enzymes: causes and clinical significance. Am J Med Technol 1983; 49: 241–245.

112. Neuman MG, Ishay JS, Eschar J. Bile aids in rat serum as indicators of hepatotoxicity by hornet venom. Proc Soc Exp Biol Med 1990; 195: 279–281.

113. Niblock AE, Leung FY, Henderson AR. Serum aspartate aminotransferase storage and the effect of pyridoxal phosphate. J Lab Clin Med 1986; 108: 461–465.

114. Nikopoulos A, Giannoulis E, Doutsos I, Grammaticos P, Tourkantonis A, Arvanitakis C. Elevation of [^{14}C] aminopyrine breath test, peripheral clearance of [99m TC] EHIDA, and serum bile acid levels in liver function and disease. Dig Dis Sci 1992; 37: 1655–1660.

115. Nyberg A, Engstrom-Laurent A, Loof L. Serum hyaluronate in primary biliary cirrhosis— a biochemical marker for progressive liver damage. Hepatology 1988; 8: 142–146.

116. O'Grady JC, Williams R. Present position of liver transplantation and its effect on hepatological practice. Gut 1989; 29: 566–570.

117. O'Grady JG, Alexander GJM, Haylak K, Williams R. Early indicators of prognosis in fulminant hepatic failure. Gastroenterology 1989; 97: 439–445.

118. Oellerich M, Burdelski M, Lautz HU, Schulz M, Schmidt FW, Herrmann H. Lidocaine metabolite formation as a measure of liver function in patients with cirrhosis. Ther Drug. Monit 1990; 12: 219–226.

119. Pauwels A, Mostefa-Kara N, Florent C, Levy VG. Emergency liver transplantation for acute liver failure: Evaluation of London and Clichy criteria. J Hepatol 1993; 17: 124–127.

120. Penn R, Worthington DJ. Is serum γ-glutamyltransferase a misleading test? Br Med J 1983; 286; 531–535.

121. Peters T Jnr. Serum albumin. In: Putnam FW, ed. The plasma proteins. Vol i. New York: Academic Press, 1975: 133–181.

122. Plaa GL, Hewitt WR. Detection and evaluation of chemically induced liver injury. In: Hayes AW. ed. Principles and methods of toxicology. 2nd Ed. New York: Raven Press, 1989: 599–628.

123. Posen S. Alkaline phosphatase. Ann Intern Med 1967; 67: 183–203.

124. Pugh RNH, Murray–Lyon IM, Dawson JL, Pietroni MC, Williams R. Transection of the oesophagus for bleeding oesophageal varices. Br J Surg 1973; 60: 646–649.

125. Reichen J, Widmer T, Cotting J. Accurate prediction of death by serial determination of glactose elimination capacity in primary biliary cirrhosis: a comparison with the Mayo model. Hepatology 1991; 14: 504–510.

126. Reichling JJ, Kaplan MM. Clinical use of serum enzymes in liver disease. Dig Dis Sci 1988; 33: 1601–1614.

127. Roberts WM. Variations in the phosphatase activity in the blood in disease. Br J Exp Pathol 1930; 11: 90–95.

128. Rosario J, Sutherland E, Zaccaro L, Simon FR. Ethinylestradiol administration selectively alters liver sinusoidal membrane lipid fluidity and protein composition. Biochemistry 1988; 27: 3939–3946.

129. Rydning A, Schrumpf E, Abdelnoor M, Elgjo K, Jenssen E. Factors of prognostic importance in primary biliary cirrhosis. Scand J Gastroenterol 1990; 25: 119–126.

130. Sahdev P, Garramone RR Jr, Schwartz RJ, Steelman SR, Jacobs LM. Evaluation of liver function tests in screening for intraabdominal injuries. Ann Emerg Med 1991; 20: 838–841.

131. Samuelson K, Aly A, Johansson C, Norman A. Evaluation of fasting serum bile acid concentration in patients with liver and gastrointestinal disorders. Scand J Gatroenterol 1981; 16: 225–234.

132. Samuelson K, Aly A, Johansson C, Norman A. Serum and urinary bile acids in patients with primary biliary cirrhosis Scand J Gatroenterol 1982; 17: 121–128.

133. Schaeffer MC, Rogers QR, Buffington CA, Wolfe BM, Strombeck DR. Long-term biological and physiological effects of surgically placed portocarval shunts in dogs. Am J Vet Res 1986; 47: 346–355.

134. Setchell KDR, Matsui A. Serum bile acid analysis. Cline Chim Acta 1983; 127: 1–17.

135. Shapiro JM, Smith H, Schaffner C. Serum bilirubin: a prognostic factor in primary biliary cirrhosis. Gut 1979; 20: 137–140.

136. Sherman KE. Alanine aminotransferase in clinical practice. Arch Intern Med 1991; 151: 260–265.

137. Stacey NH. Effects of ethinylestradiol on substrate uptake and efflux by isolated rat hepatocytes. Biochem Pharmacol 1986; 35: 2495–2500.

138. Stacey NH and Kotecka B, Inhibition of taurocholate and ouabain transport in isolated rat hepatocytes by cyclosporin A. Gastroerology 1988; 95: 780–786.

139. Stacey NH, Cook R, Priestly BG. Comparative stability of alanine aminotransferase in rat plasma and hepatocyte suspensions. Aust J Exp Biol Med Sci 1978; 56: 379–381.

140. Stacey NH, Haschek WM, Winder C. Systemic Toxicology. In: Stacey NH. ed. Occupational Toxicology. London: Taylor and Francis, 1993: 37–76.

141. Starzl TE, Demetris AJ, Van Thiel DH. Liver Transplanttion [first of two parts]. N Engl J Med 1989; 321: 1014–1022.

142. Stolz A, Kaplowitz N. Biochemical tests for liver diseases In: Zakium D, Boyer TD, eds. Hepatology: a textbook of liver disease. Philadelphia: Sunders WB, 1990: 637–667.

143. Stone BG, Udani M, Sanghvi A, Warty V, Plocki K, Bedetti CD, Van Thiel DH. Cyclosporin A-induced cholestasis. The mechanism in a rat model. Gastroenterology 1987; 93: 344–351.

144. Tagesson C. Liver damage and laboratory diagnostics. Scand J Work Environ Health 1985; 11 (suppl 1): 101–103.

145. Takahashi Y, Kumada H, Shimuzu M, Tanikawa K, Kumashiro R, Omata M, Ehata T, Tsuji T, Ukida M, Yasunaga M, Okita K, Sato S, Takeuchi T, Tsukada K, Obata H, Hashimoto E, Ohta Y, Tada K, Kosaka Y, Takase K, Yoshiba M, Sekiyama K, Kano T, Mizoguchi Y. A multicenter study on the prognosis of fulminant viral hepatitis: early prediction for liver transplantation. Hepatology 1994; 19: 1965–1071.

146. Tamburro CH, Greenberg R. Effectiveness of federally required medical laboratory screening in the detection of chemical liver injury. Environ Helth Prespect 1981; 41: 117–122.

147. Thalhammer T, Kaschnitz R, Mittermayer K, Haddad P, Graf J. Organic solvents increase membrane fliuidity and affect bile flow and K$^+$ transport in rat liver. Biochem Pharmacol 1993; 46: 1207–1215.

148. Thornton JR, Lobo AJ, Lintott DJ, Axon AT. Value of ultrasound and liver function tests in determining the need for endoscopic retrograde cholangiopancreatography in unexplained abdominal pain. Gut 1992; 33: 1559–1561.

149. Villeneuve JP, Infante-Rivard C, Ampelas M, Pomier-Layrargues G, Guet PM, Marleau D. Prognostic value of the aminopyrine breath test in cirrhotic patients. Hepatology 1986; 6: 928–931.

150. Visser JJ, Bom-van Noorloos AA, Meijer S, Hoitsma HFW. Serum total bile acids monitoring after experimental orthotopic liver transplantation. J Surg Res 1984; 36: 147–153.

151. Wang G, Staey NH, Earl J. Determination of individual bile acids in serum by high performance liquid chromatography. Biomed Chromatogr 1990; 4: 136–140.

152. Wang G, Stacey NH. Elevation of individual serum bile acids on exposure to trichloroethylene or α-napthylisothiocyanate. Toxicol Appl Pharmacol 1990; 105: 209–215.

153. Westaby D, Mc Dougall BRD, Williams R. Improved surivival following injection sclerotherapy for esophageal varices: final analysis of a control trial. Hepatology 1985; 5: 827–830.

154. Whicher J, Spence C. When is serum albumin worth measuring? Ann Clin Biochem 1987; 24: 572–580.

155. Wienser RH, Grambsch PM, Diskson ER, Ludwig J, Mac Carty RL, Hunter EB, Fleming TR, Fisher LD, Beaver SJ, LaRusso NF. Primary sclerosing cholangitis: natural history, prognostic factors and survival analysis. Hepatology 1989; 10: 430–436.

156. Wiesner RH, Porayko MK, Dickson ER, Gores GJ, LaRusso NF, Hay JE, Wahlstrom, Krom RAF. Selection and timing of liver transplantation in primary biliary cirrhosis and primary sclerosing cholangitis. Hepatology 1992; 16: 1290–1299.

157. Willson RA, Hart JR, Hall T. Chlorpromazine administered in vivo and in vitro inhibits the efflux of bile acids in freshly isolated rat hepatocytes. Pharmacol Toxicol 1989; 64: 454–458.

158. Wilson JW, Inherited elevation of alkaline phosphatase activity in the absence of disease. N Engl J Med 1979; 301: 983–984.

159. Woodman DD. Hepatic dysfunction in laboratory animals. In: Blackmore DJ, ed. Animal clinical biochemistry—The future. Cambridge: Cambridge University Press, 1988: 151–160.

160. Yaari A, Sikuler E, Keynan A, Ben–Zui Z. Bromosulfophthalein disposition in chronically bile duct obstructed rats. J Hepatol 1992; 15: 67–72.

161. Ziegler K, Frimmer M. Cyclosporin A and a diaziridine derivative inhibit the hepatocellular uptake of cholate, phalloidin and rifampicin. Biochim Biophys Acta 1986; 855: 136–142.

162. Zimmerman HJ. Hepatotoxicity. New York: Appleton-Century-Crofts, 1978.

Liver and Environmental Xenobiotics
S.V.S. Rana and K. Taketa (Eds)
Copyright © 1997, Narosa Publishing House, New Delhi, India

15. Hepatic Bilirubin Metabolism: Physiology and Pathophysiology

Yukihiko Adachi and Toshinori Kamisako*

Third Department of Internal Medicine, Faculty of Medicine
Mie University, Tsu 514, Japan

*Second Department of Internal Medicine, Kinki University School of Medicine
Osakasayama 589, Japan

Bilirubin Metabolism Under Physiological Conditions

Bilirubin is a final product of heme degradation after opening of the porphyrin ring by heme oxygenase. The 70-80% of bilirubin is derived from hemoglobin of senescent erythrocytes and the rest from ineffective erythropoiesis in the bone marrow (heme not used for hematopoiesis), and rapid hepatic metabolism of heme and hemoproteins such as cytochrome P450 [1]. Heme oxygenase is distributed in the liver, spleen, bone marrow, renal parenchyma, and reticuloendothelial system and is induced by heme substrates [2]. Bilirubin produced by heme oxygenase is released into the blood, where the majority is bound to albumin and transported to the liver. About 20% of physiological bilirubin production in the body is from hepatic heme, about a half of it is excreted into bile, and the rest contributes to the blood bilirubin turnover [3].

After transfer into the space of Disse from the sinusoids, a small quantity of bilirubin unbound to albumin is taken up into the hepatocytes by transport proteins on the hepatocellular membrane [4]. Reported transport proteins include bilitranslocase and organic anion-binding protein (OABP), which implement potential-dependent transport, and bilirubin/BSP-binding protein (BBBP), which transports the protonated form of bilirubin [5, 6,]. Recently, expression cloning in the *Xenopus laevis* oocyte system has identified a 71 kDa BSP-transporting protein, designated organic anion transporting polypeptide (oatp) [5, 6]. Since chloride ion (Cl^-) promotes dissociation of bilirubin from albumin, there is an apparent Cl^--dependency of hepatocellular bilirubin uptake as observed for OABP and oatp. The substrate specificities overlapped among these transporters and the relationship among these different transporters is still not well understood. The process of hepatocellular bilirubin uptake is thought to be energy-independent.

In the hepatocytes, bilirubin binds to ligandin (glutathione S-transferase 1-1 and 1-2 in the supernatant fraction of the liver) and is transported to endoplasmic reticulum (ER) [7]. It has also been suggested that bilirubin is transferred rapidly via the intracellular membrane structure before transportation into the ER [8]. Z protein, which is an another bilirubin-binding protein in hepatocytes, inhibits bilirubin reflux into the blood but plays no apparent role on intracellular transport [9].

After transfer into the ER from the cytoplasm, hydrophobic bilirubin undergoes glucuronidation to form hydrophilic bilirubin monoglucuronide (BMG) and then bilirubin diglucuronide (BDG) (the hydrophilicity of the latter is higher) in a process mediated by bilirubin UDP-glucuronosyl-transferase (BUGT). These bilirubin glucuronides can be secreted into the bile canalicules and are collectively referred to as conjugated bilirubin. Two families of UDP-glucuronosyltransferases (UGT) (UGT1 and UGT2) perform glucuronidation of not only bilirubin, but also steroid hormones and xenobiotics including exogenous carcinogens to make their biliary excretion possible [10]. UGT1 isozymes have sugar chains and a molecular weight of 48, 000–56, 000. They reside in the membrane of the ER and their active sites are on the inner side of the membrane [11]. The UGT1 gene *(UGT1)* is composed of 5 exons, with exon 1 (consisting of at least exons 1A to 1G) on the N terminal side specific to each isozyme and exons 2 to 5 on the C terminal side common to all isozymes (Fig. 1) [12]. Seven UGT1 isozymes varying in substrate specificity can be expressed by the one gene complex *(UGT1)* through differential splicing. BUGT is expressed from exons 1A and 2–5 and designated as UGT1*1. UGT1*6 and UGT1*7 expressed from exons 1F and 2–5 and exon 1G and 2–5, respectively, are phenol UDP-glucuronosyltransferases.

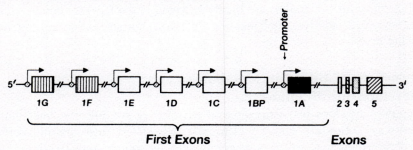

Fig. 1. Schematic diagram of *UGT1* gene encoding the human BUGT and phenol UGT isozymes. Locus of the *UGT1* gene complex is located on 2q37 and spans at least 95kb. Each specific exon 1 (1A-1G) encodes 289 out of 533 amino acids of its specific isozyme, which determine the substrate specificity, and a *cis*-positioned promoter is present for each exon 1. Exons 2–5 encode 246 amino acids in the carboxyl terminal region of all isozymes. Hence, the *UGT1* gene complex encodes at least 7 isozymes. UGT1*1 produced from exons 1A and 2–5 is BUGT, and UGT1*6 and UGT1*7 produced from exons 1F and 2–5 and exons 1G and 2–5, respectively are responsible for phenol glucuronidation UDP1*4 glucuronidates amines. However, the physiological significance of the other isozymes is yet to be determined.

Conjugated bilirubin is transferred across the microsomal membrane into the cytoplasm, binds to ligandin again and is transported to the canalicular membrane. Then, it is secreted into the bile canaliculus, through electrogenic transport [13], which is accelerated by bicarbonate ion, as well as ATP-dependent active transport [14]. The protein involved in ATP-dependent active transport is referred to as the canalicular multispecific organic anion transporter (MOAT) and differs from the ATP-dependent bile salt transporter (BST), the MDR1 which transports cationic and neutral drugs (such as daunomycin), or the MDR3 transports phospholipid [15]. These ATP-dependent transporters are called ATP-binding cassette (ABC) transporters. Recently, Mayer et al [16] reported that MOAT is homologous to the multi-drug resistance-associated protein (MRP) and MRP-immunoreactivity is defective on the canalicular membrane of the hepatocytes of the jaundiced mutant TR⁻ and Groningen yellow rats.

In addition, it has been found that ATP-dependent transport of pravastatin, an organic anion, is accelerated by an upward pH gradient (from cytoplasm to bile canalicular lumen) [17]. The above-mentioned main pathway of bilirubin transport in hepatocytes is completely different from that for bile salts. However, in the presence of excess bilirubin load, alternative vesicular transport also works for intracellular conjugated bilirubin transfer, which is shared by bile salts [18]. A schematic diagram of hepatocellular bilirubin metabolism is shown in Fig. 2.

Conjugated bilirubin secreted into bile is retained temporarily in the gallbladder and then secreted into the duodenum. Subsequently, it is reduced to urobilin compounds (such as urobilinogen) by enteric bacteria. The majority of the urobilin compounds are finally excreted in the feces, although some is reabsorbed and re-secreted into bile (entero-hepatic circulation) or excreted in the urine.

Disorders of Bilirubin Metabolism and Development of Jaundice

Jaundice develops by disturbance of any part of the bilirubin metabolic pathway. Jaundice can be clinically classified into unconjugated hyperbilirubinemia, which is predominantly due to unconjugated (indirect) bilirubin with ≤ 20% direct bilirubin, and conjugated hyperbilirubinemia which is predominantly due to conjugated (direct) bilirubin (although unconjugated bilirubin also increases in some occasions). Serum conjugated bilirubin consists of delta bilirubin, BDG, and BMG. Delta bilirubin is produced by the covalent bonding of conjugated bilirubin, especially BDG and albumin in the blood [19]. Because it is neither filtered through the renal glomeruli nor taken up by the liver, the half-life of delta bilirubin in the blood is long, as is the case with the albumin. Unconjugated hyperbilirubinemia is attributable to disturbance in bilirubin metabolism

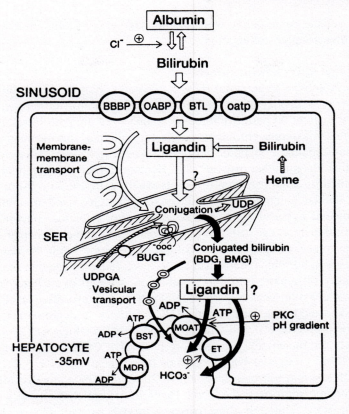

BILE CANALICULUS

Fig. 2. Schematic presentation of hepatocyte bilirubin metabolism. Four different transporters have been proposed for hepatocellular uptake of bilirubin: BTL (bilitranslocase, Mw 37 kD), BBBP (bilirubin/bromosulfophthalen-binding protein, Mw 55 kD), OABP (organic anion-binding protein, Mw 55 kD) and oatp (organic anion transporting polypeptide, Mw 80 kD). BBBP, OABP and oatp are reported to be involved in electrogenic transport, whereas BTL is involved in electroneutral transport. Chloride ion stimulated transport by OABP and oatp, probably by stimulating dissociation of bilirubin from serum albumin. For bile salt uptake, the sodium-dependent different transporter is responsible. Active site of BUGT is located in the lumen of endoplasmic reticulum (ER), and transpot of UDP-glucuronic acid (UDPGA) from the cyotoplasm into the lumen is carrier-mediated. However, the mechanism of bilirubin transport through the ER membrane is not yet elucidated. Conjugated bilirubin is bound to ligandin and transported to the canalicular membrane. When the load of conjugated bilirubin increases, the alternative vesicular transport system works additionally. At canalicular membrane, an ATP-dependent multispecific organic anion transporter (MOAT), which may be stimulated by protein kinase C (PKC) and/or transmembrane pH gradient and bicarbonate-stimulated electrogenic transporter are present for conjugated bilirubin excretion. At the least three other ATP-dependent transporters are reported on the canalicular membrane; BST (bile salt transporter), MDR1 (multidrug resistant transporter) and MDR3 (phospholipid transporter).

prior to hepatic conjugation, while conjugated heperbilirubinemia is due to its disturbance after conjugation.

Unconjugated Hyperbilirubinemia

Hemolytic anemia (congenital or acquired) and shunt hyperbilirubinemia (primary or secondary) are caused by increased bilirubin production. Secondary shunt hyperbilirubinemia is observed in pernicious anemia porphyria, thalassemia, chronic myeloblastic leukemia, aplastic anemia, iron deficiency anemia, congenital dyserythropoietic anemia, lead poisoning, exsanguination and other diseases [20]. Hepatocellular bilirubin uptake may be inhibited by administration of agents which compete with bilirubin for hepatic uptake (such as flavaspidic acid, rifampicin and bunamiodyl). Unconjugated hyperbilirubinemia occurring after hepatitis (post-hepatitis hyperbilirubinemia) can also be attributable to disturbance of hepatocelular bilirubin uptake. A few cases of Gilbert's syndrome might be due to an abnormality in bilirubin metabolism at this level. Jaundice due to a congenital abnormality of hepatic bilirubin metabolism, without overt hemolysis, is known as constitutional hyperbilirubinemia and is classified as Crigler-Najjar syndrome type I (in which BUGT activity is defective), Crigler-Najjar syndrome type II and Gilbert's syndrome (in which BUGT activity is severely and moderately decreased, respectively). Crigler-Najjar syndrome type 1 (Table 1): Crigler-Najjar sydrome type I manifests at 1–3 days after birth with a serum bilirubin level above 20 mg/dl. Unconjugated bilirubin is the predominant form in the blood. Death from kernicterus usually occurs during infancy, although some patients survive to adolescence without neurological involvement. BUGT activity is lost due to a homozygous point mutation (mainly nonsense mutation) or deletion of nucleotides in the *UGT1*1* gene (autosomal recessive inheritance) (Table 2 [21–25]). Since the enzyme cannot be induced by drugs such as phenobarbital, plasma exchange or phototherapy is performed for treatment. Hepatic transplantation is the only effective measure. Crigler-Najjar syndrome type II (Table 1 [26]): In Crigler-Najjar syndrome type II, the serum bilirubin level commonly ranges from 6 to 27 (usually 6 to 20) mg/dl and unconjugated bilirubin is predominant in the blood. There is a characteristically marked decrease in BDG (12.9 ± 6.0% vs. 76.5 ± 4.8% in healthy individuals) and marked increase in BMG (64.5 ± 7.8% vs. 9.8 ± 2.5% in healthy individuals) in the duodenal bile (Fig. 3. [27]). BUGT activity is reduced markedly to about 10% of normal [28], mainly by a homozygous point mutation (missense mutation) of *UGT1*1* gene (autosomal recessive inheritance) (Table 2) [24, 25, 29, 30]. Crigler-Najjar syndrome type II can be discriminated from type I by the fact that hyperbilirubinemia can be improved by administration of hepatic enzyme-inducing drugs (e.g. phenobarbital). Patients usually grow up without neurological symptoms and can lead a normal life. No treatment is necessary (although enzyme-inducing drugs may be used for diagnostic and cosmetic reasons). The progenosis is thus, good.

Table 1. Principal features of the inherited unconjugated hyperbilirubinemia

	Gilbert's syndrome	Crigler-Najjar syndrome type II	Crigler-Najjar syndrome type I
Pathogenesis	Missense mutation in the BUGT gene (*UGT1*) or additional TA in the promoter region of exon 1A	Missense mutations in the *UGT1* gene	Nonsense or missenense mutations or deletion of nucleotides in the *UGT1* gene
Mode of Inheritance	Autosomal dominant or recessive	Autosomal recessive (dominant in some)	Autosomal recessive
Prevalence	2–7% of population	Rare	Rare
Serum bilirubin	1–6 mg/dl	6–20 mg/dl	Above 20 mg/dl
BUGT activity in liver microsome	Reduced to about 30% of normal	Reduced to about 10% of normal	Absent
Reduction of serum bilirubin by phenobarbital	Yes	Yes	No
Biliary bilirubin	Increase in proportion of BMG	Marked increase in proportion of BMG	Trace amount (unconjugated bilirubin, about 90%)
Routine liver function test	Normal	Normal	Normal
Gross and histologic appearance of the liver	Normal	Normal	Normal
Kernicterus	None	Rare	Common
Treatment	Not needed	Not needed	Phototherapy; plasma exchange; liver transplantation
Prognosis	Good	Good	Poor due to kernicterus

Gilbert's Syndrome (Table 1 [26]): In patients with Gilbert's syndrome, the serum bilirubin level is commonly below 6 mg/dl and unconjugated bilirubin is a predominant form. There is a characteristically moderate decrease of BDG ($55.4 \pm 4.7\%$) and an increase of BMG ($28.6 \pm 5.3\%$) in bile (Fig. 3) [27]. BUGT activity is decreased to about 30% of that in healthy individuals [28]. The low calorie diet test and nicotinic acid test are used for diagnosing this type of hyperbilirubinemia. Patients usually show a two-fold or greater increase in the serum bilirubin level when fed a low calorie diet (400 cal/day) for 2 days [31]. In the nicotinic acid test, the serum bilirubin level increases markedly from 0.38 ± 0.12 mg/dl increment in normal patients to 1.73 ± 0.21 mg/dl increment in patients with Gilbert's syndrome 3–5 hr after the intravenous administration of 50 mg of nicotinic acid [32]. The incidence of Gilbert's syndrome is high, being in the range of 2–7% in the population. A heterozygous point mutation (missense mutation) of *UGT1*1* with autosomal dominant inheritance is commonly seen [33] (Table 2). Since BUGT activity is only about 30% (and not about 50%) of that in healthy individuals, despite the heterozygous state, a dominant negative mutation has been suggested as the etiology [34]. However, a homozygous mutation in the promoter region of *UGT1*1* has also been suggested as the etiology of this type of jaundice [35]. Administration of a hepatic enzyme-inducing agent (e.g. phenobarbital) can improve hyperbilirubinemia, but it is used only for diagnostic purpose since the prognosis is favorable in Gilbert's syndrome.

Decreased hepatic BUGT activity is also detected in the following pathological conditions:

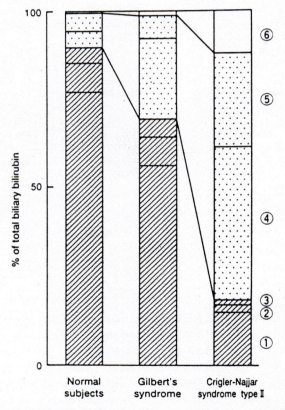

Fig. 3. Composition of biliary bile pigments in normal subjects, and patients with Gilbert's syndrome and with Crigler-Najjar syndrome. 1: BDG, 2: bilirubin monoglucuronide monoglucoside diester, 3: bilirubin monoglucuronide monoxyloside diester, 4: C_8–BMG, 5: C_{12}–BMG, 6: unconjugated bilirubin. Bilirubin diconjugates (1–3) decreased and bilirubin mono-conjugates (4 and 5) increased by steps in Gilbert's syndrome and Crigler-Najjar syndrome type II in this order.

Table 2. **Reported *UGT1* gene mutatins in hereditary unconjugated hyperbilirubinemia**

(1) Crigler-Najjar syndrome type I

No.	Zygosity	Mutation DNA	Mutation Protein	References
1.	homo	3 base pair-deletion exon 1A (508–510)	Phe 170 deletion	Ritter et al. (1993) Seppen et al (1994)
2.	home	missense, G to C, exon 1A (826)	Gly276→Arg	Seppen et al (1994) Ciotti et al. (1995)
3.	home	nonsense, C to A exon 1A (840)	Cys280→Stop	Aono et al. (1994)
4.	hetero	missense, T to C, exon 1A (529)	Cys177→Arg	Seppen et al. (1994)
		& 14 base pair-deletion, exon 2 (879–892)	Frameshift	
5.	homo	deletion, exon 2		Seppen et al. (1994)
6.	homo	13 base pair deleti- tion exon 2 (880–94)	72 aa unrelated 240 aa missing	Ritter et al. (1992)
7.	home	missense, G to A, exon 2 (923)	Gly308→Glu	Erps et al. (1994) Labrune et al. (1994)
8.	homo	nonsense, C to T exon 2 (991)	Gln331→Stop, exon 2 skipping	Bosma et al. 1992)
9.	homo	missense, C to T, exon 2 (872) &	Ala291→Val	Labrune et al. 1994)
		missense, A to G, exon 4 (1282)	Lys426→Glu	
10.	homo	nonsense, C to T exon 3 (1021)	Arg341→Stop	Morghrabi et al. (1993)
11.	homo	nonsense, C to T exon 3 (1069)	Gln357→Stop	Bosma et al. (1992)
12.	homo	missense, A to G, exon 3 (1070)	Gln357→Arg	Labrune et al. (1994)
13.	homo	missense, G to A, exon 3 (1005)	Trp335→Stop	Labrune et al. (1994)
		& missense, G to A, exon 4 (1105)	Ala401→Thr	
14.	homo	missense, G to A, exon 3 (1002)	Trp335→Stop	Labrune et al. (1994)
		& insetion of G exon 4 (after 1223)	Frameshift	
15.	homo	missense, C to T, exon 3 (1069)	Gln357→Stop	Labrune et al. (1994)
		& missense, G to C, exon 4 (1201)	Ala401→Pro	
16.	homo	missense, C to T exon 4 (1124)	Ser375→Phe	Bosma et al. (1992)
17.	homo	missense, C to T exon 4 (1130)	Ser375→Phe	Seppen et al. (1994)

(Contd)

No.	Zygosity	Mutation DNA	Mutation Protein	References
18.	homo	missense, C to G, exon 4 (1143)	Ser381→Arg	Labrune et al. (1994)
19.	homo	missense, G to C, exon 4 (1201)	Ala401→Pro	Labrune et al. (1994)
20.	homo	missense, G to C. exon 4 (1201)	Ala401→Pro	Labrune et al. (1994)
		& missense, A to T, exon 5 (1308)	Lys437→Stop	

(2) Crigler-Najjar syndrome type II

No.	Zygosity	Mutation DNA	Mutation Protein	References
1.	homo	mossense, T to C, exon 1A (209)	Arg209→Trp	Seppen et al. (1994)
2.	homo	missense, C to T, exon 1A (625)	Arg209→Trp	Bosma et al. (1993)
3.	hetero	missense, T to A, exon 1A (524)	Leu175→Glu	Seppen et al. (1994)
		& deletion of a nucleotide exon 2 (973)	Frameshift	
4.	homo	missense, G to A, exon 1A (211) &	Gly71→Arg	Aono et al. (1993)
		missense, T to G exon 5 (1456)	Tyr486→Asp	
5.	homo	missense, A to G, exon 2 (992)	Gln331→Arg	Moghrabi et al. (1993)

(3) Gilbert's syndrome

No.	Zygosity	Mutation DNA	Mutation Protein	References
1.	hetero & homo	missense, G to A, exon 1A (211)	Gly71→Arg	Aono et al. (1995)
2.	hetero	missense, C to A, exon 1A (686)	Pro229→Gln	Aono et al. (1995)
3.	hetero	missense, C to G, exon 4 (1099)	Arg367→Gly	Aono et al. (1995)
4.	hetero	missense, T to G exon J (1456)	Tyr486→Asp	Sato et al. (1996)
5.	homo	additional TA in the TATA box (promotor region)	(–)	Bosma et al. (1995)

*In this patient homozygous additional TA was found in the promotor region of exon 1A (Sato et al. unpublished data).

Neonatal Jaundice: Unconjugated hyperbilirubinemia occurring within 24 hr of birth is called neonatal jaundice. The level of unconjugated bilirubin in the serum reaches a peak at 12.8 ± 3.6 mg/dl around 5–6 days after birth in Japanese neonates. The peak bilirubin level is higher and occurs later in Japanese neonates than in Caucasians. Many factors are involved in the etiology of neonatal jaundice including excessive bilirubin production, reduced hepatic bilirubin uptake, reduced bilirubin conjugation due to immature BUGT activity, and increased enterohepatic bilirubin circulation which occurs from the deconjugation of enteric conjugated bilirubin, low production of urobilin compounds because of the paucity of enteric bacteria [36]) and the resultant increase in unconjugated bilirubin reabsorption.

Breast Milk Jaundice: Breast milk-related unconjugated hyperbilirubinemia is classified into two types: (1) the early onset type occurs in breast-feeding infants within 1 week of birth with a peak serum bilirubin level occurring at 1–2 weeks and (2) the second type of jaundice reaches its peak 1–2 weeks after birth and persists for 2–3 months. The early onset type has been suggested to be ascribable to insufficient breast milk intake and the low calorie content of breast milk. The second type, classical breast milk-related jaundice, is suggested to be caused by an increased enterohepatic circulation of bilirubin which results mainly from increased deconjugation of enteric conjugated bilirubin by β-glucuronidase in breast milk [37, 38].

Drugs and Hormones: Unconjugated hyperbilirubinemia can be induced by administration of drugs that inhibit BUGT activity such as novobiocin and gentamycin [39]. It has also been reported that glucuronidation and biliary excretion of bilirubin and other organic anions are decreased in rats given drugs such as salicylamide and diethylether [40, 41] which reduce intrahepatic UDP-glucuronic acid content. However, the clinical implications of this finding are not clear. Thyroid hormones and testosterone decrease hepatic bilirubin conjugation, whereas BUGT activity increases by a combination of progestational and estrogenic steroids [39].

Hepatocellular Damage: Hepatitis and liver cirrhosis generally induce increase of both conjugated and unconjugated bilirubin in the blood. However, the biliary bilirubin fractions do not change remarkably. Suggesting that bilirubin glucuronidation may not decrease remarkably [42].

Conjugated Hyperbilirubinemia
Constitutional jaundice is classified into Rotor's syndrome which may be associated with a defect abnormality of hepatocellular ligandin, and Dubin-Johnson syndrome which is associated with a defect in the transport of conjugated bilirubin across the bile canalicular membrane. Except for conjugated hyperbilirubinemia, these syndromes show no abnormalities in liver funcion tests including serum bile acid levels. In addition, diseases with congenital abnormalities of bile acid metabolism have been reported.

Dubin-Johnson syndrome (Table 3 [26]): Dubin-Johnson syndrome is characterized by mild to moderate conjugated hyperbilirubinemia (1–7 mg/dl in 91% of patients) as well as re-elevation of the serum BSP level after

60–180 min in the BSP test. Routine liver function tests reveal no abnormalities. Oral cholecystography shows poor gallbladder visualization and hepatobiliary scintigraphy reveals a marked delay of hepatic excretion of the scintilant. In addition, there is an increase of coproporphyrin (CP) isomer I (by $\geq$ 80%; normal range 20–45%) with a normal total urinary CP level and coarse black-brown granules in the hepatocytes (black liver). These changes are thought to be attributable to a defect in the transport of bilirubin and other organic anions across the hepatocyte canalicular membrace. *In vivo* biliary secretion of various anionic drugs, such as cefpiramide, cefodizyme and pravastatin, may be severely reduced in the jaundiced rat models. In patients who develop hepatitis, the hepatic pigment granules disappear. Jaundice can be worsened by female hormones and requires careful monitoring. The natural course is generally favorable and treatment is not indicated.

Table 3. **Principal features of the inherited conjugated hyperbilirubinemia**

	Dubin-Johnson syndrome	Rotor's syndrome
Pathogenesis	Defective transport of conjugated bilirubin across the canalicular membrane of hepatocytes (Defect of MOAT)	Defect of ligandin (glutathion S-transferase 1–1 and 1–2)
Mode of inheritance	Autosomal recessive	Autosomal recessive
Prevalence	Relativelty rare	Rare
Serum bilirubin (In most patients)	1–7 mg/dl	3–10 mg/dl
BSP test	Initial clearance: normal, Secondary rise after 60 min (mainly composed of conjugated BSP)	Initial clearance: markedly delayed, marked decrease in hepatic storage capacity
ICG test	Almost normal	Initial clearance: markedly delayed
Routine liver function tests	Normal	Normal
Clinical feature	Asymptomatic jaundic	Asymptomatic jaundice
Gross and histologic appearance of the liver	Black liver; coarse brown pigment granules in the hepatocytes	Normal
Oral cholecystography	usually unvisualized	Visualized
Hepatobiliary scintigraphy	Marked delay in biliary excretion	Marked delay in hepatic accumulation
Urinary CP	Normal amount; increased CP isomer I ($\geq$ 80%)*	Increased; Increased CP isomer I (< 80%)*
Treatment	Not introduced; Avoid using estrogens	Not introduced
Prognosis	Good	Good

MOAT: Canalicular multispecific organic anion transporter; BSP: sulfobromophthalein; ICG: indocyanine green; CP: coproporphyrin.
*Normal range: 20-45%.

Rotor's Syndrome (Table 3 [26]): Rotor's syndrome is associated with moderate conjugated hyperbilirubinemia (3–10 mg/dl in 87% of patients). Both the 15 min-plasma retention of indocyanine green (ICG) (ICG R_{15}) and the 45 min-retention of BSP (BSP R_{45}), indicate marked bilirubin retention in the blood, with the values being 72.9 ± 12.8% and 38.5 ± 12.5%, respectively. However, routine liver function tests and liver biopsy reveal no abnormalities. An increase of total urinary CP and urinary CP isomer I (by < 80%) are noted. Hepatobiliary scintigraphy reveals marked delay of hepatic accumulation of the scintilant. Oral cholecystography shows good gallbladder visualization. Since a marked decrease in the activity of glutathione S-transferase toward chloro-dinitrobenzene and negative immunohistochemical staining of the enzyme have been reported in patients with Rotor's syndrome, this disease is considered to be due to a ligandin defect [43, 44]. Although no current therapy is effective for this type of hyperbilirubinemia, the patients have a favorable prognosis.

Congenital abnormalities of bile acid metabolism: Lack of biliary secretion of primary bile acids has been reported in Byler disease [45]. Impairment of primary bile acid production can be caused by loss of 3 β-hydroxy1– Δ^5-C_{27}-steroid dehydrogenase isomerase or Δ^4–3-oxosteroid-5 β-reductase. In either case, marked intrahepatic cholestasis is observed during infancy.

Conjugated hyperbilirubinemia is caused by miscellaneous acquired abnormalities of bilirubin metabolism.

Cyclosporin A is known to inhibit canalicular transport of organic anions by MOAT and is thought to induce jaundice by inhibiting the bilirary secretion of bilirubin [46]. Hepatitis and liver cirrhosis disturb various steps of hepatic bilirubin metabolism. These liver diseases generally cause conjugated hyperbilirubinemia as a resut of impaired bilirubin secretion into the bile canaliculi, with an increase in serum unconjugated bilirubin level to a variable extent by impaired hepatic uptake and conjugation of bilirubin. Unlike constitutional jaundice, conjugated hyperbilirubinemia arising from an acquired abnormality of bilirubin metabolism is usually associated with an increase in the blood bile acid levels. Persistent conjugated hyperbilirubinemia is referred to as chronic intrahepatic cholestasis. Intrahepatic cholestasis of primary biliary cirrhosis is represented by chronic nonsuppurative destructive cholangitis. Obstructive jaundice can be caused by inflammation, biliary calculus formation and cancer of the intra- and extra-hepatic bile duct system. Actin filaments play a role in acceleration of biliary discharge through contraction of the bile canaliculi. Thus, loss of actin filaments caused by administration of actin inhibitors, such as phalloidin or cyclosporin B, is associated with cholestasis because of decreased and abnormal canalicular contraction and expansion of the canaliculi [47, 48].

During the exacerbation of obstructive jaundice, BDG and BMG levels in the blood surpasses that of delta bilirubin [delta bilirubin/(BDG + BMG +

delta bilirubin) ratio = 32.9 ± 6.6 (SD)%] and during the recovery phase this ratio increases to 78.2 ± 15.7% [49]. An experiment in rats demonstrated cessation of biliary secretion and reflux of bilirubin and bile acids into the blood when the intra-luminal pressure in the biliary tract exceeded 20 mmHg in obstructive jaundice [50]. These changes were reversible in the acute stage. In the rat study of Kountouras et al [51], bile flow increased when bile duct ligation was released after 5, 10, 15, and 28 days and the increase in flow was proportional to the period of ligation. However, the biliary bilirubin concentration decreased with time during bile duct ligation and total bilirubin secretion also decreased after 28 days of bile duct ligation. Evidence of liver cirrhosis was noted histologically after 15 days of ligation. These findings suggest that abnormal bilirubin metabolism during bile duct obstruction is induced by liver cirrhosis or liver damage resulting from sustanined cholestasis. Also in clinical medicine, prolonged jaundice is often observed without recovery of the biliary bilirubin concentration after the release of biliary obstruction.

References

1. Berk, P.D., Howe, R.B., Bloomer, J.R., Berlin, N.I. (1969). Studies on bilirubin kinetics in normal adults. J Clin Invest 48: 2176–2190.
2. Tenhunen, R., Marver, H.S., Schmid, R (1970). The enzymatic catabolism of hemoglobin: stimulation of microsomal heme oxygenase by hemin. J Lab Clin Med 75: 410–421.
3. Berk, P.D., Blaschke, T.R., Scharschmidt, B.F., Waggoner, J.G., Berlin, N. I. (1976). A new approach to quantitation of the various sources of bilirubin in man. J Lab Clin Med 87: 767–780.
4. Sorrentino, D., Zifroni, A., Van Ness, K., Berk, P.D. (1994). Unbound ligand drives hepatocyte taurocholate and BSP uptake at physiological albumin concentration. Am J Physiol 266: G425–432.
5. Ostrow, J.D., Mukerjee, P., Tiribelli, C. (1994). Structure and binding of unconjugated bilirubin: relevance for physiological and pathophysiological function. J Lipid Res 35: 1715–1737.
6. Oude Elferink, R.O.J., Meijer, D.K.F., Kuipers, F., Jansen, P.L.M., Groen A.K., Groothius, G.M.M. (1995). Hepatobiliary secretion of organic compounds; molecular mechanisms of membrane transport. Biochem Biophys Acta 1241: 215–268.
7. Mannervik, B. (1985). The isozymes of glutathione S-transferase. Adv Enzymol 57: 357–417.
8. Whitmer, D.I., Russell, P.E., Gollan, J.L. (1987). Membrane-membrane interactions associated with rapid transferase: relevance for hepatocellular transport and biotransformation of hydrophobic substrates. Biochem J. 244: 41–47.
9. Theilmann, L., Stollman, Y.R., Arias, I.M., Wolkoff, A.W. (1984). Does Z-protein have a role in transport of bilirubin and bromosulfophthalein by isolated perfused rat liver? Hepatology 4: 923–926.
10. Burchell, B., Nebert, D.W., Nelson., D.R., Bock, K.W., Iyanagi, T., Jansen, P. L.M., Lancet, D., Mulder, G. J., Roy Chowdhury, J., Siest, G., Tephly, T. R.,

Mackenzie, P.I. (1991). The UDP glucuronosyltransferase gene superfamily: suggested nomenclature based on evolutionary divergence. DNA Cell Biol 10: 487–494.

11. Shepherd, S.R.P., Baird, S.J., Hallinan, T., Burchell, B. (1989). An investigation of the transverse topology of bilirubin UDP-glucuronosyltransferase in rat hepatic endoplasmic reticulum. Biochem J 259: 617–620.

12. Owens, I. S., Ritter, J.K. (1992). The novel bilirubin/phenol UDP-glucuronosyltransferase *UGT1* gene locus: implications for multiple nonhemolytic familial hyperbilirubinemia. Phramacogenetics 2: 93–108.

13. Adachi, Y., Kobayashi, H., Kurumi, Y., Shouji, M., Kitano, M., Yamamoto, T. (1991). Bilirubin diglucuronide transport by rat liver canalicular membrane vesicles: Stimulation by bicarbonate ion. Hepatology 14: 1251–1258.

14. Nishida, T., Gatmatioan, Z., Roy-Chowdhury, J., Arias, I.M., (1992). Two distinct mechanisms for bilirubin glucuronide transport by rat bile canalicular membrane vesicles. Demonstration of defective ATP-dependent transport in rats (TR-) with inherited conjugated hyperbilirubinemia. J Clin Invest 90: 2130–2135.

15. Meier, P.J., Stieger, B. (1993). Canalicular membrane adenosine triphosphate-dependent transport systems. Progr Liver Dis 11: 27–44.

16. Mayer, R., Kartenbeck, J., Buchner, M., Jedlitschky, G., Leier, I., Keppler, D. (1995). Expression of the MRP gene-encoded conjugate export pump in liver and its selective absence from the canalicular membrane in transport-deficient mutant hepatocytes. J Cell Biol 131: 137–150.

17. Adachi, Y., Okuyama, Y., Miya, H., Matsushita, H., Kitano, M., Kamisako, T., Yamanoto, T. (1996). Pravastatin transport across the hepatocyte canalicular membrane requires both ATP and a transmembrane pH gradient. J Gastroenterol Hepatol 11: 580–585.

18. Crawford, J.M., Gollan, J.L. (1988). Hepatocyte cotransport of taurocholate and bilirubin glucuronides: role of microtubules. Am J Physiol 255: G121–G131.

19. Adachi, Y., Kambe, A., Yamashita, M., Yamamoto, T. (1991). Bilirubin diglucuronide as a main source for in vitro formation of delta bilirubin. J Lab Clin Anal 5: 331–334.

20. Bosma, P.J., Roy Chowdhury, N., Goldhoorn, B.G., Hofker, M.H., Oude Elferink, R.P.J., Jansen, P.L.M., Roy Chowdhury, J. (1992). Sequence of exons and the flanking regions of human bilirubin-UDP-glucuronosyltransferase gene complex and identification of a gene mutation in a patient with Crigler-Najjar syndrome type I. Hepatology 14: 941–947.

21. Aono, S., Yamada, Y., Keino, H., Sasaoka, Y., Nakagwa, T., Onishi, S., Mimura, S., Koiwai, O., Sato, H. (1994). A new type of defect in the gene for bilirubin uridine 5'-diphosphate-glucuronosyltransferase in a patient with Crigler-Najjar syndrome type I. Pediatr Res 35: 629–632.

22. Erps, L.T., Ritter, J.K., Hersh, J.H., Blossom, D., Martin, D.C., Owens. I.S., (1994). Identification of two single base substitutions in the UGT1 gene locus which abolish bilirubin uridine diphosphate glucuronosyltransferase activity in vitro. J Clin Invest 93: 564–570.

23. Labrune, P., Myara, A., Hadchouel, M., Ronchi, F., Bernard, O., Trivin, F., Roy Chowdhury, N., Roy Chowdhury, J., Munnich, A., Odievre, M. (1994). Genetic heterogeneity of Crigler-Najjar syndrome type I: a study of 14 cases. Hum Genet 94: 693–697.

24. Seppen, J., Bosma, P.J., Goldhoorn, B.G., Bakker, C.T.M., Roy Chowdhury, J., Roy Chowdhury, N., Jansen, P.L.M., Oude Elferink, R.P.J. (1994). Discrimination between Crigler-Najjar type I and II by expression of mutanta bilirubin uridine diphosphate-glucuronosyltransferase. J Clin Invest 94: 2385–2391.

25. Burchell, B., Coughtrie, W.H., Jansen, P.L.M. (1994). Function and regulation of UDP-glucuronosyltransferase genes in health and liver disease: report of the seventh international workshop on glucuronidation, September 1993, Pitlochry, Scotland. Hepatology 20: 1622–1630.

26. Adachi, Y., Nanno, T., Yamamoto, T., (1992). Constitutional jaundice. Jpn J Clin Med Suppl. 647: 677–685.

27. Yamashita , M., Adachi, Y., Yamamoto, T. (1987). Analysis of billirubin conjugates in human bile by column liquid chromatography—changes in their composition in hepatobiliary diseases. J Gastronenterol Hepatol 2: 181–190.

28. Adachi, Y., Yamashita, M., Nanno, T., Yamamoto, T. (1990). Proportion of conjugated bilirubin in bile in relation to the hepatic bilirubin UDP-glucuronyltransferase activity. Clin Biochem 23: 131–134.

29. Bosma, P. J., Goldhoorn, B., Oude Elferink, R. P. J., Sinaasappel, M., Oosta, B.A., Jansen, P.L.M. (1993). A mutation in bilirubin uridine 5'-diphosphate-glucuronosyltransferase isoform 1 causing Crigler-Najjar Syndrome type II. Gastroenterology 105: 216–220.

30. Aono, S., Yamada, Y., Keino, H., Hanada, N., Nakagawa, T., Sasaoaka, Y., Yazawa, T., Sato, H., Koiway, O. (1993). Identification of defect in the genes for bilirubin UDP-glucuronosyltransferase in a parient with Crigler-Najjar syndrome type II. Biochem Biophys Res Comm 197: 1239–1244.

31. Lundh, B., Jojanson, M.B., Mercke, C. (1972). Enhancement of heme catabolism by caloric restriction in man. Scand J Clin Lab Invest 30: 421–427.

32. Ohkubo, H., Musha, H., Kotoda, K., Okuda, K. (1978). The effect of nicotinic acid on bilirubin metabolism and its diagnostic significance as nicotinic acid test in various liver disorders. Jpn J Gastroenterol 74: 645–654.

33. Aono, S., Adachi, Y., Uyama, E., Yamada, Y., Keino, H., Nanno, T., Koiwai, O., Sato, H., (1995). Analysis of genes for bilirubin UDP-glucuronosyltransferase in Gilbert's syndrome. Lancet 345: 958–959.

34. Sato, H., Adachi, Y., Koiwai, O. (1995). The genetic basis of Gilbert's syndrome. Lancet 347: 577–578.

35. Bosma, P.J., Roy Chowdhury, J., Jansen, P.L.M. (1995). Genetic inheritance of Gilbert's syndrome. Lancet 346: 315–316.

36. Yamauchi, Y. (1994). Neonatal nonhemolytic unconjugated hyperbili- rubinemia—physiological and pathophysiological jaundice. Jpn J Neonatal Care 7 (Suppl. No. 87) : 85–96.

37. Gourley, L.M., Arend, R.A. (1983). β-glucuronidase and hyperbilirubinemia in breast-fed and formula-fed babies. Lancet i : 644–646.

38. Alonso, E.M., Whitington, P.F., Whitington, S.H., Rivard, W.A., Given, G. (1991). Enterohepatic circulation of nonconjugated bilirubin in rats fed with human milk. J Pediatr 118: 425–430.

39. Roy Chowdhury, J., Roy Chowdhury, N. (1992). Bilirubin metabolism and its disorders. in Liver and Biliary Diseases, ed. by Kaplowitz N, Williams & Wilkings, Baltimore, pp. 131–147.

40. Gregus, Z., Watkins, J.B., Thompson, T.N., Klaassen, C.D. (1983). Depletion of hepatic uridine diphosphoglucuronic acid decreases the biliary excretion of drugs. J Pharm Exp Ther 225: 256–262.

41. Kamisako, T., Adachi, Y., Yamamoto, T., (1990). Effect of UDP-glucuronic acid deletion by salicylamide on biliary bilirubin excretion in the rat. J Pharmacol Exp Ther 254: 380–382.

42. Yamashita, M., Adachi, Y., Yamamoto, T. (1987). Analysis of bilirubin conjugates in human bile by column liquid chromatography—changes in their composition in hepatobiliary diseases. J Gastroenterol Hepatol 2: 181–190.

43. Adachi, Y., Yamamoto, T. (1987). Partial defect in hepatic glutathione S-transferase activity in a case of Rotor's syndrome. Gastroenterol Jpn 22: 34–38.
44. Abei, M., Matsuzaki, Y., Tanaka, N., Osuga, T., Adachi, Y., (1995). Defective hepatic glutathione S-transferase in Rotor's syndrome. Am J Gastroenterol 90: 681–682.
45. Jacquemin E., Dumont, M., Bernard, O., Erlinger, S., Hadchouel, M. (1994). Evidence for defective primary bile acid secretion in children with progressive familial intrahepatic choliestasis (Byler disease). Eur J Pediatr 153: 424–428.
46. Bohme, M., Buchler, M., Muller, M., Keppler, D. (1993). Differential inhibition by cyclosporins of primary-active ATP-dependent transporters in the hepatocyte canalicular membrane. FEBS Lett 333: 193–196.
47. Watanabe, S., Miyairi, M., Oshio, C. (1993). Phalloidin alters bile canalicular contractility in primary monolayer culture of rat liver. Gastroenterology 85: 245–253.
48. Watanabe, S., Philips, M.J. (1986). Acute phalloidin toxity in living hepatocyte—evidence for a possible disturbance in membrane flow and for multiple function for actin in the liver cell. Am J Pathol 122: 101–111.
49. Adachi, Y., Inufusa, H., Yamashita, M., Kambe, A., Yamazaki, K., Sawada, Y., Yamamoto, T., (1988). Human serum bilirubin fractionation in various hepatobiliray diseases by the newly developed high performance liquid chromatography. Gastroenterol Jpn 268–272.
50. Richards, T.G., Thomson, J.Y. (1961). The secretion of bile against pressure. Gastroenterology 40: 705–707.
51. Kountouras, J., Sheuer, P.J., Billing, B.H. (1995). Effect of prolonged bile duct obstruction in the rat on hepatic transport of bilirubin. Clin Sci 68: 341–347.

Liver and Environmental Xenobiotics
S.V.S. Rana and K. Taketa (Eds)
Copyright © 1997, Narosa Publishing House, New Delhi, India

16. Hepatotrophic Activities of HGF in Liver Regeneration after Injury and the Clinical Potentiality for Liver Diseases

Uichi Koshimizu, Kunio Matsumoto and Toshikazu Nakamura

Division of Biochemistry, Biomedical Research Center, Osaka University
Medical School, Suita, Osaka 565, Japan

Introduction

One of an intriguing, unique property of mammalian liver is its matchless ability to regenerate following injury and to preserve its own optimal size (reviewed in [1]). When 70% of the rat liver is resected, the original liver mass and their functions are almost restored within 10 days. Although there were few cells (no less than 0.1%) undergoing DNA synthesis in the intact liver, hepatocytes begin to proliferate actively when the liver is subjected to several kinds of injury, such as hepatoectomy, ischemia, and hepatitis. It had long been postulated that quiescent hepatocytes were induced to grow by a humoral factor, but its molecular nature remained unknown. We identified and purified a potent mitogenic factor for adult rat hepatocytes, named hepatocyte growth factor (HGF)[2–4]. Molecular cloning of both human and rat HGF cDNAs was achieved in 1989-1990, showing that HGF was a novel growth factor distinct from other known cytokines [5–7]. From our concurrent studies, HGF is now recognised as long-sought, genuine hepatrophic factor functioning in liver regeneration (reviewed in [8–11]). In this chapter we present our work concerning the mechanisms of liver regeneration by HGF and the effective action of HGF for several hepatic dysfunction *in vivo*.

Molecular Nature of HGF and Its Receptor

As shown in Fig. 1, HGF is a disulfide-linked heterodimeric protein composed of a 69 kDa (α-chain) and 34 kDa (β-chain) subunit [3, 4]. The nucleotide and amino acid sequence revealed that HGF is synthesized as a single chain precursor of 728 amino acids and then it is proteolytically cleaved and processed to mature form [5–7]. Single chain HGF has no biological activities and the activation is coupled with the conversion by specific

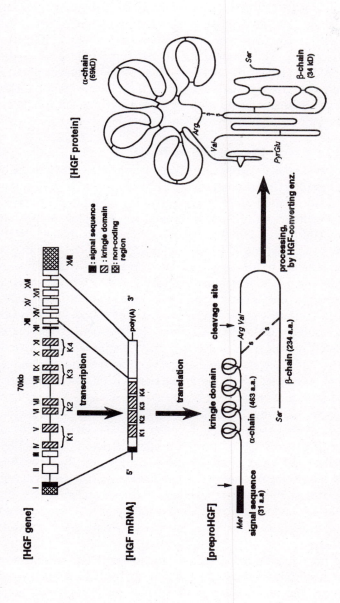

Fig. 1.   Structure of HGF Protein. Processing of prepro-HGF into mature two chain form is schematically represented. HGF gene is mapped on chromosome 7 (7q11.2-21) in human and chromosome 5 in mouse. In human, the 6 Kb of cDNA consists of a single open reading frame of 2184 nucleotides. N-terminal hairpin loop domain and the first or second kringle domain are essential for the binding of HGF to c-Met/HGF receptor. More precise informatin about the molecular nature and structure of HGF (and its receptor) is previously reviewed elsewhere [9, 12, 16].

extracellular serine-protease, HGF-converting enzyme [13, 14]. Prominent structural features of HGF are four homologous, triple-looped kringle domains in α-chain and a serine-protease like domain in β-chain. Accordingly, HGF has considerable homology (20–40%) with several kinds of proteins involved in blood coagulation and fibrinolysis, such as plasminogen, tissue- or urokinase-type plasminogen activator, and prothrombin, though HGF has no protease activity [13]. The receptor for HGF is proved to be a *c-met* proto-oncogene product [15]. The *c-met* encodes a 190 kDa transmembrane protein with a putative tyrosine kinase domain in their intracellular region, and an unique extracellular domain which is distinct from that of other growth factor receptor families (reviewed in [16]).

Enhancement of Liver Regeneration by HGF

HGF is the most potent mitogen for mature hepatocytes heretofore discovered; it is several times as effective as epidermal growth factor and transforming growth factor-α in stimulation of DNA synthesis of mature rat hepatocytes in culture [3, 4]. Furthermore, it has been proved that HGF has mitogenic activity on hepatocytes *in vivo*. For example, when human recombinant HGF (hrHGF) was administered in partial-hepatoectomized rat, the DNA synthesis of hepatocytes in remnant tissues was stimulated and the liver weight was increased in a dose-dependent fashion, indicating that HGF acted as a mitogen for hepatocytes and hepatotrophic (liver regenerative) factor [17].

The hepatitis-like injury can be induced in rodents by some chemical agents, such as carbon tetrachloride (CCl_4) and D-galactosamine, and these experimental models are useful to study liver regeneration. CCl_4 is a well known hepatotoxin which causes rapid damage via lipid peroxidation in the plasma membrane. When CCl_4 was administered into rats, acute hepatic necrosis was induced, and many liver cells undergo DNA synthesis and proliferate with a peak during 24–72 hours (hr) after treatment, although mitotic cells are scarcely observed in intact liver [17, 18]. HGF activity in the liver increased markedly 12 hr after CCl_4 administration, followed by the rapid and drastic induction of HGF mRNA expression. Reciprocally, HGF receptors on plasma membranes of the injured liver were down-regulated and decreased to almost undetectable level after 12 hr of injection. Similar transitions were also found in liver after administration of D-galactosamine, which reduces hepatic uridine phosphate content and thereby induces severe metabolic dysfunction.

By using cell fractionation technique, we found that HGF mRNA was detected only in non-parenchymal cell fraction, and not in parenchymal hepatocyte fraction, and the expression of HGF is much higher in non-parenchymal cells isolated from CCl_4-treated rat liver than in those from intact animals [18]. Furthermore, *in situ* hybridization analysis of CCl_4-treated rat liver precisely showed that HGF mRNA was mainly expressed in Kupffer cells and sinusoidal endothelial cells [19]. In contrast, *c-met* mRNA and their products are expressed in hepatocytes. Accordingly, regenerative growth of hepatocytes following injury may be mainly triggered by HGF produced from the surrounding liver cells, that is, through a paracrine system.

In the case of partial hepatoectomy, however, there is no direct damage to hepatocytes in the residual liver, which differs from the case of CCl_4 or D-galactosamine-induced hepatitis-like injury. After partial hepatoectomy in rats, HGF mRNA expression in the remnant liver was not so rapidly and markedly increased as it was in CCl_4-treated rats [20]. Interestingly, the plasma level of HGF increased as early as 3 hr after operation, followed by the extensive cell growth. These results suggested that HGF derived from blood flow may be a trigger for liver regeneration after partial hepatoectomy. Such an increase of HGF activity in the blood seems to be due to a rapid and marked induction of HGF expression in distal, non-injured organs, such as lung, spleen, and kidney.

Consequently, HGF may act as a inducer for liver regeneration through, at least, two mechanisms (Fig. 2); one is a paracrine system in which HGF is produced by adjacent non-parenchymal liver cells. The other is an endocrine mechanism through which HGF is supplied from extrahepatic organs via blood circulation. In this case, the presence of humoral factors, which are secreted from injured liver and induce HGF expression in distant intact organs, is postulated. We partially purified and named it "injurin", and further identified several known factors showing the ability to induce HGF production, including interleukin-1, tumor necrosis factor-α, prostaglandins, and so on [8, 9].

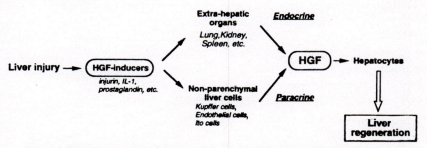

Fig. 2. **Paracrine and endocrine mechanisms of the initiation of liver regeneration by HGF.**

Anti-Hepatitis/Cirrhosis Action of HGF

We have further obtained evidence that HGF exerts anti-hepatitis action *in vivo*. In mice, intraperitoneal administration of α-naphthylisothiocyanate (ANIT) induces necrosis of the bile ducts eithelia and hepatocytes and mechanical obstruction of intralobular bile ducts with necrotic endothelial debris, which result in intrahepatic cholestasis. Therefore, in ANIT-injected mouse liver, HGF-producing cells such as sinusoidal endothelial cells and Kupffer cells are predominantly damaged, and there were few hepatocytes undergoing DNA synthesis (regeneration) [17]. When the exogenous hrHGF were administered, however, replication of hepatocytes were remarkably stimulated and, more importantly, the degree of hepatocyte necrosis was not prominent as it was in mice not given rhHGF. Furthermore, the elevations of cytosolic enzymes (such as alanine aminotransferase, lactate dehydrogenase, and alkaline phosphatase) and bilirubin in the sera were drastically suppressed. Accordingly, HGF prevented the onset of severe hepatitis and cholestasis caused by ANIT-administration, suggesting anti-hepatitis action of HGF *in vivo*.

In the case of chronic hepatic injury (hepatitis), repeated and prolonged tissue destruction and repair lead to hepatic fibrosis/cirrhosis, which are characterized by hyper-accumulation of connective tissue and hepatic necrosis. In patients with liver cirrhosis, there is high co-incidence of portal hypertension, esophageal varices, hypo-alubuminemia, and hepatocellular carcinoma. However, a few therapeutically effective methods for these diseases are established at present. Recently, we found that administration of HGF suppressed the onset of hepatic fibrosis/cirrhosis. Repeated administration of low doses of dimethylnitrosamine (DMN) into rats led to typical hepatic fibrosis/cirrhosis [21]. In DMN-treated rat liver, the extracellular matrix components were exclusively accumulated and the structure of the liver lobules was severely destroyed. However, when rats were given hrHGF, mitogenic action of hepatocytes was elicited and the structure of liver lobules remained intact even after repeated injection of DMN [22]. Moreover, hepatic collagenase activity was also stimulated by HGF-treatment and then fibrous tissue components were remarkably reduced. When DMN was repeatedly administered, almost all of rats died of severe hepatic failure within 6 weeks. On the contrary, hrHGF apparently prevented the onset/progression of cirrhosis and completely abrogated lethal hepatic dysfunction. For example, HGF-administration significantly suppressed the increase of cytosolic enzyme activities (such as GOT and GPT) caused by DMN-treatment, and restored prothrombin time (minimum time undergoing blood coagulation) to normal level.

The over-expression of TGF-β1 is thought to be a predominant cause of hepatic fibrosis/cirrhosis [23, 24]. TGF-β1 is a growth inhibitor for hepatocytes [25] and also is a most potent enhancer for extracellular matrix deposition [26, 27]. Moreover, we recently found that TGF-β1 is a strong suppressor of gene expression of HGF [28]. Based on this, we postulated possible pathogenetic mechanisms of hepatic fibrosis/cirrhosis as described below (Fig. 3). Transient hepatic injury would cause transient induction of HGF mRNA followed by TGF-β1 mRNA, which leads to normal liver regeneration. However, if hepatic injury is prolonged or repeated, as is the case in chronic hepatic diseases, TGF-β1 would suppress the induction of HGF expression, and yet it would still enhance deposition of extracellular matrix and fibroblast growth, which results in impairment of hepatocyte proliferation and in

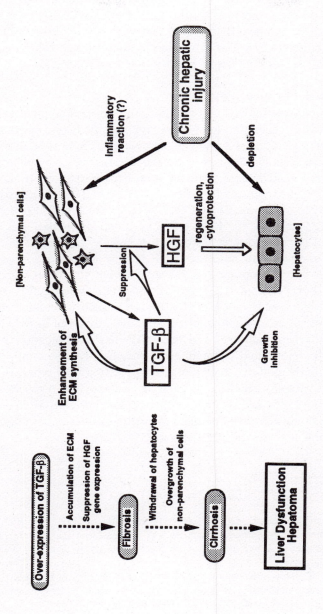

Fig. 3. Putative mechanism of onset of liver fibrosis/cirrhosis caused by over-expression of TGF-β. During chronic injury in liver, it is well known that the expression of TGF-β is remarkably and persistently up-regulated. Such a condition, via the suppression of HGF production, accumulation of extracellular matrix deposition and so on, results in the drastic replacement of cell population in liver, being largely inclined toward overgrowth of non-parenchymal cells and withdrawal of hepatocytes.

hepatic fibrosis. Prolonged depletion of HGF as well as prolonged expression of TGF-β1 would lead to withdrawal of parenchymal hepatocytes and overgrowth of stromal fibroblasts with the accumulation of extracellular matrices, and then hepatic cirrhosis would occur. Not only over-expression of TGF-β1 but also impaired HGF expression may be directly linked to hepatic fibrosis/cirrhosis, and thus exogenously administrated HGF would prevent the onset and progression of hepatic fibrosis/cirrhosis.

Conclusion and Perspective

In the present paper, we showed that administration of recombinant HGF accelerated hepatic regeneration, and more importantly it prevented the acute and chronic hepatic dysfunction. Accordingly, in future, HGF may become an effective agent for treatment of hepatic diseases, including ischemic injury after surgery, liver transplantation, partial hepatectomy for removal of tumor tissue, hepatitis induced by drugs or viruses, and hepatic fibrosis/cirrhosis. Moreover, as elevated blood HGF levels were noted in patients with hepatic diseases [29, 30], HGF levels in blood or tissues may be potentially useful for diagnosis and prospect of hepatic diseases.

Finally, it is important to note that HGF is now considered to be a pleiotropic factor that acts on not only hepatocytes but also other various types of cells. For example, HGF exerts mitogenic, motogenic, and morphogenic roles for a wide variety of epithelial cells, such as keratinocytes, renal tubular cells, bronchial epithelium, and so on (reviewed in [8–11]). Furthermore, our recent study showed that HGF may also function as a renotrophic and pulmotrophic factor in renal and lung regeneration [31–34]. Together with the findings that HGF targets a various cell types, HGF may function as a naturally occurring "organotrophic factor" for regeneration of various tissues [8, 35] and we predict that application of HGF and its gene may well become effective treatment for various diseases and injuries in different organs, as "growth factor therapy".

References

1. Fausto, N. and Webber, E.M. (1994). Liver regeneration, In *"The Liver: Biology and Pathobiology, 3rd Edition"*, eds. Arias, I.M., Boyer, J.L., Fausto, N., Jakoby, W.B., Schachter, D.A. and Shafrots, D.A., Raven Press, New York, pp. 1059–1084.
2. Nakamura, T., Nawa, K. and Ichihara, A. (1984). Partial purification and characterization of hepatocyte growth factor from serum of hepatectomized rats, *Biochem. Biophys. Res. Commun.*, Vol. 122, pp. 1450–1459.
3. Nakamura, T., Teramoto, H. and Ichihara, A. (1986). Purification and characterization of hepatocyte growth factor from rat platelets for mature parenchymal hepatocytes in primary cultures, *Proc. Natl. Acad. Sci.* USA, Vol. 83, pp. 6489–6493.

4. Nakamura, T., Nawa, K., Ichihara, A., Kaise, N. and Nishino, T. (1987). Purification and subunit structure of hepatocyte growth factor from rat platelets, *FEBS Lett.*, Vol. 224, pp. 311–318.

5. Nakamura, T., Nishizawa, T., Hagiya, M., Seki, T., Shimonishi, M., Sugimura, A., Tashiro, K. and Shimizu, S. (1989). Molecular cloning and expression of human hepatocyte growth factor. *Nature,* Vol. 342, pp. 440–443.

6. Tashiro, K., Hagiya, M., Nishizawa, T., Seki, T., Shimonishi, M., Shimizu, S. and Nakamura, T. (1990). Deduced primary structure of rat hepatocyte growth factor and expression of the mRNA in rat tissues, *Proc. Natl. Acad. Sci.* USA, Vol. 87, pp. 3200–3204.

7. Seki, T., Ihara, I., Sugimura, A., Shimonishi, M., Nishizawa, T., Asami, O., Hagiya, M., Nakamura. T. and Shimizu, S. (1990). Isolation and expression of cDNA for different forms of hepatocyte growth factor from heman leukocytes, *Biochem. Biophys. Res. Commun.,* Vol. 172, pp 321–327.

8. Matsumoto, K. and Nakamura, T. (1993). Roles of HGF as a pleiotropic factor in organ regeneration, In *"Hepatocyte Growth Factor-Scatter Factor (HGF-SF) and the C-MET Receptor"*, eds. Goldberg, I.D. and Rosen, E.M., Birkhauser Verlag, Basel, Switzerland, pp. 225–249.

9. Matsumoto, K. and Nakamura, T. (1994). Structure, pleiotropic actions, and organotrophic roles of hepatocyte growth factor, In *"Liver Carcinogenesis: The Molecular Pathways"*, NATO ASI Seires, Springer Verlag, pp. 33–53.

10. Boros, P. and Miller, C.M. (1995). Hepatocyte growth factor: a multifunctional cytokine, *Lancet*, Vol. 345, pp. 293–295.

11. Zarnegar, R. and Michalopoulos, G.K. (1995). The many faces of hepatocyte growth factor: from hepatopoiesis to hematopoiesis, *J. Cell. Biol.*, Vol. 129, pp. 1177–1180.

12. Mizuno, K. and Nakamura, T. (1993). Molecular characteristics of HGF and gene, and its biochemical aspects, In *"Hepatocyte Growth Factor-Scatter Factor (HGF-SF) and the C-MET Receptor"*, eds. Goldberg, I.D. and Rosen, E.M., Birkhauser Verlag, Basel, Switzerland, pp.1–29.

13. Mizuno, K., Tanoue, Y., Okano, I., Harano, T., Takada, K. and Nakamura, T. (1994). Purification and characterization of hepatocyte growth factor (HGF)-converting enzyme: Activation of pro HGF, *Biochem. Biophys. Res. Commun.,* Vol. 198, pp. 1161–1169.

14. Miyazawa, K., Shimomura, T., Naka, D. and Kitamura, N. (1994). Proteolytic activation of hepatocyte growth factor in response to tissue injury, *J. Biol. Chem.,* Vol. 269, pp. 8966–8970.

15. Bottaro, D.P., Rubin, J.S., Faletto, D.L., Chan, A.M.-I., Kmiecik, T.E., VandeWoude, G.F. and Aaronson, S.A (1991). Identification of the hepatocyte growth factor receptor as the c-met proto-oncogene product, *Science*, Vol. 251, pp. 802–804.

16. Comoglio, P.M. (1993). Structure, biosynthesis and biochemical properties of the HGF receptor in normal and malignant cells, In *"Hepatocyte Growth Factor-Scatter Factor (HGF-SF) and the C-MET Receptor"*, eds. Goldberg, I.D. and Rosen, E.M., Birkhauser Verlag, Basel, pp. 131–166.

17. Ishiki, Y., Ohnishi, H., Muto, Y., Matsumoto, K. and Nakamura, T. (1992). Direct evidence that hepatocyte growth factor is a hepatotrophic factor for liver regeneration and has potent antihepatitis effects in vivo, *Hepatology*, Vol. 16, pp. 1227–1235.

18. Kinoshita, T., Tashiro, K. and Nakamura, T. (1989). Marked increase of HGF mRNA in nonparenchymal liver cells of rats treated with hepatotoxins, *Biochem. Biophys. Res. Commun.*, Vol. 165, pp. 1229–1234.

19. Noji, S., Tashiro, K., Koyama, E., Nohno, T., Ohyama, K., Taniguchi, S. and Nakamura, T. (1990). Expression of hepatocyte growth factor gene in endothelial and Kupffer cells of damaged rat liver, as revealed by *in situ* hybridization, *Biochem. Biophys. Res. Commun.,* Vol. 173, pp. 42–47.

20. Kinoshita, T., Hirao, S., Matsumoto, K. and Nakamura, T. (1991). Possible endocrine control by hepatocyte growth factor of liver regeneration after partial hepatectomy, *Biochem. Biophys. Res Commun.,* Vol. 177, pp. 330–335.

21. Jenkins, S.A., Grandison, A., Bazter, J.N., Day D.W., Taylor, I. and Shields, R. (1985). A dimethylnitrosamine-induced model of cirrhosis and portal hypertension in the rat, *J. Hepatol.,* Vol. 1, pp. 489–499.

22. Matsuda, Y., Matsumoto, K, Ichida, T. and Nakamura, T. (1995). Hepatocyte growth factor suppresses the onset of liver cirrhosis and abrogates lethal hepatic dysfunction in rats, *J. Biochem.,* Vol. 1, pp. 643-649.

23. Czaja, M.J., Weiner, F.R., Flanders, K.C., Giambrone, M., Wind, R., Biempica, L., Zern, M.A. (1989). In vitro and in vivo association of transforming growth factor-β1 with hepatic fibrosis, *J. Cell Biol.,* Vol. 108, pp. 2477–2482.

24. Nakatsukasa, H., Nagy, P., Everts, R.P., Hsia, C.-C., Marsden, E. and Thorgeirsson, S.S. (1990). Cellular distribution of transforming growth factor-β1 and procollagen types I, III, and transcripts in carbon tetrachloride-induced rat liver fibrosis, *J. Clin. Invest.,* Vol. 85, pp. 1833–1843.

25. Nakamura, T., Tomita, Y., Hirai, R., Yamaoka, K., Kaji, K. and Ichihara, A. (1985). Inhibitory effect of transforming growth factor-β on DNA synthesis of adult rat hepatocytes in primary culture, *Biochem. Biophys. Res. Commun.,* Vol. 133, pp. 1042–1050.

26. Ignotz, R.A. and Massague, J. (1986). Transforming growth factor-b stimulates the expression of fibronectin and collagen and their incorporation into the extracellular matrix., *J. Bio. Chem.* Vol. 261, pp. 4337–4345.

27. Weiner, F.R., Giambrone, M.-A., Czaja, M.J., Shah, A., Annoni, G., Takahashi, S., Eghbali, M. and Zern, M.A. (1990). *Hepatology,* Vol. 11, pp. 11–117.

28. Matsumoto, K., Tajima, H., Okazaki, H. and Nakamura, T. (1992). Negative regulation of hepatocyte growth factor gene expression in human lung fibroblasts and leukemic cells by transforming growth factor-β1 and glucocorticoids, *J. Biol. Chem.,* Vol. 267, pp. 24917–24920.

29. Tsubouchi, H., Niitani, Y., Hirono, S., Nakayama, H., Gohda, E., Arakaki, N., Sakiyama, O., Takahashi, K., Kimoto, M., Kawakami, S., Setoguchi, M., Shin, S., Arima, T. and Daikuhara, Y. (1991): Levels of the human hepatocyte growth factor in serum of patients with various liver diseases determined by enzyme-linked immunosorbent assay. *Hepatology,* Vol. 13, pp. 1–5.

30. Shiota, G., Okano, J., Kawasaki, H., Kawamoto. T. and Nakamura, T. (1995). Serum hepatocyte growth factor levels in liver diseases: Clinical implications, *Hepatology,* Vol,. 21, pp. 106–112.

31. Nagaike, M., Hirao, S., Tajima, H., Noji, S., Taniguchi, S.L, Matsumoto, K. and Nakamura, T. (1991). Renotropic functions of hepatocyte growth factor in renal regeneration after unilateral nephrectomy, *J. Biol. Chem.,* Vol. 266, pp. 22781–22784.

32. Kawaida, K., Matsumoto, K., Shimazu, H. and Nakamura. T. (1994). Hepatocyte growth factor prevents acute renal failure and accelerates renal regeneration, *Proc. Natl. Acad. Sci. USA,* Vol. 91, pp. 4357–4361.

33. Yanagita, K., Matsumoto, K., Sekiguchi, K., Ishibashi, H., Niho, Y. and Nakamura, T. (1993). Hepatocyte growth factor may act as a pulmotrophic factor on lung regeneration after acute lung injury. *J. Biol. Chem.,* Vol. 268, pp. 21212–21217.

34. Ohmichi, H., Matsumoto, K., and Nakamura, T. (1996). In vitro mitogenic action of HGF on lung epithelial cells: pulmotrophic role in lung regeneration, *J. Am. Physiol.*, Vol. 270, pp. L 1031–1039.

35. Matsumoto K., Nakamura T. (1994). Hepatotrophic and renotrophic activities of HGF in vivo: Possible application of HGF for hepatic and renal diseases, In *"Liver Carcinogenesis: The Molecular Pathways"*, NATO ASI Series, Springer-Verlag, pp. 436–448.

Liver and Environmental Xenobiotics
S.V.S. Rana and K. Taketa (Eds)
Copyright © 1997, Narosa Publishing House, New Delhi, India

17. Apoptosis in Liver

Akira Ichihara

Department of Environmental Science, Tokushima Bunri University
Tokushima 770, Japan

Apoptosis is a cellular mechanism of "programmed death" and plays very important role in cell turnover in normal tissues, differentiation, tissue damage and immune determination [1]. It has been shown recently that the mechanism of liver injury in diseases, such as hepatitis is closely related with apoptosis. This chapter reviews recent progress in the apoptotic mechanism in liver. However, information is still fragmentary and incomplete with respect to the liver, although much is known about it in other cells such as lymphatic cells. It should also be mentioned that this review article is by no means a complete review of studies on apoptosis in the liver, rather being restricted to recent progress.

In 1970s Kerr et al reported that Councilman bodies (apoptotic bodies) were found in liver tissue in hepatitis [2]. Yonehara et al isolated an antibody called Fas antibody which induces apoptosis in some cells [3]. When the Fas antibody was injected intraperitoneally into mice, it induced massive liver cell damage like a fulminant hepatitis [4], but did not cause any liver damage in *lpr* strain mice, which lacks Fas, a member of the family of TNF/NGF receptors [5]. It is a transmembrane protein, whose extracellular part contains 3 cysteine-rich domains and whose cytoplasmic domain has 68 amino acids homologous with those of the TNF receptor (Fig. 1A) and was shown to be important for exerting a cytotoxic effect [6]. Fas is expressed mainly in the thymus, heart, liver, and ovary in mice [4, 7], but is not expressed in normal human liver. It is, however, strongly expressed in human liver in chronic C [8] and B hepatitis [9]. These observations indicate that the Fas apoptotic mechanism plays a decisive role in liver damage in hepatitis. We also found that Fas is expressed in both parenchymal and non-parenchymal cells isolated from mouse liver and that these cells die by apoptosis within 24 h on addition of Fas antibody plus actinomycin D or cycloheximide [10].

cDNA of a Fas ligand was cloned from a cytotoxic T lymphoma cell line [11]. The molecular weight of this ligand is about 31 kDa and it contains a proline-rich N-terminal domain which is supposed to be in its cytoplasmic part. Its extracellular carboxyl terminal 148 amino acids have a very similar

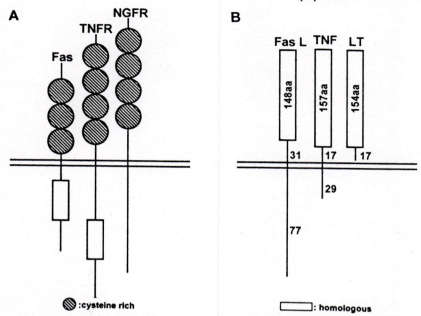

Fig. 1. (A) Fas/TNF receptor family and (B) FasL/TNF family.

sequence to those of TNF or lymphotoxin, suggesting that the ligand belongs to the TNF family (Fig. 1B). The Fas ligand is most strongly expressed in seminal vesicles, and is not expressed in tissues expressing Fas. However, in spleen cells or thymocytes, which do not express the Fas ligand, it can be induced by treatment with phorbol ester and ionomycin or IL-2 and Con A. This suggests that normal liver contains Fas but not the Fas ligand, and either that lymphocytes with the Fas ligand may infiltrate into inflammatory liver or some cells in the liver can express Fas ligand under certain conditions and cause apoptosis (Fig. 2). In the human body the Fas ligand is found in mononuclear cells in patients with hepatitis C, but not in normal liver tissue [12].

Although the involvement of the lymphatic Fas-Fas ligand system in liver injury is evident, this mechanism cannot completely explain the massive liver damage caused by this system, in which there is the possibility of participation of some humoral factor(s) such as glycocholate [13], TNF-α [14], or TGF-β [15].

Growth of hepatoma cells can be prevented by apoptosis induced by various inducers of cell differentiation, such as acyclic retinoid [16], monoterpene alcohol [17], Saikosaponin A [18] or reduction of caloric intake [19]. Some compounds induce the TGF-β receptor in hepatoma cells which may cause apoptosis [17]. It would be very useful clinically if some compounds were found to induce apoptosis of tumor cells specifically. On the contrary, prevention of normal hepatic apoptosis by various compounds

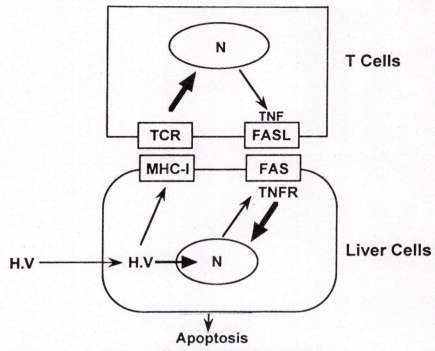

Fig. 2. Cellular mechanism of Apoptosis

may induce hepatomas [20, 21], because hepatocytes that escape from spontaneous apoptosis may become carcinogenic.

The mechanisms of intracellular signal transduction in apoptosis and apoptosis itself are still obscure. It is interesting that Fas is normally expressed in mouse hepatocytes, but addition of Fas antibody alone to these cells in culture did not induce apoptosis except in the presence of either actinomycin D or cycloheximide [10]. This finding suggests that a protein(s) with rapid turnover prevents apoptosis either by signal transduction from Fas or by apoptotic enzymes. In relation with this Leist et al suggests a putative protein [14]. The effect of TNF-α in inducing injury of mouse liver *in vivo* and *in vitro* is very similar to that of the Fas ligand-Fas system and requires actinomycin D, but the TNF-TNF receptor system is independent of the Fas ligand-Fas system. Leist et al speculated that actinomycin D may inhibit the synthesis of nitric oxide synthase induced by TNF and that liver damage by TNF may not be prevented by nitric oxide. Recently, introduction of oncogene bcl-2 into transgenic mice was shown to protect against hepatic apoptosis induced by injection of Fas antibody [22]. Bcl-2 is a gene for chromosomal translocation and the product protein is found in various membranes including the nuclear envelope. The mechanism of the protective effect of Bcl-2 against apoptosis is still unknown, but Bcl-2 may be useful in future for gene therapy of liver damage. Bcl-2 is also reported to be related with a protease in IL-1β–converting enzyem (ICE) family [23], but how this enzyme is related with apoptosis is unknown. Similarly, we found that Fas related apoptosis in cultured hepatocytes is enhanced by inhibitors of protein kinase C[10]. This is well accord with the fact that the action of protein kinase C inhibits apoptosis [24]. Again, how phosphorylation is related to hepatic apoptosis cannot be explained exactly. Various other factors may also be involved, such as oxygen radicals, nitric oxide, and various transcriptional factors (NF_kB, Myc, Fos and Jun). RelA/p65 is a subunit of NF_kB, that is related with liver regeneration [25], and deficiency of Rel A prepared in transgenic mice caused massive apoptotic degeneration of embryonic hepatocytes [26]. These factors may eventually cause increase in the intracellular Ca^{2+} concentration, followed by activation of endonuclease, poly (ADP ribose) transferase, and transglutaminase, finally leading to formation of apoptotic bodies (Figure 1). These enzymes are activated by proteases [13, 27]. An interesting possibility is that these proteases may be related with ICE described above.

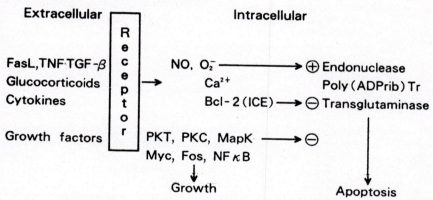

Fig. 1. Possible factors involved in apoptosis.

In summary, it is evident that apoptosis is closely involved in liver regeneration, injury and carcinogenesis. However, further studies are certainly necessary to understand hepatic apoptosis more clearly.

References

1. Nagata, S. and Golstein, P. (1995). The Fas death factor, Science Vol. 267, pp. 1449–1456.
2. Kerr, J.F.R., Cooksley, W.G.A., Searle, J., Halliday, J.W., Halliday, W. J., Holder, L., Roberts, I., Burmett, W. and Powell, L.W. (1979). The nature of piecemeal necrosis in chronic active hepatitis, Lancet Vol. 2, pp. 827–828.
3. Yonehara, S., Ishii, A. and Yonehara, M. (1989). A cell killing monoclonal antibody (anti-Fas) to a cell surface antigen codown-regulated with the receptor for tumor necrosis factor, J. Exp. Med. Vol. 169, pp. 1747– 1756.
4. Ogasawara, J., Watanabe-Fukunaga, R., Brannan, C.I., Copeland, N.G., Jenkins,

N.A. and Nagata, S. (1993). Lethal effect of the anti-Fas antibody in mice, Nature Vol. 364, pp.806–809.

5. Itoh, N., Yonehara, S., Ishii, A., Yonehara, M., Mizushima, S., Sameshima, M., Hase, A., Seto, Y. and Nagata, S. (1991). The polypeptide encoded by the cDNA for human cell antigen Fas can mediate apoptosis, Cell Vol. 66, pp. 233–243.

6. Cleaveland, J.L. and Ihle, J.N. (1995). Contender of FasL/TNF death signaling, Cell, Vol. 81, pp.479–48.

7. Watanabe-Fukunaga, R., Brannan, C.I., Itoh, N., Yonehara, S., Copeland, N.G., Jenkins, N.A. and Nagata, S. (1992). The cDNA structure, expression and chromosomal assignment of the mouse Fas antigen, J. Immunol. Vol. 148, pp1274–1279.

8. Hiramatsu, N., Hayashi, N., Katayama, K., Mochizaki, K., Kawanishi, Y., Kasahara, A., Fusamoto, H. and Kamada, T. (1994). Immunohistochemical detection of Fas antigen in liver tissue of patients with chronic hepatitis C, Hepatology Vol. 19, pp. 1354–359.

9. Mochizuke, K., Hayashi, N., Hiramatsu, N., Katayama, K., Kawanishi, Y., Kasahara, A., Fusamoto, H. and Kamada, T. (1996). Fas antigen expression in liver tissues of patients with chronic hepatitis B, J. Hepatol. Vol.24, pp.1–7.

10. Ni, R-Z., Tomita, Y., Matsuda, K., Ichihara, A. Ishimura, K., Ogasawara, J. and Nagata, S. (1994) Fas-mediated apoptosis in primary cultured mouse hepatocytes, Exp. Cell Res. Vol. 215, pp.332–337.

11. Suda, T., Takahashi, T. Golstein, P. and Nagata, S. (1993). Molecular cloning and expression of the Fas ligand, a novel member of the tumor necrosis factor family, Cell Vol. 75, pp. 1169–1178.

12. Mita, E., Hayashi, N., Ito, S., Takehara, T., Hijioka, T., Kasahara, A., Fusamoto, H. and Kamada, T. (1994). Role of Fas ligand in apoptosis induced by hepatitis C virus infection, Biochem. Biophys. Res. Commun. Vol 204, pp. 468–474.

13. Kwo, P., Patel, T., Bronk, S.F. and Gores, G.J.(1995). Nuclear serine protease activity contributes to bile acid-induced apoptosis in hepatocytes, Am. J. Physiol. Vol 268, pp. 612–621.

14. Leist, M., Gantner, F., Jilg, S. and Wendel, A. (1995). Activation of the 55kDa TNF receptor is necessary and sufficient for TNF-induced liver failure, hepatocyte apoptosis and nitrite release, J. Immunol. Vol 154, pp. 1307–1316.

15. Sanderson, N., Factor, V., Nagy, P., Kopp, J., Kondaiah, P., Wakefield, L., Roberts, A.B., Sporn, M.B. and Thorgeirsson, S.S. (1995). Hepatic expression of mature transforming growth factor β 1 in transgenic mice results in multiple tissue lesions, Proc. Natl, Acad. Sci. USA, Vol. 92, pp. 2572–2576.

16. Nakamura, N., Shidoji, Y., Yamada, Y., Hatakeyama, H., Moriwaki, H. and Muto Y. (1995). Induction of apoptosis by a cyclic retinoid in the human hepatoma-derived cell line, HUH-7, Biochem. Biophys. Res. Commun. Vol. 207, pp. 382–388.

17. Mills, J.J., Chari, R.S., Boyer, I.J., Gould, M.N. and Jirtle, R.S. (1995) Induction of apoptosis in liver tumors by the monoterpene perillyl alcohol, Cancer Res. Vol. 55, pp. 979–983.

18. Qian, L., Murakami, T., Kimura, Y., Takahashi, M. and Okita, K. (1995). Saikosaponin A-induced cell death of a human hepatoma cell line (HUH-7), Pathol. Int. Vol 45, pp. 207–214.

19. James, S.J. and Muskhelishvili, L. (1994). Rates of apoptosis and proliferation vary with caloric intake and may influence incidences of spontaneous hepatoma in C57BL/6XC3H FI mice, Cancer Res. Vol 54, pp. 5508–5510.

20. Snyder, R.D., Pullman, J., Carter, J.H., Carter, H.W. and DeAngelo, A.B. (1995) In vivo administration of dichloroacetic acid suppresses spontaneous apoptosis in murine hepatocytes, Cancer Res. Vol 55, pp. 3702–3705.
21. Bayly, A.C., Roberts, R.A. and Dive, C. (1994). Suppression of liver cell apoptosis in vitro by the non-genotoxie hepatocarcinogen and peroxisome proliferation, nefenopin, J. Cell Biol. Vol 125, pp. 197–203.
22. Lacronique, V., Mignon, A., Fabre, M., Violet, B., Bouquet, N., Molina, T., Porteu, A., Henrion, A., Bouscary, D., Varlet, P., Joulin, V. and Kahn, A. (1996). Bcl-2 protects from lethal hepatic apotosis induced by an anti-fas antibody in mice, Nature Medicine Vol. 2, pp. 80–86.
23. Enari, M., Hug, H. and Nagata, S. (1995) Involvement of an ICE like protease in Fas mediated apoptosis, Nature Vol. 375, pp. 78–81.
24. Tenniswood, M., Taillfer, D., Lakins, J., Guenette, R., Mooibrook, M., Drehlin, L. and Welsh, J. (1994). Control of gene expression during apoptosis in hormone-dependent tissues, In "Apoptosis II: The molecular Basis of Apoptosis in Diseases", eds. Tomei, L.D. and Cope, F.O., Cold Spring Harbor Laboratory Press, New York, pp. 285–311.
25. Cressman, D.E., Greenbaum, L.E., Harber, B.A. and Taub, R. (1994). Rapid activation of posthepatectomy factor/nuclear factor κB in hepatocytes, a primary response in the regenerating liver, J. Biol. Chem. Vol. 269, pp. 30429–30435.
26. Beg, A.A., Sha, W.C., Bronson, R.T., Ghosh, S. and Baltimore, D. (1995). Embryonic lethality and liver degeneration in mice lacking the RelA component of NF-$_k$B, Nature Vol. 376, pp. 167–170.
27. Kaufmann, S.H., Dernoyer, S., Ottaviano, Y., Davidson, N.E. and Poirier, G.G. (1993). Specific proteolysis cleavage of poly (ADP-ribose) polymerase: an early marker of chemotherapy induced apoptosis, Cancer Res, Vol 53, pp. 3976–3985.